Diagnosis Made Easier

T0173094

Also by James Morrison

DSM-5-TR Made Easy: The Clinician's Guide to Diagnosis

The First Interview, Fourth Edition

Interviewing Children and Adolescents: Skills and Strategies
for Effective DSM-5 Diagnosis, Second Edition
with Kathryn Flegel

The Mental Health Clinician's Workbook:
Locking In Your Professional Skills

When Psychological Problems Mask Medical Disorders:
A Guide for Psychotherapists, Second Edition

Diagnosis Made Easier

Principles and Techniques for Mental Health Clinicians

THIRD EDITION

James Morrison

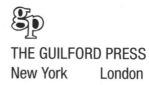

THE GUILFORD PRESS

New York   London

Copyright © 2024 The Guilford Press
A Division of Guilford Publications, Inc.
370 Seventh Avenue, Suite 1200, New York, NY 10001
www.guilford.com

All rights reserved

No part of this book may be reproduced, translated, stored in a retrieval
system, or transmitted, in any form or by any means, electronic, mechanical,
photocopying, microfilming, recording, or otherwise, without written permission
from the publisher.

Printed in the United States of America

This book is printed on acid-free paper.

Last digit is print number: 9   8   7   6   5   4   3   2   1

The author has checked with sources believed to be reliable in his efforts to
provide information that is complete and generally in accord with the standards
of practice that are accepted at the time of publication. However, in view of the
possibility of human error or changes in behavioral, mental health, or medical
sciences, neither the author, nor the editor and publisher, nor any other party
who has been involved in the preparation or publication of this work warrants
that the information contained herein is in every respect accurate or complete,
and they are not responsible for any errors or omissions or the results obtained
from the use of such information. Readers are encouraged to confirm the
information contained in this book with other sources.

Library of Congress Cataloging-in-Publication Data

Names: Morrison, James R., 1940– author.
Title: Diagnosis made easier : principles and techniques for mental health
    clinicians / James Morrison.
Description: Third edition. | New York : The Guilford Press, [2024] |
    Includes bibliographical references and index.
Identifiers: LCCN 2023037220 | ISBN 9781462553419 (hardcover) |
    ISBN 9781462553402 (paperback)
Subjects: LCSH: Mental illness—Diagnosis. | Mental health services. |
    BISAC: MEDICAL / Nursing / Psychiatric & Mental Health | PSYCHOLOGY
    / Psychotherapy / Counseling
Classification: LCC RA469 .M67 2024 | DDC 616.89/075—dc23/eng/20231016
LC record available at *https://lccn.loc.gov/2023037220*

For my editor and friend of many years, Kitty Moore

About the Author

James Morrison, MD, is Affiliate Professor of Psychiatry at Oregon Health and Science University in Portland. His long career includes extensive experience in both the private and public sectors. With his acclaimed practical books—including, most recently, *DSM-5-TR Made Easy, The Mental Health Clinician's Workbook,* and *The First Interview, Fourth Edition*—Dr. Morrison has guided hundreds of thousands of mental health professionals and students through the complexities of clinical evaluation and diagnosis.

Contents

Introduction

When I set out to write about the diagnostic process, I envisioned a text that could both complement classroom teaching and provide a guide for independent study. That was before I undertook a completely unscientific survey of practicing health care professionals, to learn how they had learned about mental health diagnosis. What I found surprised me.

For most of the practitioners I surveyed, training in the refined art of diagnosis was—well, no training at all. Most of the professional schools at which my interviewees trained presented no formal course material on diagnosis, and still do not do so. Even in medical schools, students and residents are expected to know the current diagnostic criteria, but they receive little if any exposure to a method for making diagnoses. Almost to a person, my sample endorsed the sentiment "I learned diagnosis through on-the-job training." Similarly, chapters and books that strive to teach clinicians how to perform a competent clinical evaluation focus on the product, while largely ignoring information about the process.

That process is neither simple nor intuitive, and I'd certainly never describe it as easy. But after decades of experience and long consideration, I believe it can be explained in a way that is straightforward and comprehensible—in short, we can make diagnosis easier.

In this book, I present a way of thinking about diagnostic problems. The material doesn't depend much on the vagaries of the latest diagnostic standards or code numbers. Instead, I focus on the essential characteristics of mental disorder, which have been recognized for decades. What's imperative to learn is the scientific method—yes, and the art—of evaluating patients and arriving at logical diagnoses consistent with the facts.

Part I focuses on the process of diagnosis. Learning how to diagnose accurately involves systematically applying logical, easily understood principles to information of several different types, assembled from a variety of sources. Although real life requires us to confront many diagnostic issues at once, for convenience I've divided the tasks into chapters. By the end of

Part I, you'll see how seasoned clinicians unite their experience with new information to create a working diagnosis.

The three chapters of Part II explore the social and other background data you need to understand each patient's mental health diagnosis. Of course, this is the stuff you need to have first, so you can make the diagnosis. But when learning new material, you must start somewhere, and I have judged that many (probably most) of my readers already have some familiarity with interviewing and information gathering. That's why I've presented the diagnostic method first.

Finally, in the chapters of Part III, we'll sift through a great deal of clinical material to see how the Part I methods and the Part II data apply to various clinical disorders. We won't consider every disorder, or even all the varieties of the main disorders; other manuals (including my own *DSM-5-TR Made Easy*) handle that chore. Rather, we'll concentrate on the issues and illnesses that mental health clinicians confront every day.

To illustrate the diagnostic methods, I've included over 100 patient histories. Before you read my analysis of each clinical example, I recommend that you try working through the decision trees and writing up your own list of relevant diagnostic principles. It has been amply proven that we all learn far more efficiently by actively thinking about the solution to a problem than by passively reading what someone else has written. I think you'll benefit from engaging with the histories to find the clues that will direct you to the diagnosis. And by the way, to preserve privacy while illustrating the teaching points, I have changed personal details of some patients so that their own mothers would not recognize them; but the vast majority I simply made up.

You may wonder why each decision tree endpoint reads "Consider. . . ." Why not just write down a name and move on? After much thought about these diagrams, I have decided that the more tentative wording is safer. Without being too prescriptive, I want to encourage you to avoid the trap of rushing headlong into diagnostic closure before you have all the necessary facts.

Figure 1.1 of this book (which is reproduced on the front endpaper) provides a roadmap that shows the diagnostic process graphically. The Appendix (which for convenience we've reproduced on the back endpaper) lists the diagnostic principles I consider important to apply in making a mental health diagnosis. In the interest of space and economy, I've put quite a lot of information relevant to currently recognized major diagnoses into tables in Chapters 3 and 6. Table 3.2 provides a differential diagnosis for each major diagnosis; Table 6.1 lists the illnesses that are commonly comorbid.

If, after reading this book, you still have questions about mental health diagnosis, you can email me at *morrjame@ohsu.edu*. I try to answer every email I receive.

Terminology

Throughout this edition, I've largely used the terms used by DSM-5-TR, but you'll find a few places where I haven't done so—for several reasons. (1) Some of the new terms are frankly clumsy to use. So, for example, I've continued to use *dysthymia* and *dysthymic disorder* instead of the official *persistent depressive disorder*. (DSM-5 officially allowed the shorter term as a synonym; in DSM-5-TR that is no longer the case.) (2) I've also continued to use *mood disorder* as a general term to encompass conditions described in both the bipolar and depressive disorders chapters—it's just a matter of economy of space. *Bipolar depression* serves as shorthand that I think readers will have no problem understanding. (3) I've sometimes substituted the older, shorter term *dementia* for the new, somewhat clumsy *major neurocognitive disorder*. On the other hand, I've tried to expunge terms such as *substance dependence* and *substance abuse*—in their DSM-IV meanings. If you see one of them, I mean it in the more general sense.

And here's another term that deserves explanation. I've personally continued to use the criteria for *somatization disorder,* even though DSM-5 replaced it with *somatic symptom disorder.* In its proper place (p. 111), I've explained my feelings about the new diagnostic criteria and the old; here, I will simply urge readers to pay careful note that there are two names to consider, but only one set of criteria that, to me, makes any sense. To avoid confusion, however, I've largely continued to use the new DSM-5-TR terminology—or, sometimes, a weasel expression, *somatizing disorders.*

Acknowledgments

In the end, every writer owes a debt that can never be paid to the many unseen people who provide inspiration, guidance, and courage. Of course, there are the innumerable clinicians and countless patients who have, however unwittingly, furthered my own education and helped show me the way. But among the people I can identify, I owe special thanks to my wife, Mary. Though she has midwifed each of my books, for this one she also provided prenatal checkups in the form of careful reviews of the manuscript. I also want to mention Eric Fesler, to whom I owe an unusual debt: Though not a health care professional himself, he has repeatedly sent my way notes and observations concerning mental health issues and resources. I also salute my collaborators at The Guilford Press, including (but not, as they say, limited to) Anna Brackett, who over the years has been the editorial project manager on many editions of my various books—she's the brilliant person of infinite patience who holds my hand through the final stages of publication. I truly appreciate the superb copyediting of Deborah Heimann, who has saved me from myself over and again. Carolyn Graham, in so many ways on so many occasions, has stepped in to help fix my solecisms and omissions.

Finally, and most especially, I want to thank my longtime editor and friend , Kitty Moore, to whom this book is gratefully dedicated.

Part I

The Basics of Diagnosis

1 The Road to Diagnosis

Carson

Years ago I evaluated Carson, a 29-year-old graduate student in psychology. He had always lived in the town where he was born, supported by numerous relatives and friends. Through a long history of repeated depressive episodes, he had taken antidepressant medications on and off for a decade. At one time or another he had complained of trouble concentrating on his studies, of worries that he wouldn't be able to find a job, and of fears that he would become chronically depressed like his maternal grandmother.

When Carson's mood was at its nadir (usually in the late fall), he had trouble sleeping and eating, so he was pretty thin by the time Christmas rolled around. Each spring his mood picked up, and he invariably felt well the entire summer and early fall, though he admitted that he was prone to be "sensitive to the minor vicissitudes of life." This meant, his wife told me, that he sometimes felt down when things weren't going well.

As a teenager, Carson had experimented with both alcohol and drugs. Once, when withdrawing from a 3-day run of amphetamine use, he had briefly become depressed, but his mood had lifted spontaneously within a few days. His girlfriend had agreed to marry him only on the condition that he "clean up his act"; now he swore he had been completely clean and sober for the 4 years they had been together. He had never had symptoms of mania, and he thought his physical health was excellent.

Medication had helped Carson get through college, after which he had spent the summer searching for a graduate fellowship. Finally, though the economy was depressed and few positions were available in the social sciences, he was offered a graduate fellowship with a generous stipend in a well-regarded department. Despite this triumph, his celebration was muted: His new university was nearly 2,500 miles away, in a part of the country where he'd never lived before.

On a Friday afternoon in late June, at his regular clinician's request, Carson appeared for an emergency evaluation. He sat slumped uneasily in his chair, with one knee jumping up and down and his gaze downcast. He complained of severe anxiety: His wife was pregnant with their first child; the following day they would start driving across the country to the site of his new job, in a city he'd never even visited. The previous afternoon he had become "almost panicky" when he was asked to sign a routine extension of his student loan.

As Carson described his fears for the future, his eyes reddened and he brushed away tears. Though he didn't think he was depressed, he feared that he "couldn't go through with it"—that he felt abandoned and alone. "I'm falling apart," he said, and broke down in sobs.

A Roadmap to Diagnosis

As you can imagine, a lot rides on an evaluation like Carson's. If you were his clinician, you would need to answer many questions in the effort to determine what's wrong. Is it the same as his previous problems with depression? Does he need treatment at all? If so, what's most likely to help? Should he have more medicine, or a different antidepressant, or psychotherapy? What should you tell Carson and his wife—should they postpone their move? What should Carson tell his new boss? The answer to each of these important questions would depend on your assessment of his condition. To be helpful, it must be based on information that will assist you in finding a road to the future. Reaching the initial destination on that road— we can call it a diagnosis—is what this book is all about.

The word *diagnose* means "to recognize," as a disease from its characteristic symptoms; its origin is Greek, meaning "to know." Beyond the word itself, the concept of distinguishing one disease from another is crucially important to patients and medical scientists alike. As British psychiatrist R. E. Kendell wrote decades ago, without diagnosis our journals would print only case reports and opinions.

When a person goes to a medical doctor with a physical complaint, in most cases the diagnosis conveys three sorts of information: the nature of the problem (symptoms, signs, and history), its cause, and the physical changes that consistently occur as a result. Any disorder that clearly meets these criteria can be called a *disease*. Take pneumonia, for example. This term tells us that the patient will feel weak and tired, and that this person will likely experience the symptoms of shortness of breath, fever, and a cough that produces sputum. But only after we learn the results of sputum cultures and other tests can we know that the cause of the pneumonia is bacteria growing in the patient's lungs, causing the air sacs to fill with fluid and cells, producing shortness of breath. Then we can say that the patient has the disease of pneumococcal pneumonia.

The clinical symptoms and other information establish coordinates on the roadmap a doctor follows in prescribing treatment and predicting outcome. I'm somewhat geographically challenged, so whether I enter a destination on my car's GPS or log onto Google maps, I like to have both driving directions and a graphic depiction of the route for my trip. Having both verbal and pictorial guidance is a belt-and-suspenders approach that helps me arrive at the right place, on time. In the list below, we'll take a brief overview of the "driving directions" for mental health diagnosis. I've indicated the page numbers where you can find discussions of these parts of the evaluation. (In Figure 1.1, I've drawn them as a map so you can see just where we're going. For convenience, you'll find the same graphic inside the front cover.) Don't worry if some of the terms seem unfamiliar—we'll define them as we go.

- *Level I*. Gather a complete database, including history of the current illness, previous mental health history, personal and social background, family history, medical history, and mental status examination (MSE). Obviously, you must first have material that describes your patient as fully as possible. Most of it will come from interviews with the patient and, very often, with other informants. You'll discover a lot about these building blocks in the Part II database quarry. Pages 89–125.
- *Level II*. Identify syndromes. *Syndromes* are collections of symptoms that go together to produce an identifiable illness. Major depression is a syndrome; so is alcoholism. Page 9.
- *Level III*. Construct a differential diagnosis. *Differential diagnosis* is just a collective term for all the disorders you think that a patient could have. You don't want to overlook any possibilities, however unlikely, so at first you must cast a very wide net. Page 14.
- *Level IV*. Select the most likely provisional diagnosis for further evaluation and treatment. (You might want to use a decision tree for help.) Page 19.
- *Level V*. Identify other diagnoses that could be comorbid (coexist) with your principal diagnosis. Arrange multiple diagnoses according to the urgency of their need for treatment. Page 58.
- *Level VI*. Write a formulation as a check on your evaluation. This brief statement of your patient summarizes your findings and conclusions. Page 81.
- *Level VII*. Reevaluate your diagnoses as new data become available. Page 82.

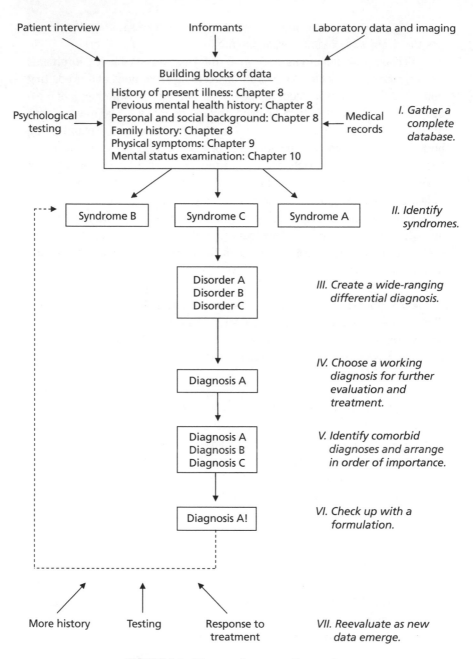

FIGURE 1.1. The roadmap to diagnosis.

2 Getting Started with the Roadmap

Most often, the information the patient provides at the initial interview starts you on the road to diagnosis. As with Carson (see Chapter 1), relatives and friends can provide additional details. I cannot emphasize too strongly the importance of this collateral information to the overall clinical picture. Patients don't usually mislead us on purpose, but often they lack the advantage of perspective on their own situations. I have frequently found that friends, relatives, and other clinicians provide information crucial to my appraisal. At the very least, such information adds color and depth to the emerging portrait of a new patient. When available, old records can sometimes save hours of digging for background information; at times they've saved me from a calamitous misdiagnosis.

The clinical history usually begins with the problem that was immediately responsible for bringing the person to clinical attention—the *history of the present illness*. Perhaps this was an acute episode of depression, the recent onset of hearing voices, a bout of heavy drug use, or serious conflict within a personal relationship. Woven through will be information that helps you understand how the life of the patient, relatives, and close associates have been affected. You'll also begin to pick up *previous mental health history,* which includes information about other mental or emotional problems, or earlier episodes of the current problem, which can also be important in determining what's currently wrong.

In the movies, in novels, and on the stage, far more is involved in storytelling than a simple narrative. Any but the simplest Dick-and-Jane story conveys information about the main character's surroundings, culture, family, and social milieu. Sometimes this material has occurred before the main action; then it's called the *back story,* and it provides texture and layers of meaning that illuminate the motives, actions, and emotions of the characters. So it is with patients—all of whom have their back stories, too, which in the clinic we call *personal and social history.* For the same reasons that a play is more compelling when we understand what motivates its characters, this information is not only interesting but often highly relevant, even vital, to diagnosis. This material is so important that I've devoted Chapter 8 to discussing childhood background, current living situation, and *family history,* especially of mental disorder. Medical background (Chapter 9) is another important part of your evaluation. Finally, you'll make use of the MSE (Chapter 10)—though perhaps not quite as much use as you might think. Throughout Part I of this book, we'll be examining these various aspects of the mental health assessment and how we can use them to create a diagnosis.

In the real world, patients, like Shakespeare's sorrows, tend to come not as single spies but in battalions. As a result, you may not have enough time to gather all the material you need for a complete initial evaluation. That's OK. The task here is to learn how the job is done when conditions are ideal; with practice, you will later become able to accomplish the same thing in the course of a busy office day or frantic evening in the emergency room.

Symptoms and Signs

In Chapter 3 we'll discuss the basic plan for making a sound diagnosis. But before we get there, we need to define some terms that relate to the raw materials for any health care diagnosis. Technically, *symptoms* are what patients complain of, whereas *signs* are what clinicians notice. The patient with pneumonia I described in Chapter 1 complained of several relevant symptoms, including a cough, shortness of breath, and feeling tired. Symptoms are the indicators of disease that are perceived by patients or their friends and relatives; they are the issues that patients mention when they talk to their care providers. In the mental health field, symptoms can include a tremendous variety of emotions, behaviors, and physical sensations. At one time or another, Carson's symptoms included feeling depressed, trouble concentrating on his studies, panicky feelings, trouble sleeping, and poor appetite. Hallucinations and delusions are symptoms. So are "nervousness," fear of spiders, and ideas of suicide.

Of course, circumstance and degree play important roles in determining what is and what is not a symptom: Many people don't care for spiders, and doctors normally wash their hands frequently, so as not to spread germs from one patient to another. So we should understand that symptoms are always more or less subjective; they depend on a person's perspective. Signs, on the other hand, are far more objective clues to illness. Usually patients and informants don't complain of signs; rather, the clinician

Symptom: A subjective sensation, discomfort, or change in functioning that a patient or informant complains about. Examples include headache, abdominal pain, itching, depression, and an itching sensation in the nose.

Sign: An indicator of abnormality that can be noticed by others. Examples include lump on the head, abdominal tenderness to touch, skin rash, weeping, and sneezing.

identifies them from a patient's appearance or behavior. The patient with pneumonia would probably show the signs of fever, increased heart rate, and perhaps altered blood pressure, and someone with a stethoscope would hear crackling sounds of fluid in the lungs as that patient struggled to breathe. Carson's signs of mental illness included tearfulness and slumped posture.

The sets of signs and symptoms sometimes intersect. At times in this book, I may talk about a sign that could be a symptom (see the sidebar "Symptoms and Signs"). You'll have to put up with that ambiguity; it's part of the clinical mystique. So why, you may ask, do we need to note that there is a difference? The reason is that signs are more objective than symptoms, and so are more reliable indicators of disease. And so, a bit later on we'll say that "signs trump symptoms" is one of our diagnostic principles. It doesn't hold always, but it holds often enough to justify noting the differences between signs and symptoms. For example, despite his doubt that he felt depressed (symptom), Carson's tearfulness and slumped shoulders (signs) suggested otherwise.

Symptoms and signs are useful in two ways. First, like Carson's panic attack, they signal that something is wrong. In the same way, suicidal thoughts, poor appetite, or hearing voices can indicate the need for a mental health assessment. The second use of signs and symptoms is to set us on the path to an appropriate diagnosis: Repeated public intoxication suggests alcohol use disorder; an arrest for shoplifting should prompt questions concerning kleptomania; and an anxiety attack when watching a war movie might motivate a combat veteran to seek attention for posttraumatic stress disorder (PTSD).

Why We Need Syndromes

By themselves, signs and symptoms are not sufficient to make a usable diagnosis. Our physical medicine patient with cough, shortness of breath, and weakness could have COVID, but the same symptoms could indicate an

Signs and Symptoms

Mental illness doesn't have a lot of signs, but here are a few: weeping, sighing, pacing, weight loss, tattered clothing, and poor hygiene. Some indicators can be either a sign or a symptom, depending on who notices. Carson wouldn't have complained about his own slumped posture, but his wife or a next-door neighbor might notice it and mention it to a clinician. Depending on circumstances, nearly any behavior that can be observed by others and that is usually treated as a sign could be a symptom instead.

Until about 1850, clinicians didn't discriminate between signs and symptoms; now whole books are devoted to the concept. Recently, however, there have been a few indications that we may once again be blurring the boundary, at least in the United States. In the late 1990s, concern that medical people too often ignored patients' pain led to calling pain a "fifth vital sign." The intent was to encourage the evaluation and documentation of pain at every clinical visit, along with the four classical (and undeniable) vital signs—temperature, blood pressure, pulse, and respiration rate. Technically, however, pain is a complaint that, because of its innate subjectivity, can only be a symptom.

Sometimes we clinicians get careless in our speech and forget the very real difference between signs and symptoms. After decades of experience, I've decided that there's no winning this battle. But we should never forget that there is a difference, and that we can use it to help us evaluate our patients.

ordinary cold—or lung cancer. For a diagnosis we can use to make predictions, we must consider the circumstances surrounding the signs and symptoms we have identified.

Although many normal people worry about what lies in the future, worry can also be a symptom of an anxiety disorder or depressive episode. If you buy a handgun, you may be interested only in improving your marksmanship for a shooting competition. But if mental depression has you believing that life's no longer worth living, the purchase carries ominous implications. If I break down in tears during a professional meeting, it could mean that I am depressed and need treatment. But suppose I've just received a text message that my sister has unexpectedly died; then I'm only reacting normally in the context of appalling news.

> *Syndrome:* Symptoms, signs, and circumstances occurring in a defined pattern that indicates the existence of a disorder.

And so we come to the *syndrome,* a Greek term first used nearly 500 years ago that means "things running or occurring together." More than just a collection of symptoms and signs, it should be more fully understood as symptoms, signs, *and circumstances,* all of which occur in a recognizable pattern that implies the existence of a particular disorder. Thus a syndrome includes such diverse features as rapidity of onset, age at onset, occurrence of precipitants, history of previous episodes, duration of current episode, and the extent to which a person's work or social life is disrupted. Each of these features restricts the meaning of the syndrome and helps identify a uniform group of patients. An obvious feature of Carson's recurring depression is that it regularly began and ended at a certain time of year. The combination of this one piece of historical evidence with his mood symptoms defines the syndrome of seasonal affective disorder.

A syndrome is an excellent starting point for disease identification, but we mental health professionals still have a long way to go before we reach a diagnosis. Internal medicine categorizes illness according to its cause. Pneumonia, as we've noted, can be caused by bacteria (a great variety of them), viruses (many to choose from here, too), or even chemicals (someone who has swallowed gasoline can develop breathing problems that are very similar to infectious types of pneumonia). The virtue of a cause-based diagnosis is that it accurately directs the clinician to the best treatment. Unfortunately, we've managed to identify very few mental health diagnoses by cause. Indeed, current diagnostic schemes remain proudly "atheoretical," using criteria written so as not to force clinicians to choose among competing hypotheses about how and why mental disorders develop. Perhaps this facilitates communication between clinicians who endorse different schools of thought—for instance, a behaviorist and a psychoanalyst can amicably discuss Carson's diagnosis—but it won't help them agree about treatment.

Creating a collection of symptoms, signs, and other features that reliably identifies homogeneous groups of patients is only a part of disease identification. The next phase is to see whether the selection process can help predict the future—that is, whether it is *valid* (see the sidebar "Validity and Reliability"). Here's how it is done. Researchers follow up patients from the group being studied to learn their outcomes: After several years, do they continue to have similar symptoms and respond uniformly to treatment, or do various diagnoses become apparent with time?

A good illustration of this process occurred during the middle years of the 20th century, when the term *hysteria* was still in common use as a diagnosis. By tracking down patients who had been diagnosed with hysteria,

Validity and Reliability

Validity and *reliability* are two words often used to describe findings in all fields of health care. They have meanings that are distinct from one another, yet they are sometimes used interchangeably in everyday speech and writing. Here is the important distinction: A *valid* finding has been demonstrated through scientific study to be solid, well established. A *reliable* finding is one that, regardless of its basic truth, may be replicated from one time or individual to another.

Take weather patterns, for example. If many writers state that the temperatures around the globe are warming, these reports might seem reliable because they are so often repeated. But this claim would only be validated when investigators verify it by recording actual evidence of year-on-year temperature elevations at various locations. Similarly, if severely depressed patients repeatedly complain that they awaken early in the morning and cannot get back to sleep, we can say that early morning insomnia is a reliable characteristic of depression. But not until double-blind sleep studies, possibly using electroencephalograms (EEGs), affirm the observation would we call it validated.

researchers learned that, years later, some were completely well whereas others now had a physical illness that could explain the symptoms their doctors had once thought to be emotional in origin. Oh yes, and quite a few still seemed to have symptoms that were, well, hysterical in origin. The researchers concluded that hysteria is not a valid diagnosis because it does not predict a uniform outcome. From this realization sprang the concept of *somatization disorder,* which is far better than hysteria at predicting the outcome for patients. Unhappily, recent editions of the *Diagnostic and Statistical Manual of Mental Disorders* (now, DSM-5-TR) state markedly revised criteria for this diagnosis—and not for the better, in my estimation. It is now lumped together with other former somatoform disorders into the *somatic symptom disorder* chapter. I will continue to advocate for the older diagnostic criteria where appropriate, and I'll have a lot more to say about this in Chapter 9.

Because we know that many, perhaps most, mental illnesses run in families (Carson's grandmother also had depression), another check on the validity of a diagnosis is to learn how likely relatives of the patient are to have had the same or similar illnesses. We'll discuss this more fully in Chapter 8.

A meaningful diagnosis for Carson's disorder would help you as his clinician decide whether to treat him with antidepressant medication, mood stabilizers, or cognitive-behavioral therapy—or possibly all three. Accurate labeling would also help avert the harm that ineffective treatments might cause by delaying the use of effective ones. In addition, you would anticipate the course of Carson's illness and advise him whether to use a treatment that would help protect against future episodes, whether to obtain additional health care insurance, and whether his siblings and children might develop a similar illness. Finally, carefully defined syndromes facilitate research into new treatments. And the more narrowly we define the syndromes, the better will be the predictions we base on them.

Ultimately, we would like to know that a syndrome can be supported by laboratory or imaging findings that are similar to those for pneumonia. But so far, almost no objective laboratory tests have been devised for the mental health field. Without definitive testing, it is hard to attribute causation, and in the absence of cause we cannot really say that we have identified a mental *disease*. *Syndrome* remains the dominant conception of mental disorder, and it is likely to stay that way far into the future. But that's OK— carefully applied, the concept works well. And besides, there is simply no good alternative.

Of course, there's a lot more to diagnosis than just identifying syndromes. Otherwise, you'd now be finishing a pamphlet rather than beginning a book. In Chapter 11 you can find a fuller discussion of Carson and his problems, which turned out to be a little more complicated than they first appeared. Now, however, we'll move on to a discussion of a diagnostic method that many experienced clinicians use, often without realizing it.

3 The Diagnostic Method

Even an experienced clinician sometimes stumbles when making a mental health diagnosis, so what hope can there be for a newbie? Fortunately, a number of scientific studies have confirmed the value of two important behaviors that all clinicians should employ. The first of these is, right from the first meeting with a new patient, to consider alternative diagnoses. When we clinicians formulate several hypotheses early in our diagnostic decision making, we are more likely to include the one that is correct. The second behavior is, early on to sift systematically through all the possible diagnoses, allowing us to reject those that are wrong in favor of those that are correct.

In this chapter we'll talk about two devices that can help us generate and evaluate alternative hypotheses. The differential diagnosis is the best way I know to ensure a comprehensive listing of all the possible causes of a patient's condition; we'll discuss it just below. The decision tree is a systematic method for sifting through the possibilities in that list. Regardless of our level of experience as clinicians, all of us can exploit these two keys to thinking about the diagnostic process.

> **Two behaviors are vital for accurate diagnosis:**
>
> 1. **Beginning early in the process, consider all alternatives—think differential diagnosis.**
> 2. **Systematically sift through all possible diagnoses. Climb the decision tree.**

The Differential Diagnosis

The *differential diagnosis* (this term is often shortened to *differential*) is a comprehensive list of conditions that could account for a patient's symptoms. For example, the possible diagnoses for a 23-year-old who hallucinates would include psychotic depression, medication toxicity, mania, schizophrenia, alcohol misuse, and medical conditions such as epilepsy or a brain tumor. If you've had little experience with the symptom at hand, you'll need some help with creating such a list; in Part III of this book, I've provided many examples. If you are a seasoned clinician, you'll have encountered dozens of patients who hallucinate, and you'll be able to rattle off many possible disorders that could be responsible. However, even highly experienced clinicians occasionally need to be reminded of the possibilities in difficult or unusual cases. From my own experience, I know how important a glance at a list of differential possibilities can be. As an example, here is a patient with a baffling case of dementia.

> For several months, 58-year-old Alvin, a certified public accountant, has been having problems with his memory. At first he couldn't recall the latest changes in tax law; later he forgot appointments and blanked on the names of clients. As a result, he had to take leave from his job with a national tax preparation firm. Within a few months, the ages of his children have escaped him; eventually he can't even remember *their* names. Now he can no longer care for himself, and his wife has to employ a home care nurse several hours a day just to cope with his bathing, feeding, and other activities of daily living.
>   Alvin's doctor has diagnosed Alzheimer's disease and is on the verge of recommending nursing home placement, when Alvin is hospitalized for pneumonia. There a consulting neurologist puts together several important observations: Alvin's relatively young age, a negative family history for Alzheimer's, his shuffling gait when he walks, and the unmistakable odor of urine clinging to his clothes. The problem with walking and the loss of bladder control are the classic symptoms of normal-pressure hydrocephalus (NPH), a potentially correctable condition. When imaging studies confirm the diagnosis, a shunting procedure drains excess fluid from his brain. Alvin's symptoms improve.

Had Alvin's first doctor worked through a careful differential diagnosis of dementia, the nightmarish gradual deterioration might have been avoided. Started soon enough, effective treatment for NPH can restore much of a person's lost cognitive ability. Although it accounts for as many as 10% of all dementia cases (today, rather than *dementia* we'd record the official diagnosis of *major neurocognitive disorder*), NPH is much less common than other causes of dementia—including Alzheimer's disease and cerebrovascular accidents—so it is easily overlooked.

The Safety Hierarchy

Alvin's close brush with tragedy illustrates that even experienced clinicians sometimes must be reminded about unusual conditions that may be treatable. There is more to creating a differential list than simply collecting diagnoses; how we arrange them makes a big difference. Think of it as you would a list of home repair jobs—paint the porch railing, sweep the garage, mend the pipe that's just burst in the basement. You don't just select a job at random to do first. Rather, you prioritize: "Hmm, maybe I really ought to deal with my flooded basement first."

So at the top you place emergencies, such as the ruptured pipe or a fire on the cooktop. Further down the list will be those matters that are important but less urgent, such as mending a hole in the roof or exterminating the carpenter ants. Toward the bottom are the jobs that can wait until the other, higher-up tasks have been attended to—the patching, plastering, and painting that constitute aspects of routine maintenance. Note that what we put at the top won't necessarily be the most likely to occur: Defective pipes are pretty rare, especially compared with the amount of touching up that any house requires. In effect, we've created a *safety hierarchy* for home repairs.

And this is exactly what we need for our differential diagnosis—a way to list the possible diagnoses so as to expose our patients to the least possible risk from such perils as inadequate or downright erroneous treatment, inaccurate prognosis, social stigma, and inappropriate living arrangements. A safety hierarchy places at the top those conditions that are most urgent to treat, are most likely to respond well to treatment, and have the best outcome. For me, a safe diagnosis is the one that I'd prefer for myself or for a member of my family. Such a diagnosis, if it turns out to be correct and treatment is effective, could restore sanity, cure a threatening physical illness, or even save a life.

> *Diagnostic Principle:* **Arrange your wide-ranging differential diagnosis according to a safety hierarchy.**

At the bottom go conditions that treatment seems unlikely to help—that have a terrible prognosis. Everything else goes somewhere in the middle. We'd probably get pretty good consensus among experienced clinicians as to what belongs in the top and bottom categories, but the exact order for the middle layer could be debated forever (and probably will be).

> *Diagnostic Principle:* **Physical disorders and their treatment can cause or worsen mental symptoms.**

Now our list has become a tool with which we can wring some sort of order out of the chaos that so often confronts us when we evaluate a new patient. And with the safety hierarchy, we arrive at our first diagnostic principle: List the items of your differential diagnosis according to a safety hierarchy, such as that in Table 3.1.

> *Diagnostic Principle:* **Substance use, including prescribed and over-the-counter medications, can cause a variety of mental disorders.**

I need to mention one other issue here—well, two, really. The safety hierarchy sets us up for a couple of additional diagnostic principles. Notice what we put right at the top of the safety hierarchy: disorders that are due to a physical disease (you'll find quite a number of them listed in Table 9.1) or that are due to the effects of substance use (Tables 9.2 and 9.3). I'll have quite a lot more to say about these in Chapter 9, but for now

---

TABLE 3.1. Hierarchy of Conservative (Safe) Diagnoses

Most desirable (most dangerous, most treatable, best outcome)
   Any disorder due to substance use or a medical illness
   Recurrent depression
   Mania or hypomania

Middle ground
   Alcohol use disorder
   Panic disorder
   Phobic disorders
   Obsessive–compulsive disorder
   Anorexia nervosa
   Adjustment disorder
   Substance (other than alcohol) use disorder
   Borderline personality disorder

Least desirable (hard to treat, poor outcome)
   Schizophrenia
   Antisocial personality disorder
   AIDS-related dementia
   Alzheimer's dementia

Note. Adapted from *Boarding Time: The Psychiatry Candidate's New Guide to Part II of the ABPN Examination* (4th ed.) by James Morrison and Rodrigo A. Muñoz (American Psychiatric Press, 2009). Copyright © 2009 the American Psychiatric Association. Adapted by permission.

let's just note that these two classes of conditions belong at the top of every differential diagnosis we create.

More about Carson

To see a differential diagnosis in action, let's revisit Carson, whom we met at the beginning of Chapter 1. For the moment, we'll limit ourselves to the possible causes of his depression. Even an abbreviated list should include several of what I (mostly) continue to call *mood disorders,* following DSM-IV rather than DSM-5-TR; these include bipolar disorders, major depressive disorder, persistent depressive disorder, depression due either to a physical illness or to substance misuse, and seasonal affective disorder. I would also include adjustment disorder with depressed mood and some sort of personality disorder. As I have indicated above, we don't just write down what we consider *likely,* but also the "barely possibles." We include them all because every so often a real long shot comes in first, and we want to be alert and receptive when that happens. Even so, some of the conditions on this list appear a bit far-fetched. With a previous history of good health, the risk that Carson's depression is due to a physical illness such as a brain tumor or endocrine disorder would be pretty small. On the other hand, though we haven't read any evidence that suggests a personality disorder, there's no proof of its absence, either.

 Although as Carson's clinicians we would have to contend with quite a long and complicated list of mental disorders, we'll use the safety hierarchy to create some order.

Depression related to a medical illness Substance-related depression	Treatable disorders that can quickly have a profound effect on a patient's health
Bipolar depression Major depressive disorder Seasonal affective disorder Dysthymic disorder	Disorders that are serious, but a little less urgent to treat
Adjustment disorder Personality disorder	Disorders that are chronic, have no specific treatment, or have a poor prognosis

In Table 3.2 I've listed differential diagnoses for the more common mental disorders. That is, for each mental disorder listed in the left-hand column, I have indicated with an "×" each diagnosis that should be considered in the differential for that disorder—because they share at least one criterion or other important characteristic. The degree of similarity is strong in many cases (e.g., dysthymia with major depression). In others, the similarity is weak (e.g., schizophrenia with major depression, which includes psychotic symptoms only in extreme cases). Nonetheless, the purpose of a differential diagnosis is to list each real possibility, however remote. I've included physical and substance use causes everywhere— a reminder whenever you use the table to consider first these important causes of mental symptoms.

Of course, diagnoses on a list are only the first part of the exercise; they'll do you no good at all until you discriminate among them. To that end, the differential lists I've included in most of the Part III chapters contain brief definitions for each disorder. Your differential could grow to include quite a lot of possibilities, and you may need to explore more than one decision tree. And that brings us to this next section.

The Decision Tree

A *decision tree* is a device that guides the user through a series of steps to arrive at some goal. For a patient, that would be a diagnosis or treatment. On paper, it does look something like a tree, if you think of trees as growing upside down. You use it by answering a series of yes–no questions; each answer determines which branch to take next. The word *algorithm* is another way that this concept is commonly expressed.

I first ran across decision trees in biology, where they are used to identify unfamiliar plants. Whole books are devoted to keying out grasses, bushes, and other wildlife from various parts of the world. Perhaps without realizing it, you may have used a similar device to help make commonplace life choices. For example, let's consider a decision about where to have supper:

> "For a big occasion, and depending on my financial health, I'd like to have a really nice meal—the Ritz, if I can get a reservation, or Figaro's, which just opened, so it isn't crowded. Otherwise, I might go to the Sea Grotto, unless Mom comes along—she hates fish. Then we could try Chiquita's for tacos (unless it's Monday, when they're closed). But if

TABLE 3.2. Differential Diagnosis by Diagnosis

Use these → diagnoses in the differential diagnosis for these ↓ disorders	Physical causes	Subst. intox./withdr.	Intellectual disability	Autism spectrum dis.	Delirium	Dementia	Schizophrenia	Schizoaffective dis.	Schizophreniform dis.	Delusional dis.	Major depression	Dysthymia	Mania (bip. I)	Hypomania (bip. II)	Cyclothymia	Panic dis.	Agoraphobia	Specific phobia	Social anxiety dis.	Separation anx. dis.	OCD	PTSD	GAD	Somat. dis.	Somat. pain dis.	Illness anxiety dis.	Body dysmorphic dis.
Intellectual disability	×	×	—		×																						
Autism spectrum dis.	×	×	×	—			×												×			×					
Delirium	×	×			—	×	×	×	×	×	×		×														
NCD dementia	×	×	×		×	—	×	×	×		×																
Subst. intox./withdr.	×	—		×																							
Schizophrenia	×	×		×	×		—	×	×	×	×		×														
Schizoaffective dis.	×	×		×	×	×	×	—	×	×	×		×														
Schizophreniform dis.	×	×		×	×	×	×	×	—	×	×		×														
Delusional dis.	×	×					×	×	×	—	×		×									×				×	×
Major depression	×	×					×	×	×	×	—	×	×	×	×												
Dysthymia	×	×										—															
Mania (bip. I)	×	×					×	×	×	×			—	×	×												
Hypomania (bip. II)	×	×					×	×	×	×			×	—	×												
Cyclothymia	×	×									×	×	×	×	—												
Panic dis.	×	×									×					—	×	×	×		×	×	×				
Agoraphobia	×	×														×	—	×	×			×					
Specific phobia	×															×	×	—	×								×
Social anxiety dis.	×		×				×				×		×			×	×	×	—	×							×
Separation anx. dis.	×		×				×	×	×	×	×					×	×		×	—			×				
OCD	×	×								×							×	×			—		×			×	×
PTSD	×	×			×		×				×											—					
GAD	×	×									×					×			×	×	×	×	—	×		×	
Somat. dis.	×	×					×	×	×															—			
Somat. pain dis.	×	×									×													×	—		
Illness anxiety dis.	×	×					×				×										×	×		×		—	×
Body dysmorphic dis.	×										×							×	×		×			×		×	—
Dissoc. amnesia	×	×			×	×																×		×			
Dissoc. identity dis.	×	×					×	×	×		×											×					
Depers./dereal. dis.	×	×					×	×					×			×		×	×			×					
Sexual dysfunctions	×	×									×															×	
Gender dysphoria	×						×																				
Paraphilic dis.	×	×	×				×	×					×														
Anorexia nervosa	×						×				×	×									×			×			×
Bulimia nervosa	×										×																
Binge-eating dis.	×																										
Sleep–wake dis.	×	×			×	×	×				×	×	×			×								×		×	
Intermitt. explos. dis.	×	×			×	×					×		×			×											
Kleptomania	×	×			×								×														
Pyromania	×	×	×		×	×							×														
Gambling dis.	×												×														
Trichotillomania	×						×																	×			
Adjustment dis.	×	×																							×		
Schizotypal PD	×	×					×		×																		
Antisocial PD	×	×								×																	
Borderline PD	×	×									×	×	×														
Narcissistic PD	×	×											×	×													
Avoidant PD	×	×															×		×								
Obsess.–compul. PD	×	×																									

Note. NCD, neurocognitive disorder; OCD, obsessive–compulsive disorder; PTSD, posttraumatic stress disorder; GAD, generalized anxiety disorder; PD, personality disorder.

Use these → diagnoses in the differential diagnosis for these ↓ disorders	Dissoc. amnesia	Dissoc. identity dis.	Depers./dereal. dis.	Sexual dysfunctions	Gender dysphoria	Paraphilic dis.	Anorexia nervosa	Bulimia nervosa	Binge-eating dis.	Intermitt. explos. dis.	Kleptomania	Pyromania	Gambling dis.	Trichotillomania	Adjustment dis.	Schizotypal PD	Antisocial PD	Borderline PD	Narcissistic PD	Avoidant PD	Obsess.–compul. PD	Factitious dis.	Malingering	Normal cogn. decline	Normal bereavement
Intellectual disability																									
Autism spectrum dis.																									
Delirium																						×	×		
NCD (dementia)																						×	×	×	
Subst. intox./withdr.																									
Schizophrenia																×									
Schizoaffective dis.																									
Schizophreniform dis.																×									
Delusional dis.																									
Major depression															×										×
Dysthymia																									
Mania (bip. I)																									
Hypomania (bip. II)																									
Cyclothymia																		×							
Panic dis.																									
Agoraphobia																									
Specific phobia																									
Social anxiety dis.																				×					
Separation anx. dis.																		×							×
OCD														×											
PTSD															×							×			
GAD															×										
Somat. dis.																									
Somat. pain dis.				×																		×	×		
Illness anxiety dis.																									
Body dysmorphic dis.					×		×						×						×						
Dissoc. amnesia	—	×	×																			×	×		
Dissoc. identity dis.	×	—	×																			×	×		
Depers./dereal. dis.			—																						
Sexual dysfunctions				—																					
Gender dysphoria					—	×																			
Paraphilic dis.					×	—																			
Anorexia nervosa							—	×	×																
Bulimia nervosa							×	—	×									×							
Binge-eating dis.							×	×	—																
Sleep–wake dis.																									×
Intermitt. explos. dis.										—							×	×					×		
Kleptomania											—						×						×		
Pyromania												—					×								
Gambling dis.													—				×								
Trichotillomania														—								×			
Adjustment dis.															—										×
Schizotypal PD																—	×	×	×						
Antisocial PD																	—	×	×						
Borderline PD																	×	—	×						
Narcissistic PD																×	×	×	—		×				
Avoidant PD																×				—					
Obsess.–compul. PD																×			×		—				

this sneezing fit turns into the flu, my fall-back position is to fix veggie burgers at home."

To work through these choices, you could set up a decision tree, which would look something like Figure 3.1. Of course, once you've made a decision, as a successful diner (or clinician) you should always remain alert for new information that could suggest the need for a last-minute change of plans.

Decision trees are a bit like training wheels: useful when you're learning to ride, but something you remove and store in the garage later on. If you want to see how the decision tree is used for a patient, you can skip ahead to Chapter 11, where we'll employ one to explore Carson's diagnosis further.

Before moving on, let's take a break (maybe we'll share an order of nachos from Chiquita's—I hope this isn't Monday) and recap our diagnostic method so far. We've learned to aggregate symptoms and signs into familiar groups, called *syndromes*. Because they can have many causes, we gather

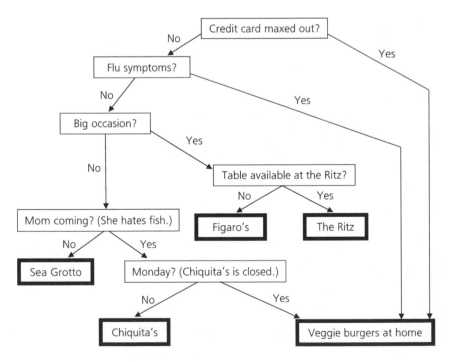

FIGURE 3.1. A decision tree for dining.

the syndromes a patient might have into a list, called a *differential diagnosis,* which we arrange into a *safety hierarchy.* Perhaps aided by the use of a *decision tree,* we'll find our working diagnosis at or near the top of that hierarchy. (See sidebar "What Is the Medical Model?")

Pass the salsa, *por favor.*

What Is the Medical Model?

If you read widely about mental health or listen to popular podcasts or watch television specials on the subject, you'll eventually come across these opinions: making a diagnosis medicalizes misery; diagnoses are subjective and don't consider individual circumstances; emotional symptoms are nothing more than understandable reactions to untoward events. You may also hear that diagnosticians just "tick boxes" to collect symptoms rather than listening carefully for the patient's individual concerns, or that the subjective criteria we use are based on social norms rather than needs and characteristics of the individual. You may even hear that telling patients they have an illness will cause them to feel hopeless about the future. These views have been around for as long as I've been a clinician, and that's coming up on quite a few years now. So let's deal with them.

I acknowledge that Yes!—our model is a medical one; and right up front I'll say, that is a good thing. It is so good that we've already discussed its foundations (see p. 5); so good that it allows us to make accurate predictions about our patients— what the outcome will be if they remain untreated (we call this the *natural history* of the condition) and how they will respond to various treatments and other interventions. (And note that the symptoms we evaluate are far from subjective: Indeed, they are based on careful scientific study that has been widely published and replicated.)

But this is not to devalue our patients as individuals. We acknowledge that they are troubled people who often cannot see the way forward. Because each has the usual collection of habits, traits, and quirks that illuminates their humanity, part of our job is to recognize and accommodate these individual characteristics at the same time we steer our patients onto paths that lead toward health—paths we know well because we have traveled them with so many others.

As for how the future might appear to our patients, it seems to me that having a disorder that has been studied in many other people, one for which there are proven, reliable treatments (and not just pills, either), should provide a sound basis for confidence in the method, for encouragement to see the treatment plan through, for faith in a brighter day coming. Indeed, wouldn't it be the scariest situation of all, if the issue you face is a complete unknown, a thicket of misery from which you must discover your own exit? Rather, the medical model approach adopts the view that countless others have been here before, so that no one need face their pain alone.

---

4 Putting It Together

And now is the time to put together all the material you have gathered for your patient and create a diagnosis that will guide treatment and predict outcome. The chapters of Part III focus on specific areas of diagnostic interest; this chapter covers the basics of how you can weave together the various threads of information to create an initial diagnosis. The first big issue is judging the relative value of the pieces of information you have assembled.

Sometimes, of course, everything points in the same direction:

Nedra is a 78-year-old widow whose daughter-in-law and son relate that over the past 2 years her memory has gradually worsened. At first, she seemed only to misplace things; with time, she began forgetting conversations she had just had, could not remember how to prepare certain favorite foods, and several times neglected to turn off a burner on the stove. Lifelong a cheerful, positive person who never says a word against anyone, now she appears morose and angry. Her only family history of mental disorder is in her own mother, who, after a lengthy period of decline, had been diagnosed as "senile" by the family doctor the year before she died in a nursing home.

When examined, Nedra refuses to shake hands and will respond only with the phrase "damned foolishness" when asked to identify her son. When a nursing aide walks into the room, Nedra curses and mutters racial epithets.

Nedra's diagnosis of Alzheimer's is suggested powerfully by three data sources: the recent history, the family history, and the current MSE. There's nothing that would support a different diagnosis, though data from a routine physical exam and laboratory screening should be obtained.

Such unanimity among sources isn't always the case. Consider the history of Rusty.

When he was 23, and again at 28, Rusty had been clinically depressed. His father had suffered depression off and on with his drinking—"He was a hopeless alcoholic," Rusty testified—but Rusty swore alcohol had never been a problem for him. With each episode he had responded rapidly and completely to treatment with antidepressant medication, and for several years between episodes, he had required no medication.

Now 36, he has just remarried and for the third time has become depressed. This time, however, there is a difference: Whereas during his two previous episodes he complained of rather severe terminal insomnia, now he feels "forever tired" and sleeps 12 hours a day. His clinician refers Rusty to an internist, who finds that his thyroid is severely underperforming. Within a week of starting thyroid replacement hormone as his only medication, Rusty is on his way back to normal.

Rusty's past history tells one story; his family history tells another. And then along comes a third episode—with a subtle difference in symptoms. When one line of information contradicts another, determining what weight to give the various lines of evidence can pose problems.

When Information Sources Conflict

Fortunately, a number of diagnostic principles can help sort out the confusion that can result from conflicting information sources.

History Beats Current Appearance

We clinicians need to keep reminding ourselves that accurate diagnosis depends heavily on the previous history of mental illness. Take delusions as an example: What does it really mean when Jerome says that a scanning radio has been implanted in his brain? Of course, he could have schizophrenia, which is what we often (and often mistakenly) think of first when considering any psychotic symptom. But delusions can also take place in the context of a substance use disorder, a physical disease, dementia, or even antisocial personality disorder. Or, they may characterize severe mood disorder.

Five years earlier, Dick was hospitalized when he became acutely excited and psychotic. Believing that he possessed the divine power of healing, he had wandered the streets, praying and placing his hands on the head of anyone using a wheelchair he met. For several weeks he was hospitalized and treated with antipsychotic drugs. Subsequent to his discharge, he developed what was called a "postpsychotic depression"; in its depths, he left his position at work and isolated himself almost completely from his family life. He later reported that several times during this period, he had nearly killed himself.

Eventually, however, Dick recovered completely and took a job even better than the one from which he had resigned. Reunited with his family, he prospered for 3 years until, while once again attending an out-of-town convention, he became acutely confused. This time, he would enter strangers' homes, where he would inform the startled residents that he was the "literal brother of Christ." Again he was hospitalized; this time, a new mental health team diagnosed him as having bipolar I disorder and treated him with antipsychotics and lithium. He recovered within 10 days and has subsequently remained well on lithium alone.

Dick's MSE suggested schizophrenia, but the historical information conveys a far different picture: abrupt onset (schizophrenia usually begins gradually) and complete recovery (schizophrenia often leaves behind some residual symptoms). Patients with schizophrenia sometimes have extremely severe and long-lasting depressions, but these are far more typical of bipolar I disorder. In other words, for Dick, as for many mental health patients, the longitudinal history shouting "bipolar I disorder" far outweighs the MSE that seems to whisper "schizophrenia." Using the course of illness as the basis for diagnosis was first described in 1852 by French psychiatrist Benedict Morel (who also coined the term *dementia praecox,* an early name for schizophrenia).

> **Diagnostic Principle:** A patient's history often provides better guidance for diagnosis than does the cross-sectional appearance (MSE).

Sorting out a delusion's true meaning requires us to focus on many elements from the patient's history, including the presence of physical health problems, severe depression or mania, and family history of mental illness. How long have symptoms been present? Do drugs or alcohol seemingly cause them to appear? Do they regress only with medication, or do they come and go spontaneously? These historical considerations, of course, apply to hallucinations and to many other symptoms that the patient presents. We'll discuss them more fully in Parts II and III.

Recent History Beats Ancient History

Here we pay homage to the fact that symptoms reported early in the course of a patient's illness may carry far less diagnostic information than does later evidence.

> When I first saw Nancy as an office patient, she was just 16 and none too delighted to be there. Her mother had insisted on the appointment, however, because of Nancy's problem with appetite. "Her weight just keeps going down," Mom said, "and she picks at her food. I'm so afraid that she has anorexia, like Julie down the street." But Nancy denied thinking that she was too fat. "I guess I do look kinda skinny," she confided, in what was just about the last complete sentence she would speak before dropping out of treatment. She told her mother that she'd try to eat more and not to bug her, and that seemed to be the end of it.
>
> At the time, I realized that Nancy could have anorexia nervosa or another eating disorder, but that depression and substance use were also possibilities. It could even turn out that her symptom was just an expression of the problems nearly all adolescents experience while becoming adults. I didn't learn the answer until one afternoon 8 years later, when Nancy returned on her own, again with loss of appetite—and a 15-pound weight loss. This time, she admitted that her mood was so low she was having trouble performing on her job as a bank junior officer. To the consternation of her fiancé, her sex interest had dropped to near zero and she was even having thoughts about suicide. Her problem this time was clearly severe depression; I suspected that, in attenuated form, this had also been her problem as a teenager.

> **Diagnostic Principle:** A patient's recent history often more accurately indicates diagnosis than does older history.

Clinicians of long experience have had similar encounters with anxiety symptoms (will they become generalized anxiety disorder [GAD], panic disorder, or a mood disorder?) and depression (will it become bipolar I or II disorder, dysthymia, or an adjustment disorder?). When older symptoms are clarified, newer ones can change diagnosis and inform treatment.

Collateral History Sometimes Beats the Patient's Own

Let's not go overboard here. Of course, diagnosis is largely driven by what your patient tells you. But some patients lack perspective on their own difficulties. An elderly widow who lives alone may not realize how forgetful she has become; a teenage boy may grow up unaware that his gang affiliations have been so troublesome. Occasionally, someone just plain lies. Even patients who try their best to provide accurate, complete information may lack access to family history or early social history, either of which can help determine a diagnosis.

A biology student at a local college, Jack complains about "indecision and lack of direction." He tells me that he fears he is developing schizophrenia, the diagnosis for which his father was institutionalized years ago. When later (with Jack's permission) I meet with his mother, she tells me in confidence that Jack is not her biological child, but the product of a brief relationship a younger sister had

> *Diagnostic Principle:* **Obtain collateral history whenever possible; it is sometimes more accurate than the patient's own.**

with her boss. Jack had been adopted at birth and never learned the truth about his origins. His legal father's diagnosis has no biological bearing on Jack's own illness.

Signs Beat Symptoms

Here we need to insist on the technical definitions of signs (what you observe about the patient) and symptoms (what the patient has noticed and can tell you). The trouble with symptoms is that they can carry two different interpretations—yours and the patient's. Some patients may not understand your interpretation; others may even misconstrue your meaning as they report it to others. In other words, the objectivity of signs may point the way to a correct diagnosis.

You've probably encountered the phenomenon yourself—perhaps when an office patient, with eyes filling quietly with tears, denies feeling hurt by a lover's abandonment. More striking denials are those of the gaunt patient with anorexia nervosa who claims to look fat, or the patient with schizophrenia who denies hallucinations but keeps glancing uneasily around the room.

> *Diagnostic Principle:* **Signs (what you observe about a patient) can be a better guide to diagnosis than symptoms (what the patient tells you).**

Imogene, a patient with somatization disorder (see Chapter 9 for my discussion of this condition), lies on a gurney in the urgent care center. Though immobilized by "complete paralysis" from the waist down, she nonchalantly chews gum and discusses with a nurse the just-played Super Bowl game. The disconnect between the sign of her emotional detachment and her physical symptom of paralysis is a classic example of *la belle indifférence*, or paradoxical lack of distress.

Be Wary of Crisis-Generated Data

When people are acutely troubled, it can affect how they view the world and their place in it. If your patient has just been jilted by a lover, fired, or bereaved, the resulting mood can color the tone of the story you hear, even to the point of affecting the patient's perspective on experiences that occurred long ago.

Diagnostic Principle: **The stress of crisis can color how a patient perceives life's experiences.**

The day after her apartment was burglarized, Jill complains that she is the unluckiest person in the world: "I never catch a break!" she moans. Her therapist, who has known her for years, decides it's time to institute a course of cognitive-behavioral therapy, in an effort to help her deal with the negative stereotypes she holds of herself.

The flip side is that a positive experience like the joy of new love can also distort a person's understanding of reality.

Objective Findings Beat Subjective Judgments

Here's a reminder that clinicians' intuitions, while sometimes uncannily accurate, should never outrank verifiable information. The "schizophrenic feel" you might experience when talking to a new patient should only prompt due diligence in your hunt for signs and symptoms. My own favorite *bête noire*, borderline personality disorder, is a diagnosis that clinicians may be tempted to make without a full evaluation.

Or take 19-year-old Jordan, whose slow, quiet speech, level gaze, and sad smile create instant sympathy in his interviewer. Although he claims not to know what triggers his anxiety attacks, just a few minutes' conversation made it seem likely that he has panic disorder. Perhaps it covers a pretty severe major depressive episode. These predictions are shattered when more history is obtained from his older sister, who has accompanied him to his appointment. She reports that he has been increasingly distressed by his feelings about his own sexual orientation. Confusion, shame, and fears that his homophobic father would become enraged have caused him to confide only in her. With the sister's additional information, adjustment disorder moves closer to the top of the differential diagnosis.

> *Diagnostic Principle:* **Resist the allure of the hunch—embrace objective data as the bedrock of diagnosis.**

Consider Family History

For decades, we've known that mental disorders run in families. Indeed, during the last half of the 20th century, a great deal of work established the fact that many (perhaps most) of the syndromes we confront every day have a strong genetic component. In Chapter 8 we'll consider the issues surrounding family history in greater detail, but for now we'll just note an example:

> Grant has always been a quiet, thoughtful boy, but not long after his 15th birthday his behavior turns erratic. For several months his family endures verbal outbursts over minor disappointments. He becomes belligerent, several times accosting total strangers on the street who he thinks "look funny" at him. One afternoon after school, he actually picks a fight with a policeman, who escorts him to the emergency room. There he talks to himself in apparent response to auditory hallucinations. After admission, he masturbates openly in the ward dayroom— twice. After a week on antipsychotic medication, he isn't much better, and the staff wonders whether he has schizophrenia. However, a consultant notes that years ago Grant's uncle (his mother's brother) had an acute psychosis and was subsequently successfully maintained on lithium. With the addition of a mood stabilizer, Grant's psychosis rapidly resolves.

Of course, it would be unwise to base your entire therapeutic strategy on a single data point, but family history can erect a useful signpost on your diagnostic path. I will qualify this assertion somewhat (and will provide a revised version of the following diagnostic principle) at the end of Chapter 8, but for the moment let us state the principle as it is given here.

> *Diagnostic Principle:* **Family history can help guide diagnosis.**

Simplify with Occam's Razor

William of Occam, a 14th-century English philosopher, stated a law that applies in many fields beyond health care. Now a mainstay of medical diagnosis (and many other areas of problem solving), it advises that if something has two possible explanations, you should choose the simpler one. Because it "shaves away" unneeded detail, it has come to be known as *Occam's razor*, or the principle of parsimony.

> At age 47, Jakob appears at the emergency room complaining of two problems: He feels terribly depressed, and he hears voices. The depression has plagued him for several months; he is "at the end of [his] tether." He fears he is close to committing suicide—the fate of his older brother, Hans, only 2 years ago. Jakob admits that his appetite has been off, and he's lost weight; he sleeps poorly; he has little interest in his usual activities (he is an avid collector of old guns and usually haunts antique shows); and his concentration at work is so poor that his boss has ordered him to take time off to "get straightened out." Jakob believes he has let everyone down, including his boss and his family, and he feels enormously guilty, deserving of death.
>
> The voices have troubled him for only a few days. He hears them just behind his left ear and, though he doesn't know their cause, they seem terribly real. At all hours of the day and through much of the night, two strangers, a man and a woman, shout that he is "a real bum" and tell him that he should use one of his weapons "for the purpose God intended them"—that is, to kill himself. Tears well in his eyes and his lip trembles as he stammers, "I feel really terrified."
>
> Although Jakob resists talking about it, he admits to drinking "a little too much, now and again." Close questioning reveals the following: Whereas for 20 years he has consumed nearly three fifths of hard liquor a week, over the past 6 months his alcohol intake had nearly doubled. A week ago, "stomach flu" caused him to vomit so often that he couldn't keep anything down, not even alcohol. It was shortly afterward that the voices began their insistent clamor.

A novice diagnostician might consider Jakob to be suffering from three different mental conditions: major depression, an acute psychotic disorder, and severe alcohol abuse. Occam's razor, however, pares the problem to its essentials: As is quite common in alcohol use disorder, Jakob's heavy alcohol use eventually induced a severe depression. When he became physically ill (was it really flu, or did his system finally rebel at so much alcohol?), he went into alcohol withdrawal and heard voices. The auditory hallucinations a person can experience in alcohol withdrawal closely mimic those of schizophrenia. Occam's razor directs us to propose that Jakob has one basic illness that has caused many symptoms and at least three mental disorders.

Such parsimonious thinking is important in part because it helps us understand what not to do. For example, Jakob's depression will probably abate once he stops drinking. Antidepressant medication would both burden his system with yet more chemicals and reinforce the idea that his depression was an independent illness that could be addressed with pills, without facing the issues of his alcohol use. The diagnosis of a psychosis due to alcohol use militates against the long-term use of antipsychotic agents: Once Jakob stops drinking, his hallucinations will surely disappear.

> *Diagnostic Principle:* **Use Occam's razor—prefer the diagnosis that provides the simplest explanation for your data.**

Zebras and Horses

The healing professions have a saying, taught to generations of students: "If you hear hoofbeats in the street, think of horses, not zebras." In other words, keep in mind the not-too-surprising fact that you are more likely to encounter common disorders than uncommon ones and adjust your diagnostic thinking accordingly. This highly useful adage is also a diagnostic principle, but it can be used in a wrong way or a right way.

The wrong way is to make it the mainstay of your diagnostic strategy, as I've seen happen, especially in regard to depression. We so often encounter what appears to be major depressive disorder that it tends to crowd out competing possibilities. Perhaps because it is readily reimbursed by insurance, clinicians often feel pressured to use this term instead of other, less well-compensated diagnoses, such as personality or adjustment disorders. Some writers have quite seriously suggested that a purely statistical approach to diagnosis (that is, always diagnose major depression, which is encountered in over 50% of mental health patients, especially in the clinic) could be a winning strategy more than half the time. Of course, what we want for our patients is to be right all the time, or as nearly so as possible.

The apparent rarity of any condition depends on the population you typically work with. If you are employed in a mental hospital, psychotic patients with schizophrenia and bipolar disorders may constitute the bulk of your practice. If you see only outpatients, you'll probably encounter many who have anxiety disorders or mild to moderate depression. Similarly (no surprise), you'll find a lot of people with drug-induced disorders in substance use treatment facilities, and patients with PTSD in Department of Veterans Affairs (VA) hospitals. It's seductive, isn't it, to think that if you see a regressed patient in a nursing home, Alzheimer's dementia will be the diagnosis? Alas, you can't rely for your diagnosis on the popularity of a given condition in your own patient population. I've encountered depression in veterans (who may also have PTSD); bipolar disorders in schoolboys (who typically have attention-deficit/hyperactivity disorder [ADHD]); and many, many instances of depression (and mania, too) in geriatric patients.

A better way to use the "horses, not zebras" principle is always to consider common diagnoses, but not to the point of ignoring other possibilities. For example (as we'll discuss in Chapter 10), when formulating a differential diagnosis I often include mood disorders, though they may not make the final cut.

> When Irwin comes to the mental health clinic, he has felt depressed for nearly 6 months. His symptoms are pretty typical, his clinician thinks—trouble sleeping, loss of appetite (though his weight had actually increased a few pounds), feelings that he is a failure, and inability to focus on his work as a kitchen remodel designer. He emphatically denies any thoughts about suicide. His boss suggested the appointment because Irwin seemed to be suffering so much. At age 38, he has never had previous emotional difficulties; he neither drinks nor uses drugs.
>
> The recent weight gain puzzles his clinician, who wonders whether, in the face of reduced appetite, the depression could have a physical cause (such as hypothyroidism or some other endocrine disorder). To be on the safe side, Irwin agrees to a checkup from his family practitioner, whom he hasn't seen for "almost longer than I can remember." In the meantime, recognizing that a physical cause for a mood disorder like Irwin's is a long shot, his clinician initiates a course of cognitive-behavioral therapy.

The diagnosis of a rare disorder is so attractive that it can seduce you into ignoring more common causes for whatever mental symptoms the patient has. Making (and reporting) such a finding is a coup; the clinician achieves instant hero status. Whereas it is vital always to keep in mind that such a thing is possible, a measured approach that also employs Occam's razor melds the benefits of accurate

Diagnostic Principle: **Horses are more common than zebras; prefer the more frequently encountered diagnosis.**

diagnosis with speedy treatment. (In the event, the concerns of Irwin's clinician were set to rest when a workup revealed no evidence of a physical cause for depression. In other words, no zebras, just an ordinary horse.)

Evaluating Your Data for a Differential Diagnosis

Putting the foregoing principles to work every day in the service of our patients may seem daunting. However, if we follow these steps for the following case histories, we'll end up with viable differential lists that lead to working diagnoses, which in each case will help us formulate a prognosis and recommend treatment. I've never met a patient whose condition required that I use all the diagnostic principles at once, but the somewhat more detailed case vignette that follows will serve to illustrate several of them.

Edna

Edna has recently become engaged, yet she has begun having anxiety episodes that she fears could make her lose her scholarship. "Could I just have a few Valiums to get me through finals?" she begs her counselor. "Maybe we should try to understand the whole picture first," comes the reply. Her story turns out to be more complicated than a few tablets can fix.

Edna had been a cheerful, somewhat roly-poly baby born to first-time parents when they were in their 40s. Her mother juggled a professional career and obsessive–compulsive disorder (OCD), which limited the time she spent with baby Edna. Her father traveled on business; when home, he spent much of his free time attending Alcoholics Anonymous (AA) meetings to maintain his rather tenuous sobriety. As a result, Edna was reared by a succession of housekeepers whose principal duties weren't child care. Left largely to her own devices, she grew up with books and television for friends, and not much in the way of social graces. A moody child to begin with, her disposition didn't improve when her menstrual periods started at age 13.

Edna had been "unnaturally shy." In fact, throughout high school she had had only one date, and that was with a second-string football player who had tried to have sex with her after the movies. "He got me down to my underwear before good judgment grabbed hold, and I got dressed." Throughout high school and her first 3 years of college, she immersed herself in study and not much else. By the fall of her senior year, she was on track to graduate a semester early, *summa cum laude* in political science.

Near Christmas, she met a young man. Always persuaded that she would never marry, she hadn't bothered much with her looks, but a roommate recently had taught her how to fix her hair and had burned the tacky pair of jeans Edna wore to class nearly every day. Perhaps the new clothes and lipstick did the trick; her young man, himself a perpetual wallflower, had pursued her vigorously and proposed on the second date. On the spot, she accepted him. "I guess I was so grateful that I just said 'Yes,'" she comments to her clinician. "It was the happiest night of my life, to coin a cliché." It was also the last truly happy day she'd enjoyed.

In the week since her engagement, Edna has spent many anxious hours. "I feel afraid—though of what, God knows—and I get short of breath and my heart beats too fast. It makes my chest hurt." In 2 days she will introduce Geoffrey to her parents, and she feels nauseated at the prospect. Now she stays up at night, trying to study, worrying that she will fail her final exams and have to remain in school an extra year. She also worries about how her parents will regard Geoffrey. Most of all, she agonizes over the prospect of getting married and perhaps having the responsibility of a family.

Edna's facial expression is lively and pleasant, though appropriately concerned; once or twice she becomes tearful, but mostly she speaks logically and in complete sentences, showing good command of her facts. Toward the end of the evaluation, Edna mentions that her roommate wants to speak with the clinician. Ann's information is brief, but telling: Edna seems just fine when she is with Ann. It's only when she is with Geoffrey, or is about to see him, or sometimes is even talking about him, that she seems flooded with anxiety.

Analysis

Here's how I'd go about mining Edna's history to create a broad-ranging differential diagnosis:

1. As in any differential diagnosis, I would first question whether there was a medical or substance use problem (two diagnostic principles that I've already mentioned, and that we'll cover further in Chapter 9). Of course, I consider medical disorder causes first—not because they are so terribly common, but because of their considerable potential for causing harm to the patient and because, often, they can be readily treated. Either the current use of a substance or withdrawal from substance use commonly

causes anxiety, and Edna had requested Valium; so a possible substance use etiology also earns its place on my list.

2. Edna's chief complaint is anxiety, so I'd then review the full spectrum of anxiety disorders, summarized in Table 12.1. She could have an incipient panic disorder or GAD, though the course of her symptoms had been very brief. The history of her present illness informs many of the choices in our differential diagnosis.

3. The family history diagnostic principle rears its head! Edna's mother had been treated for OCD, which runs in families. Genetic studies tell us that a patient with an anxiety disorder is likely to have relatives with a variety of other anxiety disorders, not just the one. (DSM-5-TR places OCD in a separate chapter, but it carries with it loads of anxiety.)

4. What wouldn't I include from the anxiety disorders list? I'd agree there's no evidence for agoraphobia, and Edna said nothing about phobias, other than whatever might be implied by the prospect of growing old without a mate. Although Geoffrey's sudden proposal preceded Edna's symptoms, it would be a real stretch to frame her story as PTSD (another former anxiety disorder that DSM-5-TR places in its own chapter).

5. Among the other items of information from the initial assessment, we note Edna's somewhat isolated childhood, which suggests the possibility of avoidant personality disorder. (However, later on we'll note a diagnostic principle that cautions us to be wary of diagnosing a personality disorder in the face of any major mental disorder.) And by the way, I'd certainly want to rule out somatizing disorders for any young person.

6. I don't mean to slight the MSE; however, rather than providing closure, its components often serve best to suggest other fields for inquiry. Edna's tearfulness does show some evidence of depression, which I nearly always include in a differential diagnosis, anyway. And yes, that is another of my diagnostic principles.

7. This vignette also demonstrates the important yet often ignored principle that collateral history can help frame the discussion of diagnosis. The information from Edna's roommate provides something that Edna seemingly cannot—perspective on timing and precipitating events. The "horses, not zebras" diagnostic principle reminds us that we should especially consider those diagnoses that occur commonly in the general population, among which are situational problems (also known as problems of living).

Considering all of the points made above, I'll propose the following differential diagnosis in evaluating Edna's problem (and leave it as an exercise to arrange these items in a safety hierarchy and determine the best diagnosis overall):

- Adjustment disorder with anxiety symptoms (problems of living)
- Anxiety disorder due to medical problem
- Avoidant personality disorder
- Depressive disorder
- GAD
- OCD
- Panic disorder
- Somatic symptom disorder
- Substance-related anxiety disorder

Dealing with Contradictory Information

When clinicians with years of experience face contradictory information, the appropriate diagnosis often seems to emerge almost by instinct. As I'll try to show with another detailed vignette, this apparent intuition is usually just a matter of noticing when clues from the history conflict with one another, or when cues from the MSE don't match up with the usual course

> *Diagnostic Principle:* Watch for contradictory information, such as affect that doesn't fit the content of thought, or symptoms that don't match the usual history of a disorder.

of a mental disorder. Resolving contradictory information is not a matter of spiritualism but of practice. I feel strongly enough about this to call it a diagnostic principle.

Tony

Tony is only 45, but as he relates his complicated history, he looks a good 10 years older. Homeless and severely depressed, he suffers from poor concentration and appetite, punishing insomnia, inability to work, and recurrent death wishes and suicidal attempts. During one such attempt, he parked his car in a remote area and ran a hose from the exhaust into the passenger compartment, started the engine, then settled down to die. That attempt failed when the gas tank ran dry before he even lost consciousness. More recently, he pointed a borrowed pistol at his head. Because several friends intervened to take it away from him, he fired all five shots into the ceiling. "It only harmed the plaster."

That episode prompted his admission to a VA hospital, where he was treated with medications. (Of all the antidepressants he has tried over the years, Prozac seemed to help the most.) While in the hospital, Tony applied for housing assistance, which was ultimately denied—he doesn't know why. Subsequently, he apparently checked himself out of the hospital; 4 days later, he found himself 200 miles away, in yet another VA hospital. He doesn't know how he traveled from one city to the other, and he cannot recall what happened during the lost time. At first, he can't even dredge up personal information such as his Social Security number, though he always knows his own name.

Tony states that besides his depression, for many years he has intermittently heard several different voices. There is his mother's voice, which laughs at him, and the voice of his dead brother. A stranger he knows only as "Cathy" pronounces his name so clearly that every time he hears it, he turns to see who might be there. He has heard none of these voices for several days prior to the current evaluation. From time to time he also has visual hallucinations of a man who stands about 12 inches tall, whom he encountered for the first time many years ago on Okinawa when serving in the Army. He also sometimes sees his mother (who is still alive) in a scene "so real I could touch her." From time to time he believes that she and other people are "laughing behind my back."

During his interview, Tony's mood appears to be about medium in quality and appropriate to the content of his thought. His affect, which is of normal lability, becomes tearful when he discusses his failed marriage. This story is that two decades ago he married a woman from Colombia, taking pains to ensure that she, her children, and her mother all became legal U.S. residents. As the result of his wife's unfounded accusations and legal chicanery, he ended up living in a hotel room while she and her relatives continued to occupy his house. He eventually abandoned all his property and moved on to become a security guard at a casino. He claims never to have used alcohol or street drugs intemperately.

As a child, Tony says, he was always depressed. Nearly friendless, he played with a rubber lizard he called "Tonto" and a number of imaginary playmates. He had a clubbed foot that was treated with a cast, which he remembers kicking through the boards of his crib when he was just a small baby.

Analysis

Some of Tony's data conflict either with one another or with common sense. For example, the repeated suicide attempts that went badly (though fortunately) awry seem exaggerated, possibly invented. In answer to his devastating marriage, he stoically abandoned his property and moved on. The visual hallucinations of his mother were more vivid than is usual for psychosis. Seeing Lilliputian people is characteristic of delirium tremens, yet he denies the use of alcohol. He gave a name to one of the voices he heard, which is unusual in psychosis. Whereas genuinely psychotic people try to ignore the hallucinations that torment them, he invariably turned to see who was talking. While in a purported fugue-like state, he traveled with apparent purpose to another VA hospital, where he was not known. Although he could have been recounting what others had told him, some statements about his own childhood seem wildly extravagant: He has "always" been depressed; he can recall kicking his crib. Finally, despite his many afflictions and sorrowful history, his mood on interview is comfortable, not depressed.

Taken one at a time, these characteristics might seem unimpressive, but in aggregate they create a reasonable suspicion of someone trying to present himself as sick and needy. This clinical picture, which also fits with a motivation for the secondary gain of being housed, places a duty upon the clinician to reject the story's face value and to investigate further before making a diagnosis and recommending treatment.

Malingering

I hate it when I'm faced with the need to diagnose malingering. Of course, if I refuse, I can't fulfill my duty as a diagnostician—but once someone's been labeled "malingerer," the cat's among the pigeons and it's hard ever again to regard that individual as anything but a manipulator and a liar. If someone admits to inventing a story, and if I can be absolutely sure of my ground, I will limit my statement to that one piece of behavior: "History of fugue state was fabricated." In other words, I label the behavior as "malingered" rather than the person as a "malingerer."

My reluctance to use these terms stems from the twin facts that, especially for mental events, malingering is terribly hard to prove, and there are no reliable criteria. A patient series that demonstrates my concern was reported from Israel by Witztum and colleagues in the journal *Military Medicine* in 1996. Of 24 individuals diagnosed as "malingerers" in the course of a year, the authors rediagnosed nearly all as having serious psychopathology, including psychosis, mental retardation, and mood disorders. All but 3 of the 24 were judged unfit to serve in the military.

The manufacture of physical symptoms is relatively easy to spot: Careful observation will reveal that the patient claiming to have kidney stones drops grains of sand into a urine specimen, or that an apparently persistent fever is the result of using the thermometer to stir coffee. Much more difficult to detect is the manufacture of mental symptoms and syndromes, which can include amnesia, PTSD, psychosis, eating disorders, bereavement, depression, mania, and even reports of stalking. I've discussed some of the warning signs in the sidebar "Recognizing Red Flag Information."

Besides the prospect of obtaining money—think insurance fraud—a variety of motives can encourage the reporting of false symptoms. Some patients want to avoid social responsibilities (such as work or child support) or dangerous assignments, especially in the military. Many clinicians have encountered patients who fake pain to obtain prescription drugs they can sell or misuse. An occasional person may minimize actual mental symptoms, "faking good" to win release from a mental hospital or regain custody of a child. And a well-known motive is to avoid punishment for a crime, through a plea of reduced capacity or insanity.

A notorious (and nearly successful) instance of blatant malingering is that of Kenneth Bianchi, one of two men who carried out the Hillside Strangler murders in the 1970s in Los Angeles and Washington State. A charming, lifelong chronic liar, Bianchi had previously set himself up as a psychotherapist with a fake diploma from Columbia University and a "doctor of psychiatry" degree from a nonexistent institution. When caught, Bianchi produced a second personality, Steven, who brazenly claimed responsibility for the murders ("Killing a broad doesn't make any difference to me"). So persuasive was this performance that several experts in multiple personality disorder (MPD, now referred to as dissociative identity disorder) pronounced him psychotic and therefore not accountable for his crimes. But Bianchi met his match when the prosecution brought in psychiatrist Martin Orne, who told him (falsely) that all cases of MPD have more than two made-up personalities. Within hours, a third personality obligingly emerged. One of the clinicians who had been taken in, after becoming a prison psychiatrist and learning that he had "no reason to believe anything they said," later recanted belief in Bianchi's MPD.

There are degrees of malingering. In the most blatant cases, patients simply make stuff up; some exaggerate actual symptoms. Still others may

Recognizing Red Flag Information

A variety of characteristics raise the red flag of warning that a patient's data cannot be accepted at face value. Before fully trusting this information, you must compare it with interview data from informants, with previous medical records, with laboratory tests—or perhaps you should test it by the simple means of further frank discussion. Especially revealing among such items of history and behavior are the following, listed in no particular order:

Memory loss in the absence of cognitive disorder. A poor memory, readily fabricated and difficult to verify, can prove irresistible for patients who have something to hide or to gain.

Spotty amnesia. Someone claims not to remember personal information but converses about contemporary issues of the day.

Use of extreme language to describe symptoms. Examples include "I lost 20 pounds in 3 days," "I sometimes go a whole week without a wink of sleep."

A patient who engages in criminal behavior while hospitalized. This may include assaults, sex with staff or other patients, and dealing drugs.

Repeated unsuccessful suicide attempts. Although many patients make multiple, sincere efforts to end their lives, others seem to be play-acting in an effort to attract attention or sympathy. The danger is that it can be hard to gauge the level of sincerity.

Unusual symptoms. Here we'd include symptoms that are excessively dramatic, rare, or severe—beyond the usual range of psychopathology. One example is Tony's behavior on hearing voices (he turned to confront them every time he heard them). Others would be claims to have schizophrenia characterized by delusions that begin or end suddenly, visual hallucinations of doll-sized people, or hallucinations that are continuous rather than intermittent. The onset of symptoms may be more sudden than is usual for the given diagnosis (full-blown delusions that develop overnight). Symptoms of many disorders beginning at the same time can sometimes be a tip-off. Of course, an especially crafty patient may have consulted textbooks to learn how mental illness typically presents.

Absence of typical symptoms. For example, most depressed people will have problems with sleep and appetite; the absence of such problems should raise suspicions.

A story that keeps changing. People who make up or exaggerate material may find it hard to keep their stories straight.

(*cont.*)

Recognizing Red Flag Information (*cont.*)

Multiple personalities. Genuine dissociative identity disorder has been well documented for decades, but so has the fabrication of "alternates" by some people to avoid detection or punishment for criminal or otherwise unwelcome behavior.

Secondary gain. Symptoms that help a person gain money or avert loss require thoughtful evaluation.

Course of illness atypical for a given mental disorder. A patient who has worked steadily for a decade yet claims a long history of schizophrenia would arouse my suspicions.

Poor cooperation. Patients who evade or outright refuse to answer questions during testing or the interview may have something to hide. I'd also worry about someone who refuses to allow consultation with informants.

Incongruous affect. Bland or even cheerful affect that doesn't match a person's serious circumstances, such as paralysis or blindness, is sometimes called *la belle indifférence*; it is often encountered in patients with somatizing disorders. (However, you may encounter a silly or otherwise incongruous affect in other disorders.)

Interpersonal manner. Research has documented clinicians' tendency to believe an assertive individual who has a pleasant facial expression and dominates the conversation. We need to be alert lest such characteristics of normalcy overwhelm our judgment of a patient's essential truthfulness.

Performance below chance on standard tests of memory, cognition, or intellect. Even random answers should be right some of the time; to score worse than chance requires planning. Some patients give blatantly false answers: "2 times 2 is 5," "Santa's suit is green," "There are 30 hours in a day."

Hospitalization in many locations. In what was classically called Münchausen syndrome (now, factitious disorder), patients move from one caregiving institution to another.

Failure of multiple normally adequate treatments. Patients who remain depressed after treatment with various antidepressants, cognitive-behavioral therapy, and a course of electroconvulsive therapy deserve a complete reevaluation rather than yet another course of therapy.

Internal inconsistencies in the patient's history. For example, a patient on welfare who talks about business deals should prompt more careful examination of other aspects of the history.

falsely attribute their symptoms to something they know is not actually the cause; for example, a patient may claim that anxiety symptoms, actually of long standing, arose after a minor industrial accident.

Whether history and behaviors are tailored from whole cloth or merely embroidered, there's more to the differential diagnosis than just malingering. One possibility is factitious disorder (most famously, persons with Münchausen syndrome who obtain admission to a succession of hospitals); another, which seems possible in the case of Kenneth Bianchi, antisocial personality disorder. You may also encounter unconsciously augmented or made up symptoms in patients with various somatizing and dissociative disorders.

5 Coping with Uncertainty

When I was a medical student, several of my teachers, in agreement rare among psychiatrists, pointed out that a well-trained mental health clinician can make a valid diagnosis after a single interview about four times out of five; on the fifth, however, the clinician can interview for hours and still be uncertain. Over the intervening decades, that figure hasn't changed much, so if you evaluate several new patients a week, you'll have to learn to cope with diagnostic uncertainty. This chapter presents some ideas on dealing with uncertainty when it arises and explains why the concept itself is so valuable to the pursuit of accurate diagnoses.

Why Aren't We Certain?

You might dream of the time when all the uncertainty will be gone from the diagnostic process, but I think that happy day is far in the future. The main reason is both obvious and inescapable: There will always be patients for whom we lack adequate, reliable information. Although patients with cognitive deficits such as Alzheimer's dementia may want very much to cooperate, they will have difficulty remembering important facts. Relatives may have been out of contact with such people too long to contribute essential information. Someone who is paranoid or who has previously had unhappy experiences with health care may be afraid to reveal facts pertinent to diagnosis.

> When Nigel first consults his new caregiver, a young woman still in training at the university clinic, he feels suddenly embarrassed about the cause of his anxiety and depression. It requires most of the first session before he finally discloses that he has been repeatedly impotent with his fiancée, who had suggested the evaluation.

Other patients may try to shield themselves or others from possible prosecution.

> Accused of destroying his neighbor's home in a futile search for money and drugs, Trevor is interviewed in jail. Professing to have a bipolar disorder, he claims to have been "blacked out" for the events in question. He refuses to allow clinicians to contact family members for additional information that could validate—or, of course, refute—his claim of a potentially exculpatory mental disorder.

Still other patients who seek to restrict information about their histories include those who have factitious or paranoid disorders. And some, for a great variety of other reasons, just plain don't tell the truth.

It happens more often than we sometimes realize that a patient's database simply will never be complete until we've obtained collateral information—usually from a relative, but sometimes from old charts or previous clinicians.

> Jeff gave a history of manic and depressive mood swings typical of bipolar illness. Although he denied that he had ever used alcohol heavily, Louise, his ex-wife, left me a voice mail message that she had often seen him in a stupor. It wasn't until I went to his house one evening, after a neighbor had called Louise to express concern about a raucous disturbance, that I saw him acutely intoxicated on both alcohol and cocaine. I persuaded him to be admitted to a hospital; the following day, he finally confessed that his mood swings had all occurred while he was under the influence.

Sometimes we clinicians must bear the responsibility for insufficient information. If in the rush to complete an assessment I omit questions about anxiety symptoms, I risk overlooking an important diagnosis. In the middle of the night, a sleepy on-call clinician who doesn't dig through a thick chart may fail to note that a psychotic patient had an abnormal EEG the year before and was successfully treated with anticonvulsants. I believe that many missed and incorrect diagnoses stem from failure to collect and use all the relevant data, although I have no data other than my years of observing interviewer performance to support this belief.

On the other hand (wouldn't you know?), sometimes extra information confuses the diagnosis. The situation can be something rather simple, as when a patient with a long history of psychosis presents features that are atypical for schizophrenia—terrific insight and well-modulated affect, perhaps. Or consider those who, in their eagerness to provide information, give positive answers to such a broad array of questions that you can't rule out anything. Then it's a matter of sifting through the facts and deciding which are most relevant to the current clinical situation. And in Chapter 4, I've described how contradictory information sources can lead to diagnostic confusion.

An issue we don't often mention is the clinician who fails to keep up to date with the explosive growth of knowledge. I've encountered any number of mental health professionals who base diagnoses of schizophrenia on their clinical intuition, rather than on the best practices informed by clinical studies. The specter of such behavior is what drives most of us—almost from the moment we complete training and embark on independent careers as health care providers—to read journals, attend conferences, and accumulate continuing education credits, all in the effort to stay current with the latest developments in diagnosis and treatment. Keeping current has become institutionalized for medical professionals, whose board certifications are now good only for a limited time (usually 10 years), after which they must sit for a recertification exam.

Of course, the myriad combinations of symptoms individual patients present can confuse even the best-trained, most up-to-date practitioners. Some well-recognized examples are even written into established criteria. In one of these, the atypical specifier for depression, appetite and sleep may be increased, not decreased as you'd expect in the usual case of depression.

Sometimes, sticking too closely to established criteria can cause a missed diagnosis.

> A rare example would be Corrine, whose magnum of red wine every day has never caused her problems. Single all her life, she lives on inherited wealth. A companion manages her financial affairs and sees to it that she gets proper nutrition and good health care. If you insist on the exact criteria for alcohol use disorder, Corrine might not qualify.

Then again, established criteria don't cover every possible manifestation of mental disease; some patients have symptoms that don't conform to conventional notions of a given disorder.

> Arvin recently moved west from Indiana, where he attended college. Now 35, his long history of mood disorder began at the age of 10, when he attempted suicide by drinking Lysol. Fortunately, he gagged

before he could get much of the liquid down and he suffered no lasting ill effects. At about that time he also took his first drink of alcohol, and thus began a long downward spiral of substance use (marijuana and amphetamines when he was 12) and depression. Because he was bright and could pass tests easily, he finished high school with his class. Then, when he was 19, he suffered his first episode of mania.

Now going forward, Arvin's depressions never last longer than about 10 days, and about half the time they are interwoven with bursts of mania. His lows and his highs meet respective criteria for major depression or manic episode, sometimes with mixed features. However, because his depressive episodes are so brief, a clinician recently refused to diagnose him with bipolar I disorder. "He told me that I had 'mood disorder not otherwise specified,' " Arvin reports in some consternation. "What does *that* mean?" Despite his diagnosis, Arvin's moods level out when he starts taking a mood-stabilizing medication.

Every experienced clinician has seen countless patients like Arvin who in some way or other don't quite fit official diagnostic criteria. Mostly, therapy proceeds just as though the criteria have been fully met, and it works out just fine. I echo the view, enshrined in the easily overlooked statements in the fine print of official criteria sets: Criteria should be viewed as guidelines, not straitjackets, and clinicians should use them with judgment that takes all the individual circumstances into account.

We must also acknowledge that some behaviors can resemble mental illness at first glance but are actually more or less "normal" (see the sidebar "What's Normal?"). Sometimes these are termed *mental illness confounds*. For example, some people will respond to a variety of situations with emotion that is more intense than average. What I'm trying to warn against is overinterpreting behavior that may differ from our own in a similar circumstance, yet still be within the boundaries of normal. Here are a few examples:

- Francine is a senior in college. Her anxiety could signal GAD or some other anxiety disorder, but it might reflect a normal response to the divorce of her parents and her impending Graduate Record Examination. Often, anxiety is perfectly normal, even expected.
- Do Oscar's feelings of intense sadness indicate mood disorder or a response to breaking up with his fiancée? Personal unhappiness is often normal.
- At 16, Winnie repeatedly shoplifts from several stores in the mall. She could have kleptomania, but might she be responding to a schoolmate's

What's Normal?

From my internet correspondents, I repeatedly hear this complaint: "The textbooks and diagnostic manuals don't tell me what's normal."

It's a fair criticism. We're so used to spelling out the abnormal that we sometimes end up defining what's normal by what we believe. That puts it into the dubious category of "I know it when I see it," as Potter Stewart, associate justice of the U.S. Supreme Court, famously defined *pornography*. Derived from the Latin *norma,* meaning "carpenter's square," the meanings of *normal* include "average," "healthy," "usual," and "the ideal." There are problems with each of these—you might be forgiven for suspecting that definitional diversity is the norm. If we define *normal* as "average," then it would mean some (if minor) degree of impairment, because so many adults are impaired by mental disorder. If it means "healthy," as in the absence of disease, then nearly half of all Americans are mentally abnormal. If it's "what's usual," then we'd consider abnormal those who drink no alcohol at all. And if it's "the ideal," then normality is a state to which we can aspire, but never attain.

We are left bobbing in a sea of ad hoc decisions concerning the illnesses we encounter. For example, we must differentiate the misuse of substances from social drinking, recreational drug use (however normal that may be), and the appropriate use of prescription drugs. We've even coined special terms for some conditions that we regard as normal and must differentiate from illness: *adult antisocial behavior,* for common criminals who lack the cachet of antisocial personality disorder; *age-related decline,* for the not-quite-dementia experienced by those of us lucky enough to survive middle age; *bereavement,* which we all (mostly) hope never to experience ourselves yet assume others will one day suffer on our behalf.

Below I've listed some mental states and symptoms, along with the normal situations from which we must differentiate them. Note that we sometimes use the words *common, ordinary,* or *everyday* as code for *normal.* This raises the interesting point that for some behaviors, the definition of what's normal is a little skewed. Consider, for example, ordinary shoplifting (as distinct from kleptomania), common criminality (vs. antisocial personality disorder), and everyday fire starting for profit (vs. pyromania).

Pathology	*Normal*
Psychosis	Dreams, imaginary playmates, *déjà vu,* and the hallucinations that occur when we are falling asleep or awakening
Depression, mania	Common sadness and joy experienced in daily life

Pathology	*Normal*
Panic attacks	Adaptive fright that helps us avoid speeding trucks, raging torrents, and crashing bores
Phobias	Realistic concerns about being embarrassed (such as someone who stutters might feel) or unable to help oneself (as perhaps a person with physical handicap might feel)
Social anxiety	Stage or microphone fright and ordinary shyness that doesn't result in clinically important distress or impairment
Obsessions, compulsions	Superstitions; checking once to see that the stove is truly turned off before we depart for the airport
Pathological worry	Legitimate concerns such as paying the rent and putting the kids through college when we've just been laid off
Somatization, hypochondriasis	Concerns about demonstrable physical disorders
Dissociation	Daydreams, reveries, and fantasies
Compulsive gambling	Professional and recreational betting
Gender dysphoria	Tomboyishness, theatrical role playing
Paraphilias	Use of fantasy to enhance sexual excitement
Personality disorder	Personality and character traits that are merely annoying (yours) or even endearing (mine)

threats to tell her religiously strict parents that she has had an abortion? Isolated bits of behavior can suggest a diagnosis, but without context, they don't constitute one.

• On the day of the big game, Gordon wears the colors of his high school's arch-rival team. He courts social disapproval and undoubtedly craves attention, but his behavior doesn't qualify him for a diagnosis. A need for individuality and recognition is part of growing up, and of the human condition in general.

- Sandy drinks and uses drugs excessively, to the point of having declining grades and an arrest for drunk driving. Does this extremely common behavior foreshadow substance use disorder, or is it simply going along with the gang?

Resolving Diagnostic Uncertainty

As I've noted earlier, only about 80% of new patients can be diagnosed on first interview. This section provides some techniques that may help you reach that percentage.

It is natural that whenever we come to a stumbling block in the diagnostic process, often our first impulse is to look for more information. Sometimes an additional patient interview, focused on the specifics of what we need to resolve our doubts, will succeed. At other times, information from another resource (such as a relative, friend, or former physician of the patient) or a review of previous health care records can make the difference. However, some histories are just plain confusing and will remain so well past the appropriate time to start treatment. Then we must look for clues that will help us arrange the possible diagnoses into a workable differential list.

Past Behavior

I've co-opted as a diagnostic principle the truism that the best predictor of future behavior is past behavior. It applies to many areas of life, but it is especially valuable in making a mental health diagnosis. It suggests that anyone who has had a syndrome or set of symptoms for months or years is likely to continue to have them far into the future. Here's an example:

Ned appears to be in his mid-40s when the police bring him to the emergency room. They found him at the entrance to a major shopping venue in the mall. Wearing a helmet made of aluminum foil, Ned was advising customers that a giant meteor was approaching the Pacific Northwest. When it struck, all life would be annihilated. He speaks rapidly, and his grandiose ideas (his ex-wife is a member of the Rockefeller family; he can control the outcome of an impending election)

> **Diagnostic Principle:**
> **The best predictor of future behavior is past behavior.**

seem to tumble one after another without logical sequence. A call to the telephone number scribbled on a piece of paper in his pocket elicit the information that for years Ned has been chronically ill with psychosis. For the evaluating clinician, schizophrenia becomes the best working diagnosis.

More Symptoms of a Diagnosis

You'd think that a patient who has a lot of symptoms would fit a given syndrome better than someone with just a few symptoms, and you'd be right— up to a point. I would certainly vote for depression in someone who has seven or eight of the usual symptoms. But in using this diagnostic principle, remember that some symptoms carry far greater weight than others. For example, depressive mood all day every day suggests major depression far more strongly than does another criterion, feeling fatigued. And a markedly limited range of emotional expression may suggest psychosis, though probably less strongly than does hearing the voice of your deceased grandfather.

Diagnostic Principle: **Having more symptoms of a disorder increases its likelihood as your diagnosis.**

As a corollary, note that the mere fact of having *serious* symptoms doesn't necessarily mean that a given disorder is present. For example, in Part II of this book we'll see that many people experiencing suicidal ideas have a primary diagnosis other than major depressive disorder.

Presence of Typical Features

If your patient has symptoms or other features you usually expect to encounter in a given disorder, you'll want to consider it strongly for your working diagnosis. Loss of interest in work and leisure activities (including sex), poor concentration, and poor appetite and insomnia point strongly to major depression. On the other hand, your diagnosis will be more secure if there aren't any symptoms

Diagnostic Principle: **Typical features of a disorder increase its likelihood as your diagnosis; faced with nontypical features, look for alternatives.**

that suggest other conditions. For example, if Serena complains of hallucinations but you notice numerous manic symptoms, schizophrenia becomes unattractive as her diagnosis.

Previous Typical Response to Treatment

Response to treatment can be tricky; a substantial number of patients with nearly any condition will improve, even on placebo—even if they *know* the pills contain no active ingredient. However, sometimes the response to treatment provides an important diagnostic clue. If you learn that Morton's earlier episode of so-called

> **Diagnostic Principle: Previous typical response to treatment for a disorder increases its likelihood as your current diagnosis.**

schizophrenia resolved completely with a mood-stabilizing drug, you will strongly suspect that the actual diagnosis is a mood disorder.

The Value of the Term *Undiagnosed*

After you have recorded all the history you can find, pursued every clue from the MSE, interviewed relatives and friends, and consulted the available records, you *still* may be unable to validate a definitive diagnosis. And that's just fine. It is important to recognize that for some patients, an immediate diagnosis simply won't be possible; for a few, uncertainty could drag on for months or years. For all of these, you have at your disposal one of the most powerful descriptions in the book: *undiagnosed*.

> **Diagnostic Principle: Use the word *undiagnosed* whenever you cannot be sure of your diagnosis.**

I'm not kidding about this. *Undiagnosed* is one of my all-time favorite diagnostic terms. I think of it as a safety valve that allows us to acknowledge that something is wrong without rushing to closure—which I would define as the point at which we too often stop thinking. It helps us avoid making a diagnosis such as schizophrenia, Alzheimer's dementia, or antisocial personality disorder that could harm someone if it turns out not to be true. This is doubly important, now that insurance companies, employers, law enforcement agencies, and patients themselves increasingly pursue the desire to review medical records.

Undiagnosed can keep you alert to data that don't quite fit. When you write it down you are saying, "This patient probably has a mental disorder, but I'm not sure which one." When you invoke this diagnostic principle, you keep yourself honest and you demonstrate that honesty to others. Every time we see the *undiagnosed* label on a patient's chart or record, it forces us to think anew: "What additional information have I obtained since the last time? What have I learned about disease that might now be relevant to this patient?" If the answers continue to be "Still not enough," *undiagnosed* stimulates further inquiry.

Some clinicians don't like to confess uncertainty: Could it reduce a patient's confidence in them? I think it far more likely to facilitate trust in a clinician candid enough to acknowledge that knowledge has its limits. Furthermore, by reducing unrealistic expectations, it could mitigate the likelihood of litigation if unforeseen difficulties should arise in the course of therapy. *Undiagnosed* can restrain you from rushing into unwarranted, possibly high-risk treatment. (For example, if you admit you don't know what's wrong, you're unlikely to recommend medications that carry the risk of serious side effects.) It should certainly bar a patient from participation in any experimental treatment trial.

I've always considered diagnosis to be a team sport, not a vehicle for individual showboating. *Undiagnosed* alerts other clinicians on your team to think deeply about this patient. This is especially important in an institutional setting, where in the course of evaluation, patients typically encounter many professionals. Even in private offices, clinicians refer patients for specialized problems and take night and weekend calls for one another— more opportunities for a hasty, incorrect diagnosis to cause harm. Perhaps a fresh set of eyes will react to the *undiagnosed* label by uncovering information or making a connection that you and I have missed. With time, additional symptoms may bring the diagnosis into focus. *Undiagnosed* forces us to shine a light on uncertainty; without it, we remain unaware that we are still in the dark.

Quite frankly, as I have gained experience with age, I have worried more about becoming too sanguine about my diagnostic ability. This is part of the reason I emphasize *undiagnosed* in my teaching and writing. One last note: *Undiagnosed* is somewhat safer than *unspecified X disorder*, which is what DSM-5-TR calls a disorder that doesn't fully meet official criteria. My concern is that *unspecified X disorder* lends an aura of finality that tends to choke off further investigation. I try to avoid it.

Why Can't We Make a Diagnosis?

Managing uncertainty can be far more complicated than simply gathering additional information—though that would be an excellent start. Here are several factors that can contribute to confusion about a given patient's diagnosis:

- Some people simply don't show enough traditional symptoms to justify a diagnosis. Perhaps it is early in the course of an illness, and the typical symptoms have not yet developed. Time will resolve this issue, but meanwhile, clinicians will struggle to create a sensible treatment plan. It raises this question: How close to the ideal patient should we require a person's symptoms to be before making a diagnosis? Here's one guidepost: Any illness close to the bottom of the hierarchy of safe diagnoses (Table 3.1) should require more symptoms and more typical symptoms than a relatively benign diagnosis.

- Some patients have so many symptoms that clinicians become confused. Although this should be simply a matter of further inquiry, sorting it out takes time and diligence. Resist the temptation to reach for the nearest likely approximation.

- Some features are uncommon. Atypical features of depression have already been enshrined in their own special criteria, but a diagnostician who insists on the "letter of the law" could be perplexed by a patient who presents with unusual symptoms.

- Perhaps this patient has an illness that hasn't yet been identified. I admit that this is a long shot, but it's hardly beyond the realm of possibility. After all, textbooks of the early 1900s discussed only a few disorders, compared to the dozens of major ones (and hundreds of variants) we now recognize. Each of these relative newcomers came from somewhere, and there could still be other conditions out there, hiding in plain sight. Successive editions of the DSM list in an appendix research criteria for half a dozen or more new disorders for further study.

- Some emotional or behavioral characteristics may not lend themselves to being counted and lumped into categories. Perhaps dimensional criteria are needed instead. An example would be personality, for which various inventories have been devised that measure each individual against a number of scales. Patterns of deviation on these scales constitute what we call *personality disorders*. The DSM-5 Task Force flirted with dimensional personality diagnoses—before finally adopting the same old system that's been used for years. DSM-5-TR has held the line, but the debate rages on with no clear end in sight. Brace yourself for further revisions. But you should be aware that other diagnostic systems may better describe some aspects of psychopathology.

- Finally, some patients simply don't require a diagnosis. These are the folks who seek help not because they are sick, but because they fear they might be. When it's because they have a problem of living, it can be as vital to diagnose *no* mental disorder as it is for others to receive the correct diagnosis of a mental disorder. In short, the ability to rule a diagnosis in or out is one of the most powerful tools the clinician can employ. Even a disorder that is fairly far down on the safety hierarchy provides the comfort of no longer having to fear the unknown. Of course, for the clinician, nothing beats the shared

> *Diagnostic Principle:* Consider the possibility that this patient should be given no mental diagnosis at all.

joy of informing a patient, "I don't find any indication of an actual mental illness. You're only experiencing the sort of thing normal people encounter from time to time, and we can work on that together."

In the history that follows, look for evidence supporting the several reasons why I would choose to defer diagnosis.

Vickie

She's only 20 years old, but already Vickie complains of "lifelong depression." She has had two prior admissions to a psychiatric hospital for suicide attempts—the first one at age 10, when she swallowed a handful of her mother's antidepressants. Now her husband's parents have just told her that they are moving to a retirement community, where they can no longer provide day care for their granddaughter.

Vickie has been under treatment for the past 3 years, during which she's tried at least six antidepressant medications. Most recently, she took venlafaxine (300 mg per day); several weeks earlier, when she was instructed to double the dose of this medication, her moods began to "fly up and down" and she was rediagnosed as having bipolar disorder. She then discontinued the drug because of hives. At interview, she describes her moods as being depressed for up to a week, followed by 2 or 3 days of "highs," by which she appears to mean "approximately normal"—she denies grandiosity, rapid thoughts, or hyperactivity that would be typical of mania. Even when she was depressed, she felt better when events distracted her ("I can be goofy at work").

She complains that her sleep has been terrible for years: "I go all night without any sleep at all, even when I take a double dose of medicine." Because her sleep is so poor, she has trouble concentrating on her usual activities, and she worries that she will be unable to keep her two jobs, both of which she needs. Although her appetite is down, she has not lost weight.

For years Vickie has heard voices in her head. She doesn't recognize them; sometimes they say mean things, though often it is "just conversation." At times, as if viewing a TV program, she can watch herself "talking to someone else." As a result of these experiences, she has been tried on several antipsychotic medications. However, she denies ever feeling that she is being harassed, spied upon, followed, or otherwise persecuted.

In the past 6 months, Vickie has felt even worse than usual. This decline was precipitated by current problems, including many bills to pay, some of which are the result of her multiple medical problems. She also has disagreements with her husband, to whom she's been married for 3 years. Some of this marital friction has been due to her working two jobs; because their work schedules never seemed to coincide, they rarely see each other. Moreover, Vickie despairs of finding another babysitter as caring (and inexpensive) as her mother-in-law.

Besides her emotional difficulties, Vickie had been told she has fibromyalgia, hypothyroidism, and asthma. However, her physical symptoms aren't extensive enough to qualify for the diagnosis of somatic symptom disorder. When she was a child, her parents both drank heavily, and her father refused to seek help for an older sister who had mental retardation (as it was then called) that resulted in problems with acting-out behavior. There is no other history of mental illness in her immediate or extended family. However, once, when she was 8, her mother's favorite brother got into bed with her when intoxicated and fondled her under her nightdress—an episode she never revealed to her parents.

Slightly overweight, Vickie appears somewhat older than her stated age. She sits quietly during the interview, is clean and neat, dressed casually in slacks and a brightly colored blouse. Her forearms are covered with red marks that appear to be healed-over scabs. She admits that she picks at herself repeatedly "because I'm so nervous," and thin white scars on her wrists mark where during her early teens she often cut herself. She speaks clearly and coherently, and her mood seems to be about medium in quality and appropriate to the content of her thought. She brightens when she talks about the city in California where she was brought up ("I'd love to move back there some day"). Although the thought of suicide "has been my constant companion," she denies that she has those thoughts now.

Analysis

Vickie presents a history of depression that she describes extravagantly—it has been "lifelong," she can go "all night without any sleep at all"—and with too few criteria to make any solid diagnosis. Although she claims to be depressed, neither her mood nor her affect is currently depressed (we can invoke the diagnostic principle about contradictory information). Her symptoms of mania seem too weak and too brief for bipolar disorder (in other words, she doesn't meet the "typical features" diagnostic principle). She admits to some psychotic symptoms (hallucinations) yet displays no delusions or abnormalities of affect or speech that would justify the diagnosis of schizophrenia. The lesions on her forearms persuade us to consider the additional possibility of excoriation disorder. There is evidence that she and her husband have interpersonal problems; these, with a history of unpaid bills and of cutting and picking at herself, would make me wonder whether she might have a personality disorder. However, as we'll discuss in the next chapter, I much prefer not to invoke a personality diagnosis early in an evaluation and especially in the presence of a possible major mental diagnosis. Vickie's multiple trials on antidepressants have been fruitless. Of course, this could simply mean that none was the right medication or in an adequate dose, but after several attempts, we begin to think how strongly Vickie's "depression" contravened the diagnostic principle about typical response to treatment. On top of all this, she comes to evaluation in the midst of a personal crisis—a diagnostic principle that we've already noted should make us careful in assessing her information. In short, I can't get close to a concrete diagnosis for Vickie; for now, I feel we would be far better off with the *undiagnosed* label.

Comment

The term *undiagnosed* is hardly a recent invention. The *Oxford English Dictionary* notes its first appearance in 1864, but not until 1917 was it first used to mean "psychosis not diagnosed" by the American Medico-Psychological Association, the forerunner of today's American Psychiatric Association.

6 Multiple Diagnoses

Among Aaron's complaints are severe depression, auditory hallucinations, trouble sleeping, bouts of drinking, and episodes of anxiety so severe that he cannot focus on his day job as a computer programmer, let alone pursue the dream of forming his own rock band. We'll discuss his case in greater detail later, but for now consider this question: As his clinician, how would you diagnose Aaron—with one illness or five?

Although you might think that multiple diagnoses would all have to be present at the same time to count, this isn't necessarily the case. And that's just one of the sometimes puzzling features of such diagnoses. Another is the fact that with some disorders (a good example is social anxiety disorder), people usually don't even appear for treatment until other problems come up, such as depression or panic attacks. In this chapter, we'll sort all of this out and discuss what we clinicians need to consider in making (or rejecting) more than one diagnosis at a time.

What Is Comorbidity?

When someone has multiple diagnoses, we speak of *comorbidity*. Some clinicians feel it should be applied to all patients in whom two distinct disorders occur together, but most would agree that truly comorbid diagnoses cannot cause one another. Just as you wouldn't say that coughs and sneezes are comorbid in a cold, the typical facial features of Down syndrome cannot be comorbid with intellectual disability (they both result from the same pathological process). Similarly, because alcohol use disorder and intoxication regularly occur together and derive from the same underlying process, we don't speak of them as being comorbid.

> True comorbidity occurs when a person has independent multiple diagnoses.

Although some illnesses appear to be highly comorbid, their relationship may simply be one of sharing many symptoms. For example, in recent years researchers have hotly debated the question of how social anxiety disorder and avoidant personality disorder are related. Some authorities argue that the two conditions are just statistical variations of one another; others insist that they are distinct conditions that often occur together. I could make a similar case for somatic symptom disorder and histrionic personality disorder.

Even when narrow definitions are used, 21st-century patients with mental disorders have an enormous risk of comorbidity (see the sidebar "Comorbidity Rates"). For some individual diseases, the comorbidity is well over 50%. In the early 1990s, the U.S. National Comorbidity Survey of persons ages 15–54 found that a whopping 48% of the general population had at some time at least one disorder, and 27% had at least two; 14% reported three or more. A little math reveals that of those with at least one disorder, over half have at least one additional disorder. Of all mental illnesses diagnosed in adults, nearly half occur in just 14% of the overall population. This enormous burden of mental illness strongly suggests that every mental health professional should work diligently to rule in (or out) multiple diagnoses. Recognizing them all presents a challenge that often goes unmet; studies have repeatedly shown that professionals who employ an unstructured clinical interview make far fewer diagnoses than are identified by an interview that systematically covers all the bases.

Why Look for Comorbidity?

Beyond the satisfaction of having the most complete picture possible of a patient's illness, searching out comorbid diagnoses has a lot to recommend it.

Comorbidity Rates

Comorbidity rates for patients will yield estimates higher than those just given for a general population. It's easy to see why. Most people who appear for a mental health assessment will have at least one disorder, with increased odds that one or more additional disorders will be found during the course of evaluation. Here's another factor that has increased comorbidity rates: Through the years, the DSMs have eliminated many exclusionary rules. For example, most of the anxiety disorders can now be diagnosed along with a mood disorder—a practice that was not allowed earlier.

1. Comorbidity helps determine the scope of treatment. It seems obvious that if you miss part of the diagnostic picture, you might also neglect aspects of treatment. If Aaron's alcohol misuse goes undetected, he might not get substance use treatment that is vital to his overall outcome. Here's another wrinkle: I've repeatedly seen it happen that someone like Aaron with, say, schizophrenia and a substance use disorder gets bounced back and forth between treatment teams. The mental health team packs him off to the substance use folks, who throw up their hands because he has a psychotic disorder. With the remedy for each condition waiting on treatment for the other, Aaron's plight becomes a classic catch-22. Obviously, he needs simultaneous treatment for both conditions, and this depends on an early, complete diagnosis. Here are two more wrinkles. First, the presence of one diagnosis may alter the course of treatment for another, especially if drugs that interfere with one another are contemplated. Second, the patient may have a physical disorder as well (such as diabetes) that could be exacerbated by the drug prescribed for a mental condition.

2. This brings up the whole issue of prognosis. Patients who have, say, bipolar I disorder comorbid with an anxiety disorder tend to get sick younger, stay sick longer, respond less well to traditional mood-stabilizing drugs, have an increased risk of suicide, and endure a poorer quality of life than someone with uncomplicated bipolar I disorder. Successfully predicting the interactions of multiple diagnoses requires that first, we must recognize that they all exist.

3. Anticipating a second disorder can guard against future complications. For example, if your patient has bipolar disorder, you know to be extra vigilant for substance use, even though there may be no current evidence for it. In a 2003 paper, Keel and colleagues found that several women with anorexia nervosa who were not drinking at the beginning of the study had developed alcoholism by the time they were followed up 7–12 years later.

4. Some writers, such as Krueger, have suggested that comorbidity indicates underlying common psychopathology. If research demonstrates this to be the case, we should begin to look for core underpinnings, rather than focusing on the separate diagnoses.

Identifying Comorbidity

Deciding when additional diagnoses are warranted isn't always easy. Such a decision relies on having a complete set of data, to which the clinician must add the knowledge of diagnostic criteria and an understanding of cause and effect. The central question is this: After the principal diagnosis has been made, has anything been left unexplained? For an example, let's consider Aaron's mental health history in more detail.

Aaron

When Aaron comes to the clinic, he is in trouble up to his nose ring. His performance at work (as a computer programmer) is being severely hampered by the worsening state of his mental health. Now 32, 7 years earlier he suffered one episode of acute psychosis. Diagnosed then as having schizophrenia, he was treated first with Haldol and later with Risperdal. His symptoms largely resolved, he continues to have lingering fears that someone from "the government" might be watching to see whether he is creating computer viruses. Even so, he has been able to hang onto his Silicon Valley job. At the suggestion of a new HMO physician, he has recently backed off his medication "to see how little I can get by on." He has been on half his previous dose for over a month, when he once again hears voices saying, "You'd better watch yourself," and "Don't trust those doctors—they don't know what they're doing." His clinician immediately increases the dose of Risperdal to its former level, and the hallucinations begin to abate.

Even as the psychosis lifts, Aaron's mood founders. He remembers those weeks he spent in a mental hospital long ago, and he fears a recurrence of medication side effects. Ruminations about the government interfere with his concentration, so that he can accomplish only a fraction of his daily work. He loses interest in his hobby (he collects the postage stamps of Denmark) and stops attending meetings of his stamp club; professional and hobby journals piled up unread. Although he thinks his appetite is about normal, he's lost weight.

Many nights, worries that a government agency is censoring his email keep Aaron awake for hours. As he's done before, he has started to drink as a sleeping aid. "Mostly it's Bloody Marys—the tomato juice makes them seem slightly healthful—but lots of Bloody Marys," he confesses. Though he telecommutes from home, many mornings he is too hung over to start work on time. His parents tell him how worried they are about his drinking. Just before returning to his mental health counselor, he begins having thoughts that he "might be better off dead."

Analysis

The evidence supporting Aaron's diagnosis of schizophrenia is rock-solid. He has a long history (satisfying the diagnostic principle concerning past behavior) of both hallucinations and delusions (typical symptoms) that responded well to the dose of antipsychotic medication commonly prescribed for this condition; when the dose is decreased, he relapses (note the diagnostic principle about typical response to treatment). But now other symptoms appear—low mood, the loss of concentration, problems with eating and sleeping, and increasing thoughts about dying. His principal diagnosis of schizophrenia would not adequately cover this group of symptoms, so we must expand his working diagnosis to include both schizophrenia *and* a depressive disorder; we shouldn't have to choose between these two conditions.

Now let's consider Aaron's drinking, which has accelerated with increasing psychotic symptoms. The drinking is extensive enough to alarm both Aaron and his parents. Even if he didn't have schizophrenia, he would probably need help to get sober and stay that way. Although substance use frequently accompanies many mental disorders, it appears nowhere among their criteria. Aaron does not appear to be dependent on alcohol (there's no evidence that he has either developed tolerance for alcohol or suffered from withdrawal), but he is clearly misusing the stuff. Some authorities claim that patients with schizophrenia or mood disorders who use substances may develop social problems, but perhaps not dependence. Using DSM-5-TR, I'd diagnose Aaron as having alcohol use disorder that is moderate or severe, depending on how many problems (criteria) we uncover. This diagnosis would establish in my mind, as well as in Aaron's, yet another issue for future reevaluation and treatment.

But is this all? What about the possibility of a sleep disorder? Here the situation is a little less clear. Insomnia is a diagnostic criterion for depression. But the diagnostic manuals also include plain old insomnia disorder, which can be comorbid with another mental disorder. We would diagnose it when insomnia is serious enough to warrant independent evaluation and treatment. Such patients often focus on sleep symptoms to the extent that they downplay or ignore the underlying illness, perhaps even blaming poor sleep for their other symptoms. However, in my opinion, Aaron's sleep complaint doesn't rise to this level, so I won't give him a fourth mental health diagnosis. The chances are excellent that his insomnia will resolve once the other problems are brought under control.

Now let's summarize what we need to consider when making a comorbid diagnosis:

1. Are the symptoms covered by the principal diagnosis? If not, then consider the additional diagnosis.
2. What will be the benefits of the additional diagnosis? That is, does the diagnosis warn of a treatable disorder that threatens the patient's well-being? Does it clarify prognosis?
3. Does the proposed additional diagnosis meet criteria for the comorbid disorder we have in mind?

> *Diagnostic Principle:* When symptoms cannot be adequately explained by a single disorder, consider multiple diagnoses.

Personality Disorder as Comorbidity

We'll discuss personality disorders further in Chapter 17, but right now I want to bring out one or two other important points.

With a cooperative patient and some collateral information, personality disorder isn't too hard to diagnose—if it's the only issue at hand, which, admittedly, isn't often the case. However, it can be pretty hard to assess personality in a person who is acutely ill with some other mental disorder. This will be especially true in the case of something serious like an acute episode of schizophrenia or a severe mood disorder. Depression, manic grandiosity, psychosis, overwhelming anxiety, and substance use are almost ideally suited to provide cover for the often subtle indicators of personality disorder.

The flip side of this argument is that many severely ill patients who have been diagnosed with a personality disorder eventually turn out *not* to have one; once the acute illness has resolved, the personality symptoms often seem to melt away. In 2002, Fava and colleagues found that of patients with major depressive disorder who had received a comorbid diagnosis of personality disorder, many no longer qualified for the personality disorder diagnosis once they had been treated with Prozac. My thoughts boil down to this: Be especially careful when diagnosing personality disorder in the face of other mental conditions. Wait until symptoms of other disorders have been reduced to their absolute minimum; then you'll more easily recognize

> *Diagnostic Principle:* Avoid personality disorder diagnoses when your patient is acutely ill with a major mental disorder.

personality disorder symptoms and less readily misinterpret them. I feel strongly enough about this to enshrine it as a diagnostic principle.

Additional Factors to Consider in Comorbidity

A patient's demographic features can affect which disorders might be comorbid with others. For a man, give extra thought to the possibility of comorbid alcoholism, which is of course much more commonly found in men than in women. Similarly, anorexia nervosa and bulimia nervosa (and to a lesser extent, binge-eating disorder) are more common in women. In Table 8.2 I've drawn up a gender comparison (p. 95). And of course, you should be alert for any disorders that you've already identified as occurring in a patient's family.

Here's another caveat about dual diagnoses that include substance use. In a 2002 study, Heilig and colleagues reported that comorbid conditions such as mood and anxiety disorders were substantially reduced once patients had been clean and sober for as little as 3 weeks. Although the finding needs to be substantiated, it suggests that we clinicians should avoid hasty comorbid diagnoses in the face of substance use problems.

Imposing Order on Comorbidity

Once you have identified your patient's various comorbid diagnoses, does it make any real difference which disorder you list first? It can, and it often does.

We are likely to pay special attention to the first diagnosis in a list, under the logical though sometimes erroneous impression that it is the most important. Perhaps we assume it even drives whatever other pathology the patient has. The order in which diagnoses are recorded can also suggest where and how to begin treatment; it may carry an implication as regards prognosis. So, if only for the purpose of signaling special attention, it makes sense to give some thought to the different ways you could impose order on your list of diagnoses.

One is to list first the diagnosis most important for the well-being of the patient. To demonstrate this strategy, let's return to Aaron—who, we eventually decided, should be given three separate diagnoses: schizophrenia, major depressive disorder, and alcohol use disorder. Going by urgency of treatment, we would list his depression first, because at the time of his reevaluation, death had begun to appeal to him. Next in order might come schizophrenia, and finally his alcohol use disorder. An obvious drawback to this strategy would be the difficulty in knowing just which diagnosis is the more urgent. Relevant to Aaron's situation, for example, is that suicidal behavior can also be associated with schizophrenia and substance use. Who could say that Aaron's growing suicidal ideas were related only to depression?

A second strategy is to list diagnoses in the order of greatest confidence that they apply to our patient. That would put more speculative conditions lower on the list, below those that seem rock-solid. Of course, this strategy suggests a touching faith in our ability to rank-order the reliability of the diagnoses. In the case of Aaron, I would feel confident in my diagnosis of schizophrenia, but I'm pretty certain that he also had a mood disorder and, for that matter, an alcohol use disorder. Now I'm back to square one. All in all, listing in order of confidence is a strategy that probably works better for thinking about a differential diagnosis than for ranking a group of comorbid diagnoses.

Another method is to list first the diagnosis that appears to be the "prime mover," the underlying cause of the other disorders. This might work pretty well, if only we can be sure about cause and effect. For Aaron, we could probably agree that schizophrenia belongs on top; as is so often true, his alcohol use could then be understood as self-medication of a chronic psychosis. But experienced clinicians will often disagree about what causes, say, a patient's depression—is it stress, or a loss, or medication effect, or does it come out of the blue? In Aaron's case, did his psychosis cause the depression? For some clinicians, this would be a tough sell.

On the other hand, it's a relative breeze to decide whether one illness begins chronologically later than another. The one that started first would be considered primary, whereas those coming afterward would be considered secondary and listed later. The question of whether a mood disorder is primary or secondary can also sometimes help direct patient and clinician to the quickest, most effective course of therapy. According to this strategy, Aaron's schizophrenia obviously should be listed first, followed by his depression and then his drinking.

Considering everything we've said above, I've written the diagnostic principle about multiple diagnoses to read that you should first address the diagnosis that is most urgent, treatable, or specific. (This reads a lot like the safety principle at the beginning of our diagnos-

> *Diagnostic Principle:* **Arrange multiple diagnoses to list first the one that is most urgent, treatable, or specific. Whenever possible, also list diagnoses chronologically.**

tic quest, but the point is well worth considering again near the end.) If possible, multiple diagnoses should also be listed chronologically. Here is a brief example:

> When she was only 16, Annie ran away from her home in suburban Chicago. After living on the streets of San Francisco for nearly 2 years, she applies to a crisis residence facility for a place to stay and for treatment of her deteriorated mental state. One clinician notes that she has heavily misused cocaine for over a year; another is concerned about her 2-month history of depression. Now she cries frequently and expresses hopelessness about the future, though she denies having suicidal ideas.

Because the depression apparently started long after Annie began using cocaine (controlling it would probably address the depression), her two clinicians agree to list the cocaine use disorder first and the mood disorder second. They will withhold antidepressant medication for now and reevaluate her mental state when she is drug-free.

Relationships of Comorbidities

Table 6.1 (pp. 68–69) is a chart that shows which diagnoses commonly occur together. If I could, I'd have given percentages to indicate the frequency of these associations, but because the relevant studies often state widely divergent figures, I decided to make do with ×'s. Because they are so relatively new or rare that they have yet to be carefully studied, some disorders in the chart have far fewer comorbidities than others. In Part III, I'll add comments about specific associations between disorders.

Here's a note about the strength of associations. Just because disorder A frequently accompanies disorder B doesn't mean that the reverse is true, so the table can be read only in one direction: You must start with a disorder in which you are interested from the left-hand column, then find the associations by reading across the row. The reason consists in the prevalence in the general population and the relative frequency of disorders. As shown in the Figure 6.1 Venn diagram, disorder B will usually occur by itself, but when you do find disorder A, it will almost always be accompanied by B.

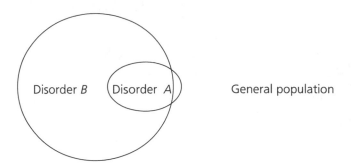

FIGURE 6.1. Relative frequencies and relationships of two mental disorders, A and B.

TABLE 6.1. Comorbid Diagnoses by Diagnosis

These diagnoses → are likely to be comorbid with these diagnoses ↓	Delirium	NCD (dementia)	Subst. intox./withdr.	Schizophrenia	Schizophreniform dis.	Delusional dis.	Major depression	Dysthymia	Mania (bipolar I)	Panic dis.	Agoraphobia	Specific phobia	Social anxiety dis.	OCD	PTSD	GAD	Somat. dis.	Illness anxiety dis.	Body dysmorphic dis.	Any anxiety dis.
NCD (dementia)	×	—																		
Subst. intox./withdr.			—	×			×		×						×		×			
Schizophrenia			×	—						×				×						
Schizoaffective dis.			×																	
Delusional dis.						—	×							×					×	
Major depression			×				—	×	×					×						
Dysthymia			×				×	—												
Mania (bipolar I)			×						—	×			×							
Hypomania (bipolar II)			×							×			×							
Cyclothymia			×																	
Panic dis.			×				×			—	×	×	×	×	×	×		×		
Specific phobia			×				×					—								×
Social anxiety dis.			×				×						—							×
OCD							×			×		×	×	—						
PTSD			×				×		×	×	×	×	×	×	—	×				
GAD			×				×	×		×		×	×			—				
Somat. dis.			×				×			×							—			
Somat. pain dis.			×				×													×
Illness anxiety dis.							×											—		×
Body dysmorphic dis.						×	×						×	×					—	
Factitious dis.				×																
Dissoc. amnesia			×				×													
Dissoc. identity dis.			×				×													
Depers./dereal. dis.			×				×	×											×	×
Sexual dysfunctions							×			×	×	×		×						
Paraphilic dis.							×													
Gender dysphoria			×																	
Anorexia nervosa			×				×						×							
Bulimia nervosa			×				×	×												×
Binge-eating dis.		×			×		×											×		
Intermitt. explos. dis.			×				×		×											×
Kleptomania							×													×
Pyromania			×																	
Gambling dis.			×				×													
Trichotillomania			×				×							×						×
Paranoid PD			×	×		×	×					×		×						
Schizoid PD				×	×	×														
Schizotypal PD				×	×	×	×													
Antisocial PD			×				×											×		×
Borderline PD			×				×								×					
Histrionic PD							×											×		
Narcissistic PD			×																	
Avoidant PD							×						×							
Dependent PD							×													×
Obsess.–compul. PD												×	×	×			×			

Note. NCD, neurocognitive disorder; OCD, obsessive–compulsive disorder; PTSD, posttraumatic stress disorder; GAD, generalized anxiety disorder; PD, personality disorder.

These diagnoses → are likely to be comorbid with these diagnoses ↓	Anorexia nervosa	Bulimia nervosa	Intermitt. explos. dis.	Kleptomania	Pyromania	Gambling dis.	Trichotillomania	Adjustment dis.	Paranoid PD	Schizoid PD	Schizotypal PD	Antisocial PD	Borderline PD	Histrionic PD	Narcissistic PD	Avoidant PD	Dependent PD	Obsess.–compul. PD	Intellectual disability	Tourette's dis.
NCD (dementia)																				
Subst. intox./withdr.												×	×							
Schizophrenia									×	×	×									
Schizoaffective dis.									×	×	×		×							
Delusional dis.									×	×						×				
Major depression	×	×											×							
Dysthymia													×	×	×	×	×			
Mania (bipolar I)	×	×																		
Hypomania (bipolar II)	×	×											×							
Cyclothymia																				
Panic dis.																				
Specific phobia																				
Social anxiety dis.		×														×				
OCD	×															×	×	×		×
PTSD																				
GAD																				
Somat. dis.												×	×	×						
Somat. pain dis.																				
Illness anxiety dis.																				
Body dysmorphic dis.																				
Factitious dis.													×							
Dissoc. amnesia																				
Dissoc. identity dis.	×												×							
Depers./dereal. dis.													×		×		×			
Sexual dysfunctions																				
Paraphilic dis.																				
Gender dysphoria																				
Anorexia nervosa	—												×							
Bulimia nervosa		—											×							
Binge-eating dis.																				
Intermitt. explos. dis.			—																	
Kleptomania		×		—																
Pyromania					—															
Gambling dis.						—						×	×		×					
Trichotillomania	×						—												×	
Paranoid PD									—	×	×		×		×	×				
Schizoid PD									×	—	×					×				
Schizotypal PD									×	×	—		×			×				
Antisocial PD						×						—	×	×	×					
Borderline PD		×											—							
Histrionic PD												×	×	—	×		×			
Narcissistic PD	×								×				×	×	—					
Avoidant PD									×	×	×		×			—	×			
Dependent PD						×							×	×		×	—			
Obsess.–compul. PD																		—		

7 Checking Up

Before moving on to Parts II and III, let's pause to review the previous chapters with another vignette. To provide material for a sustained discussion of many of the points already mentioned, I've included a lot more detail than for many of the previous case examples. As an exercise, while you are reading, write down each possible diagnosis you think of. Later, you can compare your list with mine.

Veronica

Right after spring break, her parents bring Veronica to the clinic for evaluation. Their visit is occasioned by a chance encounter between mother and daughter one morning just after Veronica showered. "She always wears those baggy sweaters and pants, so I hadn't realized how thin she's become," Mrs. Harper says, dabbing at her eyes with a handkerchief. "She always promises to eat better, but she just seems to be wasting away. Now she only weighs 89 pounds, and she's five and a half feet tall."

"She looks like a stick figure!" Her father scowls and bangs his fist on the arm of his chair.

Veronica flinches, but still she doesn't relent. "There's nothing wrong with me," she insists. "Except maybe my weight."

"Now you're showing some sense, at least." Turning to the clinician, Mr. Harper adds, "She belongs in the hospital."

"I mean, I'm pudgy and gross around the middle! Besides, I'm an adult. You can't make me go there." Veronica's eyes fill with tears, and father and daughter each look to the clinician for support. Veronica's mother frowns at her husband and encircles her daughter with a protective arm. The atmosphere in the room thickens with anger and fear.

Veronica's peculiar eating behavior began in the ninth grade when she read a women's magazine article about cellulite. Suddenly fearful that she would become obese, from that time on she has dieted sporadically, though she never previously lost so much weight as now. At various times when she was in high school, both parents had noticed how she seemed to avoid eating by just pushing food around on her plate.

Her mother had uncritically accepted the excuses—she wasn't hungry, or she was stressed by school, or she was having her period— but her father was concerned to a fault. When she was younger, he would insist that Veronica sit at the table until she'd eaten what was put before her; once she sat sulking until bedtime, the lasagna congealing on her plate. With time, though, she'd learned to circumvent parental control by gobbling down what was required, then heading off to the bathroom, where she would cause herself to retch. At first this required the stimulus of a spoon or her finger down her throat, but later, she finally admitted, she had learned to vomit at will. She would mask the sound with strategic flushing.

In 11th grade, Veronica tried medications to control her appetite. Two girls who had dropped out of school the year before had introduced her to amphetamines. These worked, but she stopped after just a few weeks "because they made me feel wired." She also briefly tried laxatives, but similarly abandoned them: "That was just plain yuck."

As a young child, Veronica was very active and often inattentive— whether during a story being read to her or even watching a favorite TV show like *Sesame Street*. Despite high intelligence, she had trouble concentrating in class during her early school years. Her second- and third-grade teachers had each asked that she be evaluated for attention deficit disorder (as it was then called), but her father had refused. An attorney who specializes in malpractice litigation, he had declared, "No kid of mine is going to be drugged by some quack doctor," and that was that. Now even he admits that something is desperately wrong. Strong measures seem indicated.

Off and on, Veronica has complained about depression. For several years she has felt worst right around Christmas ("Maybe it's because I'm an atheist, and I resent all the religious stuff"). She always seems to improve again once spring sets in. During these wintertime depressed periods, she will feel tired and sleep more than usual, and her concentration suffers to the point of declining grades. Even her interest in working out will drop; she finds it hard just to drag herself off to the pool. Then, strangely, she eats more; she notes with distress how she always picks up a few pounds when she's having "the winter blahs," as she calls them.

Last winter, her doctor put her on an antidepressant; within 3 weeks her sleep returned to normal and she was once again working hard in school—and avoiding food. She finishes up her story by telling the clinician that she now feels "great" and is happy that with the return of her workout routine, her weight is settling back to what she regards as normal. She denies feeling really hungry; rather, she is just intensely interested in food. With evident pride she mentions the hundreds of recipes in her collection, which she keeps in an Excel spreadsheet. She doesn't actually cook, but she enjoys thinking about these dishes and uses them to plan weeks' worth of menus.

Despite her profound weight loss, Veronica claims to be in excellent health. She swims every day for 90 minutes before class; earlier in the year, before becoming so busy with her studies, she played on the women's volleyball team. An avid skier, she is impatient to hit the slopes—though, as her younger brother chimed in, "she looks like one of her ski poles." Her periods stopped months ago, and a trip to her family doctor last week revealed that her thyroid is functioning at below-normal level. Besides her weight, the only other physical findings are that she has lost hair from her head (though not elsewhere, she admits with a scowl in her brother's direction); her remaining hair seems finer than it used to be.

After a rocky start in the early grades, Veronica worked hard to become an A+ student. She reworks any algebra problems she's missed on an exam until she gets them right, and she devotes countless hours to extra-credit work in biology. In her senior year, she was supposed to become the student coordinator of the science fair, but she ultimately turned it down because she feared the ridicule she'd experience if she "screwed it up." She agrees that for years she has felt insecure, and her diligence in high school serves partly to avert criticism from her parents or teachers. Once she discovered that she could challenge her way up to be first chair in the school band, she practiced her clarinet a full hour every day. She also sang in the choir and had featured roles in two school operettas. For one, she slit the skirt of her costume up the side, to acclaim from the boys in the chorus.

Veronica's older sister had been bulimic when she was in college; now married, she is pregnant and very careful about what she eats. Mr. Harper admits to occasional periods of depression—but when he was in law school, he "sometimes felt so strong, so capable, so on top of the world that it seemed that if I gradually brought the tips of my index fingers together, sparks might jump between them!" He has never been evaluated for a mood disorder, but he mentions that his own father, depressed by business failure, committed suicide in his early 40s. Mrs. Harper agrees that she likes things orderly and neat: "I guess I have OCD traits myself."

Now 19 and in her second year of college, Veronica admits that she still has only one close friend, another young woman with weight issues. "I don't feel comfortable with other people," she complains. "I get sort of, you know, anxious when I'm with people. For one thing, I think that they must notice how fat I am." She also denies any history of legal problems or of physical or sexual abuse.

Later, in a private session, Veronica grouses about still living at home. "My parents don't trust me to live on campus," she asserts. She has had no boyfriends, other than Mitchell. For a time she hooked up with him for sex, but he eventually dropped her—frightened off because, though she talked mostly about eating, she seemed to be wasting away. His abandonment doesn't bother her. She has never been especially interested in sex, which doesn't even take her mind off food. "I'd just lie there and think of English muffins," she says, with the trace of a smile.

Discussion of Veronica

Note that Veronica's evaluation draws on a wide variety of information: the history of the present illness; medical history; personal and social histories as far back as childhood; family history of mental disorder, as well as some family dynamics; and Veronica's current MSE. The resources used to develop this information include an interview with the patient herself and collateral information from her family. Her clinician also had available some medical records; if there were any, psychological testing reports and material from school counselors, clergy, and social services would also be used.

Creating the Differential Diagnosis

First let's evaluate Veronica's whole history for evidence of the syndromes we should initially include in a broad-ranging differential diagnosis. Of course, an eating disorder is high on our list. Anorexia nervosa is highly suspect, but because she indulged in some bingeing and purging, we'll add bulimia nervosa. She also has evidence of depression that, depending on time course and other features, would support a diagnosis of either dysthymia (DSM-5-TR calls it persistent depressive disorder) or major depression. Though the evidence is scanty, at times she is also irritable and overactive, so we should probably squeeze in a mention of bipolar disorder. Even a few physical symptoms in a young woman suggest somatic symptom disorder, which is attractive partly because it explains so many symptoms in one diagnosis—Occam's razor at work.

Shouldn't we mention substance use? At one time, Veronica did try amphetamines to reduce her weight. And we must always consider that a medical condition could cause mood and eating disorders. Examples: Although menstruation will stop with marked weight loss, could she have a primary endocrine disorder such as hypothyroidism? Severe weight loss due to a chronic wasting disease would be only a dim possibility, especially inasmuch as Veronica has just visited her family doctor, but we should mention it if only for completeness. Because she thinks about food a great deal and keeps lists of menus, we should at least mention OCD. Scattered throughout the vignette are instances of difficulty in getting along with other people—so we'd better let personality disorder round out our list of possibilities.

With only skimpy evidence supporting a number of the conditions on this list, including them all might seem forced. However, it is a truism that you cannot make a diagnosis that you never consider, and by our rules, including a disorder doesn't brand it as a likely cause. Rather, an extensive differential diagnosis should include even those disorders that may in context seem out of the running; occasionally one will finish in the money.

All things considered, then, Table 7.1 presents the differential diagnosis I'd consider for Veronica. Notice the five conditions at the top: According to the safety principle, they are not the diagnoses you or I might consider most likely, but those that could have the greatest immediate importance for the patient's treatment and overall well-being.

TABLE 7.1. Differential Diagnosis for Veronica

Mood disorder due to hyperthyroidism
Substance-related mood disorder
Weight loss due to a medical condition (e.g., AIDS, cancer)
Weight loss due to substance use
Amphetamine use disorder
Anorexia nervosa
Bulimia nervosa
Bipolar disorders
Major depressive disorder
Somatic symptom disorder
Dysthymia
OCD
Social anxiety disorder
ADHD
Personality disorder of an unspecified type

Winnowing the Differential List

The next step will be to eliminate disorders from consideration. I've tried to explain in detail how an experienced clinician thinks about a complex patient. But by the time you've become experienced yourself, these steps will meld into a nearly seamless process that takes place within seconds, not the minutes it will take to puzzle through a diagnostic situation for the first time. Before reading on, you might want to work through Table 7.1 yourself, to see how your thinking compares with mine.

In our discussion, we could start with either depression or anxiety; indeed, the decision trees in Figures 11.1 and 12.1 could both come into play (see pp. 133 and 170). Regardless of where we begin, the top spot always belongs to the possibility that a medical or substance use problem could be causing the major symptomatology. An underperforming thyroid can cause depression and low appetite; however, seasonal hypothyroidism would be a real novelty. Of course, one should always think of serious medical conditions when presented with profound weight loss, but I think we can take the word of Veronica's family doctor that, other than the weight loss itself, she is in pretty good health. Other than absent menses and low sex interest, she apparently did not complain about multiple somatic symptoms, and somatic symptom disorder would seem unlikely. Just to be safe, however, I'd review the symptoms of that condition (see my discussion of it in Chapter 9, "Somatization Disorder: A Special Case," pp. 111–112).

Depression, anxiety symptoms, and anorexia are all notoriously associated with amphetamine intoxication and withdrawal (see Table 9.3, pp. 116–117), but the available information suggests that Veronica's substance use was (1) the result of a desire to lose weight, not the cause of it; and (2) no longer current. Furthermore, we have nothing to suggest that she used amphetamines (which might explain her mood changes) only at specific times of the year, or that she lost weight only when using them. Nonetheless, for the sake of completeness, she should have at least one blood or urine test for substances.

Having now dismissed medical and substance use etiologies in the depression and anxiety decision trees, let's further explore Veronica's numerous mood symptoms. Some were of the atypical type (increase in sleep and appetite), but atypical symptoms are often found in teenagers. Her response to previous treatment (that's a diagnostic principle, remember) would suggest an independent mood disorder. The fact that her mood symptoms recurred each year at about the same time also strongly indicates a seasonal mood disorder (another diagnostic principle: "The best predictor of future behavior is past behavior"). Listing it as such would remind future clinicians to watch for the recurrence of symptoms each winter and possibly supply prophylactic treatment. The relatively brief duration of her depressive symptoms rules out dysthymia, which lasts for years.

Should we regard Veronica's activity level and bright affect as symptoms of mania? Even coupled with her father's history of possible hypomania, such an interpretation seems far-fetched—though she and her family should certainly be alerted to watch out for possible future bipolar symptoms. (In a 2005 study, Kennedy and colleagues reported not only that women are more likely than men to have bipolar disorder, but that for such women the first episode is likely to be one of depression.) Although we've included social anxiety disorder in the differential diagnosis, Veronica wouldn't fulfill the criteria because she didn't avoid other people. There was no suggestion of panic attacks or compulsive behavior, moving other anxiety disorders and OCD lower on our list. She did have symptoms of ADHD when she was little, but she was never seen clinically at the time, and there is no suggestion that she currently had features of that disorder.

We must now carefully consider anorexia nervosa. Veronica herself hotly denies that there is anything wrong with her eating, so we must use two of our rules for evaluating competing information. First, the signs of her skeletal appearance and activity level—both typical in patients with anorexia nervosa—outweigh (!) her reported lack of symptoms. Second, her parents' statements about her eating and weight beat Veronica's own history (collateral history wins this one). Considering all the available data, we can make an excellent case for anorexia nervosa as one of Veronica's diagnoses.

Finally, what about a personality disorder? Table 6.1 suggests that personality disorders are commonly encountered with the eating disorders. At the time of the interview, Veronica had some symptoms that could suggest avoidant or histrionic personality disorder—but, as our diagnostic principle about personality disorders advises, these should be reevaluated after adequate treatment for her anorexia nervosa. For right now, a mention of personality traits is about as far as I'd care to go.

The Working Diagnosis

Careful and rather extensive pruning yields this list of working diagnoses:

- Anorexia nervosa
- Major depressive disorder, recurrent, with seasonal pattern, with atypical features
- Diagnosis deferred as regards personality disorders; avoidant and histrionic personality traits

Arranging the order of Veronica's comorbid diagnoses shouldn't prove too difficult. We have only two principal diagnoses to consider, anorexia nervosa and major depression. From a variety of studies, we know that the outlook for patients with anorexia nervosa is worrisome. About one-quarter recover, and half are much improved at 10-year follow-up; however, the rest become chronically ill, with some studies suggesting that the overall mortality rate is in the 15–20% range. Although major depression can also result in early death from suicide, Veronica's has been seasonal, she isn't depressed at the time of the interview, and she has responded well to treatment. With plenty of time to work on her mood disorder later, I'd place it as a safe second to the more urgent anorexia nervosa. Also, in all likelihood the anorexia nervosa antedated the depression by several years, so I can satisfy my desire to list disorders chronologically.

For nearly every patient, personality disorder stuff usually comes last. With the information we have at this point, I see no reason to change Veronica's personality assessment from how it is stated above, which carries only a little more information than the ever-valuable term *undiagnosed*. However, her clinician would have to remain alert for any additional data that might permit a more definitive diagnosis (or perhaps eliminate personality issues from consideration altogether).

Easily Overlooked Issues

Even with a working diagnosis in hand, you should still pay attention to these questions: "Do I still lack information, such as additional symptoms, family history; is there a gap in the history? Have I overlooked any relatively uncommon, but still possible, diagnoses? Should I consider any additional comorbid diagnoses?" As an aid to memory, I've included in this brief section issues clinicians sometimes overlook.

- *HIV and AIDS.* Of course, plenty of infectious diseases can cause mental symptoms (see Table 9.1, pp. 106–109), but HIV and AIDS are especially preventable, and treatable.

- *Substance use.* Alcohol, street drugs, and prescription drugs are probably not often overlooked when clinicians are evaluating most adult patients, but they can also present problems for geriatric, adolescent, and even child patients.

- *Schizophreniform psychosis.* The concept is simple: A patient's symptoms look like they might add up to schizophrenia down the road; during your investigation, however, not enough time has passed to be sure. I'll discuss this in greater detail in Chapter 13.

- *Intellectual disability and borderline intellectual functioning.* I suspect that we all too often ignore intellectual disability (ID), though at least 3 people of every 100 in the general population have some degree of limited intellectual functioning. Some of them will pass through your office, and most of those who do will have other mental health disorders that require attention. It is all too easy to attribute to other disorders some of the behaviors typical of people with ID: stiff affect, apparent lack of concentration, "hallucinations" that are somehow not quite psychotic, and chronic difficulty coping with work and with other people. Remember, for many such people, these behaviors are the baseline of normal, not an indicator of major mental disorder.

- *Somatic symptom disorder.* Clinicians often overlook it, yet it causes much misery. I've given it some of the attention it deserves in Chapter 9 (see "Somatization Disorder: A Special Case," pp. 111–112).

- *No mental illness.* Frankly, I don't know whether this "diagnosis" is over- or underused; you won't find a lot of research on the topic. But I do want to point out that it happens, if infrequently, that a person who comes for an evaluation truly has no mental disorder or even a relational problem—in short, nothing for the clinician to report save good news. But because the line that divides mental illness from normality isn't always sharp, we sometimes mistake for illness any of these nonpathological features: conflict with a social institution (those with long memories will recall the conscientious objector vs. the draft); a poor fit with one's social role (remember when being a nerd was considered uncool?); and any emotion that a person feels intensely, such as plain old unhappiness. I've already enshrined "no mental illness" in its own diagnostic principle.

- *Undiagnosed.* Let me mention yet again this useful term, which implies the need for further thought and investigation without prejudicing the clinician as to the direction such inquiry should take.

- *Social and environmental issues.* Too often we forget that environmental or social problems can affect diagnosis or treatment. Most such issues arise in the context of the personal and social history. They include the patient's family (for example, can parents help provide care for a person with schizophrenia?), immediate social setting (because of mental illness, does the patient face discrimination?), education, occupation, housing, financial support, access to health care, and criminal and civil legal issues. Of course, many people will have multiple problems—like Rupert, a once popular and wealthy dot-com survivor whose drinking cost him his business, health, and family support, leading to solitary living and financial ruin.

Most of these social and environmental issues will be negative ones—circumstances that work to the individual's detriment, such as poverty, a ruptured personal relationship, or being arrested. However, occasionally an issue might seem quite the opposite.

George III, King of Great Britain during America's Revolutionary War, required treatment for an acute psychosis. As you can see for yourself in the gripping film dramatization *The Madness of King George*, because he was Britain's supreme authority, it was difficult for his clinicians—let alone his servants—to detain him for treatment.

To a degree, lofty status could similarly hinder the care of a politician or corporate executive who enjoys a position of power or authority. Whereas having advanced education in the mental health field would ordinarily seem to be a plus, a patient with, say, hypomania who has training in psychology might know enough about mental disorders to enable the canny concealment of telltale psychopathology.

• *Strengths*. The flip side of stating your patient's environmental and social problems is enumerating the patient's strengths. Take Lennie, for example. He's been experiencing a major bad patch—depression, death of both parents, and loss of his job to an overseas call center—but he enjoys the advantages of a solid education, winning personality, and supportive partner. The listing of such strengths is often honored in the breach, which is a shame, for it can help clinicians stay tuned to potentially valuable resources. Although assessment of strengths isn't a required part of diagnosis, perhaps it should be.

• *Global Assessment of Functioning (GAF)*. Finally, there is the GAF, whereby we can assess the degree to which our patients' symptoms cause distress or interfere with daily activities. Alas, DSM-5-TR has dropped it completely from use. However, that doesn't mean we must give it up: I've included a full copy in my book *DSM-5-TR Made Easy* (Guilford Press, 2023). As useful as the GAF can be, it is an irony that with it, we actually measure nothing. Rather, we are supposed to make our best guess about a patient's level of functioning and assign it a number (from 1 to 100). There is value in ascertaining, if with the imprecision of a canny estimate, the degree to which illness affects our patients' own lives and those of the people close to them.

Overused Diagnoses

On the other hand, there are several conditions that clinicians tend to diagnose too often—when circumstances and criteria do not justify them, and usually when another diagnosis entirely is warranted. I'll mention just three of them here.

• *Schizophrenia.* This is (or used to be) notoriously overdiagnosed, especially by North American clinicians. This was certainly the case a couple of generations ago, when a cross-national study found that North American psychiatrists were far more likely to diagnose schizophrenia than were European clinicians. Is this practice still a problem? Though studies show that North American clinicians have tightened up their standards, it still happens. At a meeting several years ago, senior clinicians were reviewing the case of a young woman who had hallucinations without delusions. Despite the fact that she had been ill for less than a month and came from a culture where visitations from spirits were common, the diagnosis of schizophrenia was mentioned freely and without objection. Because it carries a heavy prognostic penalty, the diagnosis should only be made when amply supported by reliable criteria.

• *Dissociative identity disorder.* This also tends to be embraced enthusiastically more often by North American clinicians. Formerly called multiple personality disorder or MPD, this condition has caught the eye of more than one movie maker (*Sybil, The Three Faces of Eve*) and of at least one serial killer. It raises a question that every clinician should keep in mind: "Am I being overly influenced by my particular specialty or interests?" We must beware the tendency to see our special interests everywhere; otherwise, as time goes by, their boundaries expand to encompass far too many patients. Long ago, I treated Emma, a highly suggestible college student who, during her summer vacation away from my watchful eye, fell under the care of a clinician who had published many articles about patients with MPD. Sure enough, when Emma returned in the fall she had developed two new identities, for which she had spent her holiday in treatment.

- *Borderline personality disorder.* In my opinion, this condition continues to be diagnosed more often than is warranted. It has been well studied over the years, and from my own experience, I am certain that it exists; however, I am equally certain that many patients who receive this diagnosis don't deserve it, or at least have something else in addition. Sometimes we apply it to people we don't like—bosses and in-laws come to mind. I'm afraid that too many clinicians use it as a sort of "wastebasket" category to cover their uncertainty when the term *undiagnosed* would do just fine. As with all other personality disorders, the borderline diagnosis should be made only with a great deal of information from at least two sources, based on a thorough appraisal of the course of symptoms across the length of the patient's adult lifetime.

Checking Up with a Formulation

Once you've completed your evaluation and have the diagnosis well in mind, I would urge a quick reality check for logic and completeness, using a mental health formulation. This device can help ensure that you've covered all the relevant facts and theories of disease development. It will be a brief statement (well, it could be of nearly any length, but I recommend brief) summarizing the history, significant symptoms, possible causes, differential diagnosis, and the patient's important strengths. You can share this summary with the clinician who referred the patient for mental health evaluation, as well as with the patient. In fact, I strongly recommend this last step; it will let the patient in on your thinking and provide a chance to correct any possible misunderstanding between the two of you. With the patient's permission, it can also help the family understand your assessment. Finally, it will provide the stone from which to sculpt your treatment plan.

The traditional approach to evaluation and treatment prescription is the *biopsychosocial model,* which incorporates three sorts of information about possible influences on a patient's current symptomatology. The *biological* area includes data such as genetic heredity, physical development, childhood diseases, previous physical injuries and diseases, operations, and toxic factors in the environment. The *psychological* realm encompasses cognition, emotions, behavior, communications, and interpersonal relations, including methods for coping with adversity (or, sometimes, success). The *social* area describes how a person interacts with family, cultural groups, and various institutions (such as school, places of worship, and different levels of government), and the availability and competence of this support network.

Because each of these three areas is understood to interact with the others to produce the final mental disease state, each should be explored in your diagnostic formulation. Here is a sample, based on the evaluation of Veronica, whom we met at the beginning of this chapter:

> Veronica Harper, a 19-year-old college student, has a 5-year history of anorexia nervosa. At 89 pounds, she is at least 25% below the minimum normal body weight for her age and height; yet she believes she looks fat and she fears gaining weight. She loves physical activity and participates in a vigorous swimming schedule. Her menses stopped 5 months ago. Although she briefly tried laxatives and amphetamines, for several years she has only restricted caloric intake to achieve low weight.
>
> For several years she has also had winter depression, beginning about December and spontaneously resolving each spring. Her symptoms include low mood, increased sleep, tiredness, improved appetite, loss of interest, and lack of concentration, but never suicidal ideas. Last winter, these symptoms resolved early with antidepressant medication. Other than low weight and mild hypothyroidism, her physical health has been good.
>
> Veronica is a painfully thin though lively and cheerful young woman who cooperates with the interview. Her speech is clear and coherent; she denies delusions, hallucinations, phobias, panic attacks, compulsions, and obsessions (other than an abiding interest in food, cooking, and recipes). Her mood shows normal lability and is appropriate to the content of thought. She has only fair insight—despite obvious wasting, she believes that she is overweight—and her judgment as regards her eating behavior is poor and dangerous to her health.
>
> Contributing to her principal disorder, anorexia nervosa, could be genetics (her mother may have some symptoms of OCD, and her sister has been bulimic); social factors (Western societies famously associate slenderness with beauty); and the psychological desire to thwart the attempts at control exerted by her father. Her seasonal major depressive disorder is in part accounted for by heredity (history of mood disorder, possibly bipolar, in her father), and in part by distress at feelings of rejection by her peers. Veronica's principal strengths are good intelligence; a strong work ethic; and parents who, though controlling, are deeply concerned and, in their way, supportive.

Following Through

Clinicians err and patients change—two reasons why we must always keep alert to the need for rethinking diagnosis. Yet readjusting diagnosis in the face of new information doesn't get talked about much. Although you should *always* consider the possibility of such a change, certain situations should set the rediagnosis machinery whirring.

1. Your new patient comes with a ready-made diagnosis. A walking trap for clinicians, this situation often signals the need for a diagnostic reevaluation. Unhappily, not everyone practices scientific diagnosis, and too often a patient's fate is decided in the not-so-good old-fashioned way—by hunch or by prejudice. The start of therapy with a new patient is the ideal point to review the complete history and reassess the mental status. Once you've accepted the old diagnosis and begun treatment, it's much harder to backtrack.

2. Your own diagnosis leaves some symptoms unexplained. Examples might include an anxious patient who has depression, a depressed patient with delusions, and, to come full circle, a psychotic patient who complains of anxiety. Although for each of these, a single diagnosis might embrace all the symptoms, each represents a situation I'd watch carefully to be sure that all symptoms respond fully to treatment.

3. A patient develops new symptoms not explained by current diagnoses. If you've treated depression in someone who then develops symptoms of mania, you've obviously got serious rethinking to do. But what about a patient with dementia who becomes depressed? Or someone with PTSD who stops eating? If the new symptom fits nicely into the current diagnosis, you've got a reasonable explanation. But try hard to resist the temptation to force new data into an old schema. Your patient needs you to maintain mental flexibility, so don't cling inappropriately to a diagnosis that no longer applies.

4. Despite treatment that seems appropriate, your patient remains mired in symptoms. Of course, the therapy itself could be at fault, but have you unwittingly been focusing on the wrong diagnosis? For example, perhaps the cocaine use for which the patient has faithfully attended Narcotics Anonymous has been hiding an underlying depression.

5. Symptoms are improving, but your patient's work or family situation is deteriorating. Although behavior therapy has reduced Elisa's panic attacks, she tells of increasing fights with her husband and critical comments from her boss. A review of her history and reevaluation of her mental status reveals a supervening depression. In other patients, this might be the time to reevaluate for the presence of a personality disorder.

6. You finally meet the patient's relatives, spouse, or significant other.

This can produce additional history, new family history, and other information that could revise your working diagnosis. At the very least, you'll have a new point of view that can validate your previous diagnosis.

7. Laboratory data can add new clues. Occasionally an abnormal thyroid hormone level or imaging result triggers the reevaluation of a patient who might otherwise appear to be doing well.

8. A disease is born. OK, so new disorders don't appear all that often. But as an exercise, you might sometime scan the relevant appendix of the current DSM, just to see how many disorders are being studied for inclusion in future editions. DSM-5-TR includes six, but it's been as high as a dozen or more, and the DSMs aren't the only game in town. Even more disorders are probably waiting in the wings.

9. On the other hand, perhaps just thumbing through a book about diagnosis (ahem!) reminds you of an existing disorder that you hadn't considered for a particular patient.

The Challenge of a Changing Diagnosis

When you obtain new information, or when other issues come forward in the course of treatment, you may have to reconsider your working diagnosis. When circumstances warrant, the failure to do so can be devastating (see the sidebar "False Positives"). Here are a few suggestions for finding your way through the swamp of an evolving diagnosis:

- Don't react hastily. Proceed with caution, especially if your patient is stable and doing well. Absent a true emergency, sudden moves can muddle rather than clarify. Even with careful deliberation, you can come to grief.

Candy, a young woman I once diagnosed as having a bipolar disorder, became increasingly psychotic despite mood stabilizers, lithium, and even a course of electroconvulsive therapy. After nearly 2 years, I reluctantly began to regard her diagnosis as schizophrenia. With antipsychotic drugs she improved somewhat, but she continued ill and incapable of maintaining a job; her husband divorced her. I eventually lost track of her, but several years later we met quite by accident and paused to talk. Using a newly available mood stabilizer, another clinician was treating her for bipolar disorder; she appeared to have recovered completely. Talk about mixed emotions: I was delighted for her, but personally chagrined.

False Positives

False positives—those diagnoses that turn out to be inaccurate—are problematic enough that they deserve discussion. (The flip side, false negatives, in which a diagnosis should have been made but is not, can also be devastating; their consequences are pretty obvious.) There are a number of reasons to avoid false positives.

- One is the stigma attached to certain mental diagnoses. Unfortunately, even well into the 21st century, having a mental health diagnosis often implies social censure, accompanied by loss in self-esteem and a diminished sense of personal responsibility. Antisocial personality disorder and schizophrenia are two such diagnoses that should only be given after careful study and with full confidence.
- While chasing a false diagnosis, you might ignore others that are more accurate. False positives can provide a bogus sense of security, when you should be busily pondering the next step in your investigation.
- False positives can have two sorts of effect on the care you give: They can promote treatment that is unnecessary and delay that which is actually needed. The resulting dollar costs (insurance expenditures, time lost from work) go almost without saying.

False-positive diagnoses are especially likely when we use criteria that rest exclusively on numbers of symptoms. (Counting symptoms is easy; understanding context can be hard.) To a degree, diagnostic manuals may promote overdiagnosis by encouraging multiple diagnoses.

Patients who have suffered the consequences of a false-positive diagnosis help persuade us of the need for careful follow-up and reconsideration of the evidence. In 2005 Opal Petty (her real name: you can Google her) died after spending 51 years in a Texas state mental hospital. Probably of borderline intelligence, as a teenager she had begun behaving strangely: She wanted to go dancing and her fundamentalist parents disapproved. When a religious exorcism failed to alleviate the crisis, they had her committed. Misdiagnosed with schizophrenia, she languished in confinement until she was 67. Clinicians testifying on her behalf concluded that although she may have had a psychotic depression when first admitted, she had recovered soon afterward. A distant relative finally requested her release, and she lived the last 20 years of her life in her own home, apparently free of psychosis—and of demonic possession.

- Carefully reassess the new information. Considering both content and source, is it credible? How does it fit in with what you already know? The diagnostic principles we've already discussed can help evaluate breaking news.
- What are the possible consequences of a change in diagnosis? Before you leap, try to determine where you might land. Of course, treatment will probably change, but what about prognosis? How will the family react?
- Get help. Mental health diagnosis can be a lonely occupation, and a colleague's fresh eye can sometimes stimulate new directions for your diagnostic thinking. Just having someone to discuss a difficult or confusing patient sometimes helps me organize my thoughts. Of the meetings I attend, the most valuable are those where staff clinicians present their tough diagnostic problems to solicit new insights from colleagues.
- Rethink any objective information that might help ensure a successful outcome. Psychological and medical tests are among the sorts of material to include.
- Share your thoughts. Fully inform your patient (and, if appropriate, the family) about the new findings, your opinion as regards the need to change diagnosis, and what all of this could mean for treatment. You can best ensure compliance by helping everyone understand the situation, even (or especially) if that includes the degree to which you may be unsure of the diagnosis. I recommend candor, which of course should be couched positively, so as to avoid inducing further emotional trauma.

Part II

The Building Blocks of Diagnosis

8 Understanding the Whole Patient

If someone comes to you with symptoms of mania and a history of bipolar I disorder, the most likely diagnosis is pretty much a slam dunk. But as regards Carson (see Chapter 1) and his depression, does it make a difference that he was in the middle of a move when he contacted me that last time? Of course, the answer is an obvious "yes," and Carson's story shows the importance of environmental and historical information to our understanding of emotions and behaviors. My point is underscored by a 2005 editorial in the *American Journal of Psychiatry,* which noted that good clinical practice goes beyond (way beyond, I'd put it) the usual diagnostic checklists of symptoms to include full social and past mental health histories.

Another reason to mine every possible scrap of information is to reassure occasional patients who have no diagnosable mental illness but are afraid that they do. Take Tom, for example. His marriage is falling apart and his boss says that if he doesn't put in more overtime, the company will fold. Tom's stress and discomfort may make him worry that he has something more fundamentally wrong—perhaps that a mental breakdown is imminent. Here, a complete history does double duty, pointing out both what he lacks (a mental disorder) and what he has (multiple problems of living). Treatment for problems like Tom's is often less specific—though perhaps no less urgent—than for a diagnosable illness, so we want to be sure that we make a context-dependent diagnosis such as job stress or marital discord only after we've ruled out other, more specific causes of emotional upheaval.

Of course, even mentally ill patients often have additional, unrelated problems that we must address.

Now in her late 30s, Dorothy has been treated for schizophrenia for the past 15 years. Although she graduated from college with a major in English literature, she lives on a small disability income and what she can earn part-time bagging groceries and retrieving carts at her local supermarket. She shares rooms in an assisted-living apartment complex, does her own shopping, and keeps her own checkbook. Thanks to antipsychotic drugs, it has been a decade since she was last hospitalized, but nonetheless she feels deeply troubled.

Her roommate, Janette, neither works nor keeps house, but spends her money (and some of Dorothy's) on bowling, video games, and pizzas that she orders in. Dorothy's social life is nonexistent: Janette yells at and bullies her, and she is such a slob that having friends over is not an option. Dorothy must do any cleaning herself. Although she knows Janette uses and manipulates her, she feels powerless to do anything about it. With a long list of people waiting for an apartment, Dorothy fears that if she complains, she'll be asked to leave in favor of someone who is more compliant.

Apart from practical aspects of management, it is interesting and rewarding to know all about another person. Greater interest builds rapport, leading in turn to augmented sympathy (in both directions) and facilitation of our ability to work together. For all of these reasons, it is absolutely vital to consider the wide range of information often described under the heading of "personal and social history," along with details of the patient's family of origin. In this chapter we'll explore many items of this great building block of mental health history: the background information that can shape our understanding of symptoms and influence the diagnoses we give our patients. I've outlined this material in Table 8.1 for quick reference.

Childhood

Roland is an accountant in his early 40s whose lifelong sour attitude has prevented him from forming close relationships. Roland's mother died when he was 2, and he was taken in by an aunt who had two small children of her own. Little Roland was adequately fed and housed, but he never had a sense of belonging. At Christmas, his cousins would receive elaborate gifts while Roland received the barest tokens. One year, the other boys got Erector sets that would build a motorized parachute jump, whereas Roland's would only build a tiny truck he had to push.

Although a 2005 research report by Kessler and colleagues noted that half of all mental illnesses begin by age 14, much of the information about your patient's childhood years will go less toward diagnosis and more toward your general appreciation of what are sometimes referred to

TABLE 8.1. Outline of Personal and Social History

Childhood	Adulthood
Where was the patient born, reared?	Currently lives with whom?
Was the patient reared by both parents?	Type/source of financial support.
Number of siblings and sibship position.	Ever homeless?
Did the patient feel wanted as child?	Current support network: family, agencies.
If adopted, what were the circumstances?	
Was the adoption extrafamilial or intrafamilial?	Number of marriages.
	Marital difficulties, divorces, separations.
Relationship with parents, siblings.	Number, age, and gender of children/ stepchildren.
Were there other adults, children in home?	
	Occupation. Number of jobs lifetime?
How was health as child?	Reasons for job change.
Education: last grade completed.	Military service: branch, rank, disciplinary problems.
Scholastic, behavioral, disciplinary problems.	
	Combat experience.
Number and quality of friendships.	Legal problems: civil, arrests, violence.
Age dating began.	Current religion, attendance.
Sexual or physical abuse. Details.	Leisure activities: organizations, hobbies.
Sexual development.	Sexual preference and adjustment.
Hobbies, interests.	Age at first sexual experience. Details.
Religion as child.	Suicide attempts: methods, association with substance use, consequences.
Losses through divorce, bereavement.	
	Personality traits and evidence of lifelong behavior patterns.
Family history	Current sexual practices.
Mental disorders in close relatives.	Sexually transmitted diseases?
Current relationship with parents, siblings, children, other relatives.	Substance use: type, quantity, duration, consequences.

as "character-forming experiences." Of course, that in itself is valuable to know. But sometimes you will gain information about a person's childhood years that can help you interpret the symptoms you encounter—perhaps the fact that a person imitates a parent or other relative when responding to positive conditions of love and success or to stress from frustration or failure. Roland's second-class childhood (his relatives could have been a model for Harry Potter's horrific aunt and uncle) had set him up for a lifetime of perceived rejection and isolation.

Early Relationships

What sort of characteristics did this patient have as a child? Outgoing? Introverted? Quiet? Serious? A show-off? A history of being a loner may be followed later by chronic psychosis and personality disorder. Someone who has always been uncomfortable with others may be at risk for alcoholism. Older children must sometimes shoulder responsibility for younger siblings, which must affect their own experience of childhood and opportunities to form relationships as adolescents.

> Being "junior mom" to six younger siblings has marked Jolie's life. As an adult, she persuaded her husband to take in foster children—up to seven at a time—until their marriage foundered on the shoals of their child-rearing responsibilities.

Information about how the person interacted with parents (was there overinvolvement? distancing?), siblings, and others both in and out of the household may be especially relevant to people who, like Jolie, have no actual mental disorder.

The early social development of a patient with Asperger's disorder (now gathered by DSM-5-TR under the umbrella of autism spectrum disorder) will be marked by poor eye contact, lack of age-appropriate peer relationships, and failure to bond with peers and family. The inability to understand and empathize with the feelings and experiences of others extends into adult life.

> Despite her Asperger's, Audrey has recently formed a romantic relationship with Bert, a developmentally disabled young man. Last Thanksgiving, when the two of them were celebrating separately with their respective families, Audrey telephoned Bert to say she loved him. Then she called again, and again—a total of 11 times, though Bert and his parents repeatedly asked her to desist.

Losses

The dissolution of a relationship can be especially hard for children; the effects can endure for years.

> When his father, a teetotaling preacher, left the family, Tyler was only 12, and he spent the next 20 years in deep resentment. "I've always thought it was a big reason I started using drugs," he says during one

therapy session. "I was just so pissed off at the old man. I think that all along I've been trying to punish him."

Though the mechanisms of such associations are obscure, childhood loss of a parent through death can sometimes be reflected in adult-onset depression. Studies have also linked major depression and generalized anxiety disorder with parental divorce or separation. Loss of a father before age 14 may signal increased risk for personality disorder.

Education

Various disciplinary and scholastic problems are correlated with later behavioral difficulties.

> When 21-year-old Dudley is caught intoxicated on alcohol and burgling an apartment near where he lives with his mother, it is his third offense in a year. "First probation, then 3 months inside haven't taught him a thing," says the assistant district attorney who was prosecuting his case. "He's clearly sociopathic." The clinician brought in by defense counsel notes that Dudley had been a model student, graduating from high school with high honors, and had had no legal difficulties at all until he started drinking a year earlier. After pointing out that the very definition of antisocial personality disorder includes early conduct disorder, which Dudley had not had, the consultant offers instead a diagnosis of alcohol use disorder. The judge accepts the proposal that Dudley enter rehab.

OK, I suppose it's possible that a person with budding antisocial personality disorder might have gotten through school without disciplinary problems, but I've never encountered such a case. You can also use a patient's education history to help differentiate dementia from intellectual disability, or a learning disorder from ADHD.

Sexuality and Abuse

Toward the end of childhood comes the time of the awakening and exploration of our sexual selves. Many adult patients will have memorable experiences to relate of that embarkation.

> At 15, Josephine's physical development has far outstripped her judgment: She and her long-time boyfriend become parents when they are

still children themselves. The resulting humiliation and lost educational opportunity follows them into young adulthood, culminating in drinking, depression, and divorce.

The sexual life of many a child is a far darker story yet, commencing with aggression and betrayal. Childhood sexual abuse is painful but vital to pursue, because it is a flag for many adult mental disorders—including bulimia nervosa, depression, alcoholism, and schizophrenia, as well as dissociative, somatizing, personality (especially borderline), panic, and conduct disorders. Such an influence across a broad diagnostic spectrum makes one wonder whether childhood sexual abuse, rather than having some specific effect, instead facilitates the development of many pathology types. Whatever the possible cause–effect relationship, I use the correlation in two ways. When I encounter someone who was abused as a child, I look for one of the disorders mentioned just above. And whenever I think a patient may have one of those disorders, I take extra care when checking for hints of abuse.

Although the data are somewhat less certain, the implications of childhood physical abuse are probably similar.

Adult Life and Living Situation

You can find many pointers to diagnosis from the basic facts of an adult's current life. Here are some of the issues I consider when I evaluate a new patient.

Age and Gender

These two basic patient characteristics have extremely important implications for diagnosis. For example, the DSM-IV version of somatization disorder—we can't yet be sure about the DSM-5-TR somatic symptom disorder—is found almost exclusively in women (especially young ones), which is why I might consider this diagnosis if my patient's name is Frances, but less strongly if it is Francis. On the other hand, you'll encounter antisocial personality disorder mostly in young men, especially those living in prison. Although a few major conditions *don't* discriminate between the sexes (schizophrenia, bipolar disorders, and OCD pretty much complete the list), most mental disorders do play favorites. Table 8.2 comprises a partial listing.

TABLE 8.2. Gender Predominance for Select Disorders

Men predominate	Women predominate
Alcohol use disorder	Anorexia nervosa
Other substance use disorders	Anxiety and related disorders (except for OCD)
Antisocial personality disorder	Bulimia nervosa
Factitious disorder	Dissociative disorders
Paraphilias	Kleptomania
Gambling disorder	Major depression
Pyromania	Somatization disorder

Sexual and Marital Life and Difficulties

Changes in sex interest (up or down) are common flags for the different phases of mood disorders, and sexual behavior inappropriate for the circumstances is sometimes associated with disorders as diverse as dementia and substance use. Low sex interest is especially typical of somatizing disorders.

With changing mores, multiple partners before marriage and sex outside marriage have become so commonplace that they no longer carry the whiff of scandal they once did. Nonetheless, when I encounter someone with more than one failed marriage, it raises my suspicions about the possibility of substance use or personality disorder. Absent clear evidence of mania, I would be especially careful to evaluate for personality disorder a patient who is inappropriately seductive, especially if the behavior targets the clinician.

Most people with schizophrenia once tended to remain single, but this may be less true today for two reasons: improved treatment and a steep decline in the practice of institutionalization. However, someone with schizoid personality disorder is by definition likely to show little interest in sex with another person.

Current Environment

People survive in a wide variety of living situations. I've known many who thrive living by themselves, sometimes in circumstances that we would consider appalling. (To a question about where he lives, one man responded, "Well, the previous tenant was a Frigidaire.") Most people, however, do better with the safety and love that close friends and neighbors can bring. That's why the mental health evaluation doesn't consist solely in disease diagnosis; you must also judge whether the patient's support system is sufficient to maintain alertness for the symptoms of mania or depression, to watch for evidence of renewed drinking or other substance use, and to notify the clinician if the patient stops taking medicine that is vital for the stability of behavior and emotions.

Years ago I interviewed a young man recovering from substance use who lived alone in an apartment. When I asked about his support network, the sad truth was that he could name only his mental health care providers and his therapy group. The outlook for such a person must be far less optimistic than for one who enjoys the continuing support of friends and family. And changes in support can prove disastrous. For example, a person with agoraphobia may suddenly become housebound when a spouse or companion dies or moves away. Of course, the quality of the relationships can be as critical as their number. It is well known that patients with schizophrenia are especially likely to relapse if they have highly emotional relatives who freely shout and cast blame. I don't know of any solid data, but it stands to reason that anyone who was rearing children alone, struggling in financial straits, or teetering on the brink of a divorce would feel more vulnerable in surroundings fraught with tension.

Where your patient lives can be especially relevant to the evaluation. A classic example occurs when a person with evolving dementia must move from familiar surroundings and becomes overwhelmed by increased disorientation. A lifelong city dweller who fears snakes may never have symptoms until moving to a rural home. Even such environmental factors as time of year can have a bearing on diagnosis. As noted in Chapter 1, Carson regularly became symptomatic with depression in the fall or winter and recovered in the spring.

Working and Financial Support

Apart from the financial support it provides, work is a cornerstone of self-esteem that enables us to see ourselves as productive members of society. The type of work and the worker's perspective on it can suggest several diagnostic possibilities. Ilsa—who trained as a librarian, then spent years doing janitorial work at a large department store as she battled hallucinations and delusions—provides an example of how people with psychosis can drift downward on the occupational scale. Nick's story is similar, though it is related to substance use.

In the course of an interstate move, I asked Nick, an intelligent man with a ready wit, how he happened to fall into his current line of work carrying furniture. He said that he had formerly been pretty good at computer repair, but his fondness for beer had led to repeated suspensions of his driver's license. When it was eventually revoked, he could no longer travel to a regular job. "What I like about humping furniture," he told me, "is that they pick me up each day and drop me off at the end. And it doesn't get between me and my 12-pack of Bud every night after work."

A history of prolonged unemployment signals that something has been seriously wrong, probably for many months or years; often, the "something" is psychosis, substance use, or bipolar I disorder. (Although a disability income suggests a serious, chronic illness such as schizophrenia, I've also known patients with somatizing or substance use disorders who collected disability.) Another tell-tale pattern is the checkered job history of repeated firing and sudden resignation that is classic for antisocial personality disorder. But even a well-heeled celebrity may not be immune to the consequences of job-related behavior. At a New York Jets team reunion, former championship quarterback Joe Namath twice on camera told a reporter that he wanted to kiss her. That was his wake-up call to enter alcohol rehab.

My own long service in VA hospitals and clinics has taught me to be especially vigilant with people whose work history includes time served in the military or as firefighters or police officers. The dangers inherent in these professions warn that any symptoms of anxiety could be due to PTSD, and such symptoms should therefore prompt a careful search for evidence of psychological trauma. Those who do have PTSD are also highly likely to have depression and substance use disorders.

Legal Involvement

Whenever you encounter a patient who has had arrests or convictions, you are likely to think first of antisocial personality disorder, conduct disorder, or substance use, because legal issues are included in these criteria sets. However, law enforcement officials often take an interest in people with paraphilias (especially pedophilia and voyeurism) and with most disorders that involve control of impulses—intermittent explosive disorder, kleptomania, pyromania, and gambling disorder. (At least so far, hair pulling isn't illegal). In the throes of mania, a patient's judgment may be sufficiently erratic to create conflicts with the law. Patients with schizophrenia occasionally have a history of violence, even to the point of homicide.

Family History

Although standard diagnostic systems don't use family history as a criterion, most mental disorders do run in families. Indeed, thousands of studies have demonstrated that nearly all mental disorders can be transmitted from one generation to the next, at least partly through genetic inheritance. That's why the existence of a biological relative with a history of mental illness can serve as a flag that your patient might have the same disorder.

> A 34-year-old priest, Father Mark had spent 2 years working in the archives at the Vatican. One afternoon, in a centuries-old Latin document, he came across a mention of the Apostle Mark. "Suddenly," he later reported, "it became crystal-clear that this reference really meant me." Over the next several days, he became more and more agitated as he realized the implication: He was himself the second coming of Christ. When he reported this revelation to other priests, it caused quite a stir. Before long, loaded with sedatives and accompanied by two burly novitiates, he was hustled back to the United States for treatment.
>
> When first evaluated, Father Mark still had grandiose delusions and heard voices telling him that he was destined to save the world. Partly because his younger brother had for several years been treated for classical bipolar I disorder, Father Mark was started on lithium. His symptoms rapidly resolved, and, fully insightful that he had been ill, he resumed priestly duties. However, he was never again posted to the Vatican.

Apart from mood disorders, family relationship patterns similar to Father Mark's can be found for a wide range of mental disorders. These include schizophrenia; many anxiety disorders (especially panic disorder, phobias, and GAD); alcoholism and the use of other drugs; somatic symptom disorder; Alzheimer's dementia; anorexia and bulimia nervosa; and personality disorders, most notably antisocial. Even narcolepsy, a sleep disorder in which patients suddenly fall asleep at inopportune times (even while driving), is strongly hereditary.

I do want to sound a note of caution about using family history to evaluate a patient. OK, three notes. The first is that it is sometimes too easy for one family member's diagnosis to influence another's. It has happened to me, so I know that I must take great care not to let my knowledge of the patient overwhelm my judgment as to what a relative's symptoms signify. Researchers are well aware of this problem, which is why they developed the so-called "blind evaluation": One clinician evaluates the patient while another, unaware of the patient's diagnosis, obtains and interprets the information about the relatives. Of course, you'll hardly ever have that luxury when making your own diagnoses, so you, too, will have to practice what I preach: Be especially careful not to let prejudice affect clinical judgment.

The second cautionary note is that the diagnoses of relatives related by patients and their families could be misleading or just plain wrong. The source may be a patient who has misunderstood—or, frankly, a clinician who has erred.

> My depressed patient Julia told me that her grandfather had been hospitalized for schizophrenia. Additional history from Julia's mother revealed that in fact there were three periods during which Grandpa had become convinced that he had special "cerebral powers" whereby the force of his thought waves could alter the course of human history. After each such episode, he had gradually returned to normal and resumed work driving a city bus. Despite Grandpa's alleged diagnosis, from the history I obtained, his psychosis was not chronic but episodic—and therefore highly suspicious for bipolar I disorder. This suggested to me that Julia should be offered treatment to prevent mania.

Diagnostic Principle: Family history can help guide diagnosis, but because we often cannot trust reports, clinicians should attempt to rediagnose each family member.

The point is that whenever possible, you should obtain all the available information to allow an independent evaluation of a relative's diagnosis. This suggests that we need to modify our diagnostic principle about family history from its previously stated version in Chapter 4.

Here is the third warning: The *absence* of a family history usually tells us nothing at all about a given patient. There are at least two reasons. The history may be incomplete (informants may forget or conceal information; a patient may have been adopted and not know it). Even with good information, however, only about 10% of the parents, siblings, and children of patients with a major mental illness will have that same illness. That's why many patients will have no known close relatives who are affected. So, regard a positive family history as a straw in the wind—but realize that even in the absence of straws, the wind may be blowing anyway.

9 Physical Illness and Mental Diagnosis

Physical illness can play a vital role in creating or extending mental health symptoms. If we forget this fact, we imperil our diagnosis and our patients' health—indeed, their very lives.

James

As one of the forward party for our infantry battalion, I thought I was doing pretty well the morning I landed in Vietnam. The terror of nighttime mortar attacks, the horror of mutilated bodies, the sickening sense of vulnerability when my own battalion commander died in combat—these experiences lay weeks in the future. For the first few hours of that first day, I kept my head down and spirits up as I went about the dull routine of setting up aid stations and inspecting field kitchens for cleanliness. But as evening drew near, I became first restless, then downright jittery. I had developed the most alarming collection of symptoms, starting with, well, alarm—anxiety too intense to be ignored coupled with fatigue so great I could barely stir myself into action. I noticed that my heart was beating too fast, too hard, and too irregularly. I had trouble drawing a breath, and the sweat rolled off my forehead, though I was standing in the shade—sitting, rather, for my legs suddenly seemed too weak to support a soldier wearing a flak jacket and a steel pot helmet while toting a medical bag and an M-16 rifle.

Was I going mad, succumbing to pressure? Or was something else afoot? As the only medical authority around, I shakily reviewed the day's activity for clues to the reason for my acute unease. Suddenly, I had it: I had forgotten (declined, actually, with the arrogance of youth) to take the salt tablets we had all been issued prior to landing. As if in retribution, my copious sweating had precipitated an acute electrolyte deficiency, which the salt tablets were supposed to forestall. With a canteen of water, I washed down a couple of the pills and vowed to sin no more; within minutes, my panic attack had begun to abate.

My own wartime experience illustrates the importance of physical health and its opposite, physical illness, to the mental health diagnostic enterprise. Indeed, if we don't seize upon these concepts as building blocks, they become roadblocks to understanding our patients' illnesses. Because physical symptoms in mental disorders can be hard to get our minds around, mental health professionals who are neither physicians nor nurses sometimes feel daunted by this material. However, it is so extremely important for the patients that every clinician, regardless of discipline, should understand this element of mental health diagnosis. It is important enough that I've already awarded it diagnostic principle status.

How Physical and Mental Disorders Are Related

The effects of physical and mental disorders on one another can be complicated, but, taken in small steps, the relationships are easily understood.

Physical Disorders Can Produce Mental Symptoms

When Derek has one of his epileptic seizures, electrical impulses pulse throughout his brain. This makes him feel elated and causes him to have a visual hallucination—it's a jar of candy sitting on his desk. People with epilepsy can experience hallucinations in any of the other senses. Some will feel depressed; still others may have trouble thinking or speaking. *Déjà vu* experiences (the false feeling that one has experienced something previously) can also occur. Like Derek, patients with brain pathology as varied as tumors or multiple sclerosis or head trauma may experience mood changes. In fact, many physical diseases produce symptoms that closely mimic mental disorders.

> In his terrific novel *Saturday,* Ian McEwan describes a street thug who is in the early stages of Huntington's disease. Within a few moments, Baxter's mood can swing from boiling anger to simmering depression to bubbling euphoria, much like that of a patient in the throes of bipolar disorder. In the page-turning dénouement, the neurosurgeon protagonist operates to remove hematomas from Baxter's brain, thus saving a life the patient might have preferred to lose.

The stuff of medical legend are patients mistakenly diagnosed as having schizophrenia or depression—and sometimes treated for those disorders for years—when the real problem is a thyroid or adrenal abnormality. A 1978 study by Hall and colleagues gives substance to these tales. Of 658 consecutive patients, 9% had medical disorders that produced mental symptoms. Depression, confusion, anxiety, and memory loss were the most frequent presenting problems. Most often the cause was an infection; pulmonary or thyroid disease; diabetes; or a disease of the blood, liver, or central nervous system. Nearly half the time, neither the patients nor their physicians had previously recognized these medical illnesses.

A generation later, physical disease that causes mental symptoms still was not being adequately recognized. A study in 2002 by Koran and colleagues reported that of 289 patients, 3 had previously undetected hypothyroidism, which in 1 case caused and in 2 others worsened a patient's mental symptoms. The investigators also found that previously known physical illness caused the mental symptoms of 6 patients and made worse those of 8. Their illnesses were as varied as drug withdrawal, alcoholic dementia, epileptic psychosis, postconcussional disorder, and myocardial infarction. And, if you query PubMed for misdiagnosis of mental disorder, you'll find plenty of evidence that we are still making some of the same errors.

Physical Disease Can Worsen Existing Mental Symptoms

Even if it isn't the original cause, it's easy to see how the burden of heart disease, substance use, or AIDS could intensify the symptoms of someone who already has serious mental illness.

> Just when Gloria is recovering from her latest episode of bipolar depression, she learns that she has Addison's disease—adrenal insufficiency. "It shouldn't take Sigmund Freud to figure out that the news would drop me right back into depression," she laments. Her family doctor agrees but points out, "Don't forget that the physiological effects of a metabolic or infectious disease can directly produce mental symptoms, such as depression, psychosis, and anxiety. That means your mood could improve a lot once we get your endocrine system back under control."

Treatment for Medical Disorders Can Cause Mental Symptoms

Most medications have side effects, some of which can include mental symptoms. For example, psychosis is occasionally brought on by taking adrenal steroids, which are prescribed for illnesses as diverse as arthritis, infections, adrenal gland insufficiency (as in Gloria's case, above), lupus, and asthma. In fact, probably the majority of all medications currently in use, including those that treat mental disorders, can produce mental symptoms of one sort or another.

Physical and Mental Disorders Can Be Independent Conditions

Even when medical illness doesn't cause or worsen mental symptoms, we must recognize and address physical illness in psychiatric patients. It is incredibly easy—it has happened to me—to become so focused on a patient's mental disorder that symptoms of an independent medical illness must knock loudly and persistently before we answer the door. Hence the diagnostic strategy that every new symptom should generate this thought first: Could a physical condition be causing this?

Uncharted Waters

There are some physical findings whose meaning we don't yet understand. For instance, for decades we've known that patients with schizophrenia often have enlarged brain ventricles. The degree of enlargement isn't great, and it doesn't always occur, so the finding isn't robust enough to enable diagnosis in an individual patient. We don't know what it means, but it's real. Here's another example: Researchers have reported reduced numbers of receptors for the neurotransmitter serotonin in the brains of patients with panic disorder. What does this mean? Once again, knowledge has preceded understanding.

The great healer, we are told, is time, which can also be a pretty darn good diagnostician. What we don't understand today often becomes clear as passing time reveals new symptoms or clarifies the meaning of older ones. Even without waiting, there are a couple of ways time helps us resolve relationships between medical illness and mental symptoms: (1) if the mental symptom and the medical disorder begin at about the same time, and (2) if the patient's mental or emotional symptoms remit after the medical disorder improves.

> When Sylvia's lupus worsens and she develops kidney failure, she becomes depressed; her appetite falls and she feels weak and lethargic. After she starts dialysis, these symptoms of depression remit.

During a brief vacation trip west to California, she misses two dialysis appointments in a row; once again, her mood heads south.

If neither of these time-related guideposts obtains, you might suspect a mental symptom if it is commonly associated with a medical condition. To that end, I've listed in Table 9.1 (pp. 106–109) the mental symptoms of 60 medical conditions. I've adapted Table 9.1 from my book *When Psychological Problems Mask Medical Disorders,* which describes these conditions in greater detail. The table's purpose is to alert clinicians to the great variety of medical conditions that can lead to such symptoms. In the second column, you'll find the relative frequency with which each condition is found in the general population:

> *Common*—Most adults have at least one friend or acquaintance who has, or who will have, this condition. (Prevalence ranges to 1 in 200.)
>
> *Frequent*—A town or small city will be home to one or more of these people. (Prevalence ranges to 1 in 10,000.)
>
> *Uncommon*—At least one such person in a large city or small state has the condition. Prevalence ranges to 1 in 500,000.
>
> *Rare*—Prevalence is less than 1 in a million.

Note that these frequencies do *not* indicate how often a medical condition produces mental symptoms; such data are simply not available. The good news here is that we don't often encounter such conditions. The bad news is that relative rarity lulls us into a false sense of security. Unless we remain alert, we run the risk that we'll misinterpret the symptoms when they come calling.

Conversely, it is also important to know what physical symptoms are often associated with mental disorders. The sidebar "Physical Symptoms Commonly Linked with Mental Disorders" on pages 110–111 discusses some of these.

Clues to a Physical Cause for Mental Symptoms

Signs, symptoms, and items of historical information can suggest underlying physical illness. If you encounter any of these patient characteristics, which I've loosely based on a 1989 article by Honig and colleagues in the *British Journal of Psychiatry* and on other sources, further investigation (physical exam, laboratory data, imaging studies) may be warranted. A physical cause for mental symptoms may be especially likely if your patient:

- Is having a first episode of the mental illness. Physical causes are less likely in recurring diseases.
- Is 40 or over. Advancing age increases the likelihood that someone is developing a major medical disease.
- Has recently given birth. Postpartum hormonal changes can create mental symptoms.
- Currently has a major medical illness. For example, in diabetes, episodes of low blood sugar can cause anxiety attacks.
- Takes medicine, either prescribed or over-the-counter. This clue will be stronger if symptoms began about the time medicine was first administered.
- IIas experienced neurological symptoms. These can include weakness on one side, numbness or tingling, clumsiness, trouble walking, tremor, involuntary movements, worsening headaches, dizziness, blurred or double vision, blindness in part of the visual field, trouble with speech or memory, loss of consciousness, slowed thinking, and trouble recognizing familiar objects or following commands.
- Has had a large weight loss (10% or more); eats an unusual diet (especially one that is very limited in variety, such as tea and toast or pasta and beer); or exhibits self-neglect. Any of these can cause symptoms from vitamin deficiency.
- Has a past history of serious medical illness, including those of the endocrine system, heart, kidney, liver, lungs, or neurological system.
- Has fallen or has had a recent head injury with loss of consciousness. Even mild head injury can be associated with postconcussional symptoms and other mental disorders.
- Has a recent history of alcohol or drug misuse, with the obvious implications for falls, malnutrition, and other physical problems.
- Has a family history of a heritable disorder such as diabetes, Alzheimer's disease, or other metabolic or degenerative disease.
- Has fluctuating levels of consciousness, any impairment in thinking, hallucinations other than auditory ones, or mental symptoms interspersed with periods of lucidity.
- Has recent onset of an alarming physical symptom such as high fever, blurred vision, swelling of abdomen or ankles, jaundice, or chest pain.

TABLE 9.1. Some Medical Conditions That Can Cause Mental Symptoms

	Relative frequency[a]	Emotional/behavioral symptoms																		
		Depression	Mania	Anxiety	Panic	OCD-like behaviors	Labile emotions	Withdrawal	Catatonia	Insomnia	Hypersomnia	Hallucinations	Delusions	Depersonalization/ derealization	*Déjà vu*	Poor judgment	Suicidal ideas	PTSD symptoms	Flushing	Kluver–Bucy
Adrenal insufficiency	U	×		×				×				×	×				×			
AIDS	F	×	×	×				×				×	×				×			
Altitude sickness	U	×			×					×						×				
Amyotrophic lateral sclerosis	U	×																		
Antidiuretic excess	F											×	×							
Brain abscess	U																			
Brain tumor	F	×	×				×					×	×	×	×					
Cancer	C	×		×	×													×		
Carcinoid	F																		×	
Cardiac arrhythmia	C			×																
Cerebrovascular disease	C	×	×	×			×			×		×	×			×	×			
Chronic obstructive lung disease	C	×		×	×					×		×				×	×			
Congestive heart failure	C	×		×	×					×		×								
Cryptococcosis	F		×									×								
Cushing's	F	×	×	×						×		×	×				×			
Deafness	C	×		×								×	×							
Diabetes mellitus	C	×		×	×							×	×							
Epilepsy	C	×	×	×					×			×	×				×			
Fibromyalgia	C	×		×	×															
Head trauma	C	×	×	×						×		×								
Herpes encephalitis	U			×					×			×								×
Homocystinuria	U								×											
Huntington's	U	×	×					×				×	×							
Hyperparathyroidism	F	×					×					×	×				×			
Hypertensive encephalopathy	F												×							
Hyperthyroidism	C	×		×	×		×			×		×								

106

Disease	Frequency[a]
Hypoparathyroidism	U
Hypothyroidism	C
Kidney failure	F
Kleinfelter's	F
Liver failure	C
Lyme disease	F
Ménière's	F
Menopause	N
Migraine	C
Mitral valve prolapse	C
Multiple sclerosis	F
Myasthenia gravis	F
Neurocutaneous diseases	F
Normal-pressure hydrocephalus	F
Parkinson's	F
Pellagra	R
Pernicious anemia	C
Pheochromocytoma	U
Pneumonia	C
Porphyria	U
Postoperative states	F
Premenstrual syndrome	C
Prion disease	R
Progressive supranuclear palsy	U
Protein energy malnutrition	C
Pulmonary thromboembolism	F
Rheumatoid arthritis	C
Sickle cell disease	F
Sleep apnea	C
Syphilis	U
Systemic infection	C
Systemic lupus erythematosus	F
Thiamine deficiency	F
Wilson's	U

Note. Adapted from *When Psychological Problems Mask Medical Disorders* (2nd ed.) by James Morrison (The Guilford Press, 2015). Copyright © 2015 The Guilford Press. Adapted by permission.

[a]For relative frequency: C, common; F, frequent; U, uncommon; R, rare; N, normal. See text for clarifications of the first four terms.

(*cont.*)

TABLE 9.1 (cont.)

		Cognitive symptoms								Personality symptoms							
	Relative frequency[a]	Memory impairment	Disorientation	Minor cognitive impairment	Delirium	Dementia	Inattention	Slow thinking	Intellectual disability	Irritability	Apathy	Disinhibition	Jocularity	Impulsiveness	Tenaciousness	Aggression	Criminality
Adrenal insufficiency	U	×	×		×					×	×						
AIDS	F	×	×	×	×	×	×	×		×	×						
Altitude sickness	U	×	×		×					×							
Amyotrophic lateral sclerosis	U					×											
Antidiuretic excess	F		×		×					×							
Brain abscess	U						×										
Brain tumor	F	×				×		×			×	×		×			
Cancer	C				×												
Carcinoid	F																
Cardiac arrhythmia	C				×												
Cerebrovascular disease	C				×	×	×				×	×	×	×			
Chronic obstructive lung disease	C				×	×	×				×						
Congestive heart failure	C			×	×												
Cryptococcosis	F					×				×							
Cushing's	F	×	×		×	×	×			×							
Deafness	C																
Diabetes mellitus	C				×												
Epilepsy	C								×						×		
Fibromyalgia	C	×		×			×	×									
Head trauma	C	×	×		×	×	×	×				×		×		×	
Herpes encephalitis	U	×				×											
Homocystinuria	U					×			×								
Huntington's	U	×				×					×	×					
Hyperparathyroidism	F	×			×		×	×		×	×						
Hypertensive encephalopathy	F	×	×		×			×		×	×					×	
Hyperthyroidism	C				×					×							

Disease	Code	1	2	3	4	5	6	7	8	9	10	11	12	13	14
Hypoparathyroidism	U	×					×	×							
Hypothyroidism	C	×	×			×	×	×	×						
Kidney failure	F	×	×					×	×					×	×
Kleinfelter's	F		×			×								×	×
Liver failure	C	×				×	×	×	×					×	
Lyme disease	F	×	×												
Ménière's	F														
Menopause	N	×				×	×	×							
Migraine	C	×				×	×		×						
Mitral valve prolapse	C														
Multiple sclerosis	F	×	×					×							
Myasthenia gravis	F	×	×												
Neurocutaneous diseases	F	×				×	×	×	×				×		
Normal-pressure hydrocephalus	F	×	×					×	×			×			
Parkinson's	F	×						×	×						
Pellagra	R	×		×			×	×							
Pernicious anemia	C	×	×				×	×							
Pheochromocytoma	U														
Pneumonia	C				×			×							
Porphyria	U			×											
Postoperative states	F	×		×	×	×		×							
Premenstrual syndrome	C		×		×	×	×	×							
Prion disease	R	×			×	×	×	×							
Progressive supranuclear palsy	U											×			
Protein energy malnutrition	C					×						×			
Pulmonary thromboembolism	F				×										
Rheumatoid arthritis	C									×					
Sickle cell disease	F	×				×	×	×							
Sleep apnea	C	×	×				×	×							
Syphilis	U	×	×	×											
Systemic infection	C		×	×	×			×							
Systemic lupus erythematosus	F		×		×			×							
Thiamine deficiency	F	×	×		×	×	×	×							
Wilson's	U	×			×			×			×				

109

Physical Symptoms Commonly Linked with Mental Disorders

Some physical symptoms are actually used as criteria for mental disorders; others serve as flags that one may exist. Below are some of the physical symptoms likely to affect patients who have mental disorders.

Sleep

Because it cuts across so many diagnoses, disturbed sleep is probably the most common physical problem you'll encounter. As was true with Carson, trouble sleeping will often indicate a mood disorder. Insomnia, or sometimes hypersomnia (excessive sleep), is frequently encountered in major depression and dysthymia and serves as a criterion for each. Patients with mania—they typically experience insomnia as reduced sleep requirement—may deny that it is a problem ("Why waste time sleeping when so much needs doing?").

Trouble sleeping is also a criterion for generalized anxiety disorder (GAD), in which patients may complain of either insomnia or unrefreshing sleep. Poor sleep is one of the hyperarousal criteria for PTSD and its cousin, acute stress disorder. Inability to sleep or excessive drowsiness is also often symptomatic of drug or alcohol intoxication or withdrawal. An early hint of schizophrenia may be that the patient stays up until all hours pacing about the bedroom. We'll deal with sleep disorders at length in Chapter 16.

Appetite

A change in appetite is probably the next most frequent physical complaint of mental health patients. Decreased and increased food intake, often attended by weight loss or gain, serve as criteria for depression. Chapter 16 will also see us through a much more detailed examination of eating disorders.

Panic Symptoms

The physical symptoms of panic include chest pain, chills, a choking sensation, dizziness, heart palpitations, nausea, numbness or tingling (which are called *paresthesias*), sweating, shortness of breath, and trembling. They may be experienced by a person who has any of several anxiety disorders, including agoraphobia, specific phobia, and social anxiety disorder. Someone with GAD might complain of excessive fatigue, muscle tension, or trouble sleeping. Some of the same anxiety symptoms are often encountered during the use of illicit substances, and during withdrawal from use.

Other

Fatigue and either reduced or increased psychomotor activity are also typical of depressed people, whereas those with mania become overly active. Manic patients may become inordinately interested in sex, whereas a depressed patient may lose all such interest. Whole chapters in diagnostic manuals are devoted to such problems as sexual arousal, pain with intercourse, and erectile dysfunction.

- Has mental or behavioral symptoms that don't resolve, despite treatment that should be effective.
- Shows any evidence of worsening medical health that hasn't yet been evaluated by a physician.

Somatization Disorder: A Special Case

Each of the diagnostic building blocks is important, but some loom larger than others. Somatization disorder is a mental condition that, as described in DSM-IV, comprises exclusively physical (somatic) symptoms. Although it is common, affecting perhaps 1% of the general population, it is often overlooked by clinicians in the process of making diagnoses. Chapters 11 and 12 contain case histories; for now we'll only address those aspects that pertain to physical symptoms.

DSM-5 and DSM-5-TR have taken what I consider to be a wrong turn with this disorder. It has been renamed *somatic symptom disorder;* it now includes DSM-IV-defined pain disorder, elements of hypochondriasis, and undifferentiated somatoform disorder as well; and it has been redefined so that a single symptom (with at least 6 months of excessive concern about health) can qualify for diagnosis. My advice: Continue to use the less permissive DSM-IV criteria (reviewed below) for somatization disorder, as I have advocated throughout this book.

In somatization disorder, the problem isn't so much the exact symptoms the patient has at any one time as the twin facts that there can be so many of them and that they are so varied—and varying. They cause the patient to seek treatment or interfere with social, work, or personal functioning, and they can include the following:

- Multiple pain symptoms in such locations as head, back, abdomen, joints, limbs, chest, or rectum; or pain related to body functions, including intercourse, menstruation, and urination.

- Gastrointestinal symptoms such as nausea, abdominal bloating, vomiting, diarrhea, and food intolerances.

- Sexual symptoms that include indifference to sex, difficulties with erection or ejaculation, irregular or excessive menses, and vomiting throughout pregnancy.

- Pseudoneurological symptoms (that is, symptoms with no anatomical or physiological basis) that include poor balance or coordination, weak or paralyzed muscles, lump in throat, loss of voice, retention of urine, hallucinations, numbness, double vision, blindness, deafness, seizures, amnesia (or other symptoms of dissociation), and loss of consciousness.

It is especially important to note that these patients aren't faking their symptoms; they believe, or fear, that they are truly ill. In the typical pattern, first one symptom and later another becomes prominent as a patient visits doctor after doctor. The pattern suggests that what's important to the patient is the process of being sick, rather than the type of sickness itself. Somatization disorder is so important to many differential diagnoses and is so often forgotten that I've dedicated a diagnostic principle to it. There's more about this disorder beginning on page 158.

> *Diagnostic Principle:* **Consider somatic symptom (somatization) disorder whenever symptoms don't jibe or treatments don't work.**

For the initial diagnostic evaluation, be aware of the following: (1) These patients typically complain of a variety of somatic symptoms; (2) they often have mood and anxiety symptoms as well; (3) their symptoms respond poorly to treatment that usually works for most patients; and (4) if a symptom does improve, a new one could well appear to take its place. All of these factors explain why general health care providers often lose patience with such patients and refer them elsewhere. By the time they come to the attention of mental health professionals, they may have seen many other doctors and therapists and received much medical care—usually to their clinicians' frustration and their own detriment.

Using Physical Symptoms to Make a Diagnosis

Physical diseases won't often be the cause of your patient's mental symptoms, but when they do play a role, it is vital to find out right away. Anxiety symptoms, for example, can stem from a great variety of medical illnesses.

> After several months of couple therapy, Milt and Marjorie's therapist notes that Marjorie has become increasingly irritable. Her hands shake visibly, and she often arises from her chair to walk back and forth. She complains that the temperature is too warm in the office, even in January when others are bundled up. During a discussion of her weight loss, the therapist suggests that she should be evaluated by her family doctor. Testing reveals moderately increased thyroid activity.

To be sure, the original reason for entering therapy was probably not her endocrine disorder. But Marjorie's thyroid may well have contributed to her advancing irritability. Physical disorders like Marjorie's can often be treated effectively; if ignored, they can wreak havoc. Here's how I think about them:

1. Make sure that information about general medical health is a part of every mental health assessment. This should include material obtained from the patient, as well as summaries from hospitalizations and medical workups.

2. Ensure that each patient has had a recent general medical checkup; if your patient doesn't have a general physician, recommend one and ensure that a complete evaluation is performed. This is especially important if you note any of the indicators of medical disease suggested above in the section "Clues to a Physical Cause for Mental Symptoms" (p. 104).

3. Become familiar with somatization disorder. I may have mentioned earlier that if you don't suspect a condition, you'll never diagnose it. Somatization disorder is too prevalent and has implications too important to risk ignoring it.

4. List physical disorder etiologies at the top of every patient's differential diagnosis. Even if you consider this possibility only momentarily before moving on, keep reminding yourself that it exists for the next patient, and the next. Eventually your vigilance will pay off.

Substance Use and Mental Disorders

The use of chemical substances—alcohol, street drugs, prescription drugs, or over-the-counter medications—can produce mental symptoms. The cause–effect relationship will be especially strong if the symptoms develop after a patient has started using a substance, and if the symptoms diminish once use stops. The association will be even stronger if the patient develops symptoms with each use, if each time they are the *same* symptoms, and if the patient has never had such symptoms prior to using that substance. I've already awarded diagnostic principle status to the important relationship between substance use and mental disorder.

That principle isn't limited to street drugs. For example, the use of anabolic steroids by athletes, from the professional level down at least through high school sports, has received much publicity over the years.

> Beginning in high school, 19-year-old Efrain Marrero had injected synthetic body-building steroids to bulk up for football. When his parents discovered what he was doing, they begged him to quit. He did, but rapidly sank into depression so deep that, as *The New York Times* reported in 2005, he shot himself to death in a bedroom at home.

You will need to make a list of all substances (legal and otherwise) taken by the patient, noting when symptoms began and when each substance was first used. Compare it to Table 9.2, which lists some of the types of medications that can produce mental symptoms, and to Table 9.3, where I've listed the mental and behavioral effects of alcohol and other substances of misuse.

Once again, let's revisit Carson (yep, Chapter 1) to assess our use of the diagnostic building blocks reviewed so far in Part II. We've used the history of his present illness; his family history (his grandmother reportedly was chronically depressed); and, from his personal and social history, the fact of his impending long-distance move. Each of these areas of information is necessary to fully understand the background to his misery. The sources of information we've used include Carson and his wife; we would also look at his previous medical records to shore up our memory that his previous episodes of depression occurred in the winter and spring. We've done all these things, yet there is still one important block to discuss—his present mental status. We'll take it up in the next chapter.

TABLE 9.2. Classes (or Names) of Medications That Can Cause Mental Symptoms

	Anxiety	Mood	Psychosis	Delirium
Analgesics	×	×	×	×
Anesthetics	×	×	×	×
Antabuse		×	×	
Antianxiety agents		×		
Anticholinergics	×	×	×	
Anticonvulsants	×	×	×	×
Antidepressants	×	×	×	×
Antihistamines	×		×	×
Antihypertensives/ cardiovascular agents	×	×	×	×
Antimicrobials		×	×	×
Antiparkinsonian agents	×	×	×	×
Antipsychotics	×	×		×
Antiulcer agents		×		
Bronchodilators	×			×
Chemotherapies			×	
Corticosteroids	×	×	×	×
Gastrointestinal agents			×	×
Histamine antagonists				×
Immunosuppressants				×
Insulin	×			
Interferon	×	×	×	
Lithium	×			
Muscle relaxants		×	×	×
NSAIDs[a]			×	
Oral contraceptives	×	×		
Thyroid replacements	×			

[a]NSAIDs, nonsteroidal anti-inflammatory drugs.

TABLE 9.3. Symptoms of Substance Use

		Substance intoxication								Substance withdrawal					
		Alcohol/sedatives	Cannabis	Stimulants[a]	Caffeine	Hallucinogens	Inhalants	Opioids	PCP	Alcohol/sedatives	Cannabis	Stimulants[a]	Caffeine	Tobacco	Opioids
Social	Impaired social functioning			×											
	Inappropriate sexuality	×													
	Social withdrawal		×												
	Interpersonal sensitivity			×											
Mood	Labile mood	×													
	Anxiety		×	×		×				×	×			×	
	Euphoria		×	×			×	×							
	Blunted affect, apathy			×			×	×							
	Anger			×								×		×	
	Dysphoria, depression					×		×		×	×	×	×	×	
	Irritability											×	×	×	
Judgment	Impaired judgment	×	×	×		×	×	×	×						
	Assaultiveness, belligerence						×		×						
	Impulsivity								×						
Sleep	Insomnia, sleeplessness				×					×	×	×		×	×
	Bad dreams										×	×			
	Hypersomnia, drowsiness											×			
Activity level	Aggression	×								×					
	Agitation, increased activity			×	×			×	×	×		×			
	Tirelessness			×											
	Restlessness				×							×		×	
	Decreased activity, retardation			×			×	×				×			
Alertness	Reduced attention, concentration	×						×					×	×	
	Stupor or coma	×		×			×	×	×						
	Sensation of slowed time		×												
	Confusion			×											
	Hypervigilance			×											
Perception	Ideas of reference, persecution					×									
	Perceptual changes					×									
	Brief halluc./illusions					×				×					
	Depers./dereal.					×									
	Fears of insanity					×									
Autonomic	Dry mouth		×												
	Pupils constricted							×							
	Pupils dilated			×		×									×
	Sweating			×		×				×	×				×
	Piloerection														×
Muscle	Weakness			×			×								
	Twitching				×										
	Aches													×	×
	Rigidity								×						

[a]Such as cocaine and amphetamines.

TABLE 9.3 (cont.)

		Substance intoxication								Substance withdrawal					
		Alcohol/sedatives	Cannabis	Stimulants[a]	Caffeine	Hallucinogens	Inhalants	Opioids	PCP	Alcohol/sedatives	Cannabis	Stimulants[a]	Caffeine	Tobacco	Opioids
Neurological	Dystonia, dyskinesia			×											
	Nystagmus	×					×		×						
	Tremors				×	×				×	×				
	Blurred vision				×	×									
	Double vision					×									
	Impaired reflexes					×									
	Seizures			×					×	×					
	Numbness							×							
	Headache									×			×		
Gastrointestinal	GI upset, diarrhea				×										×
	Nausea, vomiting			×						×			×		×
	Abdominal pain									×					
	Increased appetite/weight gain		×									×		×	
	Decreased appetite/weight loss			×						×					
Motor	Incoordination	×	×			×	×								
	Unsteady gait, trouble walking	×					×		×						
	Stereotypies			×											
	Lethargy						×								
	Slurred speech, dysarthria	×					×	×	×						
Cardiovascular	Irregular heartbeat			×	×	×									
	Slow heart rate			×											
	Rapid heart rate		×	×	×	×				×	×				
	Blood pressure up or down			×						×					
General	Depressed breathing			×											
	Chest pain			×											
	Dizziness						×								
	Red eyes		×												
	Chills			×						×					
	Fever									×					×
	Reduced memory	×					×								
	Nervousness, excitability				×					×					
	Rambling speech				×										
	Hyperacute hearing							×							
	Flushed face				×										
	Increased urination				×										
	Fatigue											×	×		
	Tearing, runny nose														×
	Yawning														×

10 Diagnosis and the Mental Status Examination

And here's the final piece of the diagnostic puzzle. In general, the MSE is simply a statement of how a person looks, feels, and behaves at the moment of examination. Nearly as important are the characteristics a person *doesn't* show. For example, although Carson's (Chapter 1) MSE specifically reflected depression, feelings of panic, tearfulness, trouble concentrating, worries, and feelings of abandonment, he *didn't* have hallucinations or delusions. Findings such as these last two, which help rule out a diagnosis that seems otherwise a real possibility, are called *pertinent negatives*. They should not only be inquired after, but faithfully reported in the clinician's write-up.

We must keep in mind that, important though the MSE may be, it is only a snapshot of a patient at a single point in time. It's easy to overemphasize MSE symptoms at the expense of other building blocks of diagnosis, and clinicians sometimes yield to this temptation (see the sidebar "Is the MSE Overrated?").

Appearance

Much of the MSE requires no questioning at all, only observation of the patient during an ordinary conversation. Nearly all the material in this section and the next two ("Mood/Affect" and "Flow of Speech") falls into that category, and it will mostly be evident even to an unpracticed eye. However, though it can signal possibilities, right up front we need to remind ourselves not to let appearance alone weigh too heavily in our evaluation.

General Appearance

As Mark Twain almost said, clothes make the individual. For example, for an adult who wears tattered, bizarre, or dirty clothing or who is otherwise generally untidy, schizophrenia and other psychoses, dementia, and the

Is the MSE Overrated?

Although the mental status examination is an important part of diagnosis and the database, can it ever be overrated? I'm afraid that's sometimes the case. Traditionally coming at the very end of a full evaluation, the MSE is where too many clinicians begin. Scientific studies of diagnosis have shown that we may too quickly jump to conclusions based on a single, arresting symptom. That's because we wrongly assume that really dramatic symptoms can mean only one thing; in the case of hallucinations and delusions, for example, this would be schizophrenia.

We forget that there is probably no mental symptom that can have only one interpretation. Even a symptom as seemingly specialized as the belief that one is pregnant (when one is not) can be found in conditions as diverse as mania, depression, dementia, and substance use. Consider the case of celebrated writer Virginia Woolf: On at least five occasions throughout her life, she became acutely and severely ill with delusional ideas about her supposed guilt and the worthlessness of her work. She hallucinated voices so terrifying that she could never bring herself to describe them. Yet within weeks or months she would recover completely—each time except the last, when she weighted the pockets of her fur coat with stones and drowned herself in the icy March waters of the river Ouse. The lesson: Mental status symptoms should never put us into a box, but onto a decision tree.

Far from being the only important factor in diagnosis, the MSE often isn't even the *most* important. MSE information doesn't usually make or break a diagnosis; much of the time, the longitudinal evaluation has greater diagnostic value than does the patient's current appearance. What the MSE should do is set flags that warn of the possibilities, which we must in turn evaluate in the context of all we have learned from the patient's own history and from the information provided by relatives, old charts, and previous clinicians.

more extreme effects of substance use will come to mind. If the patient is a teenager or child, the options will be broader still. And of course, excessive thinness can signal anorexia nervosa, especially if the person is a young woman.

An office patient I once evaluated turned out to be one of the most anxious individuals I have ever known. My first clue was upon shaking hands with Douglas, when I felt a bulge of enlarged muscle at the base of his right palm. He was a draftsman, and he habitually clutched his pen as if it were trying to escape. Over the years, that muscle had grown huge from the tension of his grip.

You might find additional clues in your patient's posture, from scars, gait, jewelry, or hairstyle. Tattoos, once suggestive of lifestyle, have become so commonplace as to lose any diagnostic value.

Level of Attention

How alert is your patient? Could the person who is drowsy or inattentive be experiencing a delirium, possibly coupled to a medical disorder or a substance use? Of course, inability to sustain attention is famously associated with ADHD, which typically occurs in children and adolescents, but is increasingly found to affect adults too. More than once, ADHD has been diagnosed in a parent whose child has just been evaluated for inattention and motor restlessness.

> Inattention is perhaps more frequently encountered in someone like Lester, who accompanies his wife to counseling, though evidently not in spirit. His wandering gaze, refusal to give eye contact to anyone in the room, and frequent responses of "Huh? Oh, sorry!" clearly proclaim his lack of investment in the proceedings. He reminds me of my high school civics course, conducted—I wouldn't say taught—every spring by the baseball coach. Even when he lectured, he mostly gazed out the window that overlooked the diamond. It was crystal clear that he wished himself elsewhere, a sentiment fervently endorsed by his captive students.

On the other end of the attention spectrum is hypervigilance, in which the patient glances frequently around the room, as though trying to locate the source of voices or a threat. Hypervigilance suggests PTSD, but it is also often associated with paranoid delusions found in psychoses.

Amount of Activity

Your patient's activity level can be an important indicator of diagnosis. The most common observation is increased motor activity, such as the jiggling leg or frequent hand wringing that indicates simple tension or anxiety, perhaps even the desire to run away. Abnormal body movements can indicate that the person has been using a medication, perhaps one of the older, now less popular antipsychotic drugs such as Prolixin or Haldol; then you might suspect a psychotic disorder. The classic back-and-forth "pill-rolling" tremor, a well-known sign of naturally occurring Parkinson's disease, can also result from these medications. An involuntary movement of lips, mouth, and upper limbs referred to as *tardive dyskinesia,* and the restless inability to sit still referred to as *akathisia* (such a patient feels the need to keep quite literally on the move), are two additional movement disorders related to these drugs. Table 9.3 lists some of the motor behaviors related to substance misuse.

Although excessive motion is probably the more common finding in mental health patients, a facial expression that shows little mobility— sometimes seeming to be nearly frozen—can be found in patients suffering from dementia or severe depression. The nearly complete immobility of catatonia is now rare.

Mood/Affect

We'll define *mood* as how we feel, *affect* as how we appear to be feeling. Let's briefly discuss three qualities of mood/affect: its *type, lability* (the degree to which it changes in a given time frame), and *appropriateness.*

We tend to think of mood almost as a diagnosis: We equate euphoria with mania, sadness with major depression or dysthymia. But who among us hasn't experienced these feelings, usually without other indicators of illness? Indeed, a person's transient emotional state doesn't usually convey much about diagnosis. Anger (and its cousin, hostility), anxiety, shame, joy, fear, guilt, surprise, disgust, and irritation are emotions that can occur in mental disorders, though most of the time they are perfectly normal. Patients who worry about normal moods will often benefit from simple reassurance.

Excessive lability of mood may yield more accurate diagnostic inferences. For example, a person whose mood seems to rapidly shift between extremes (from laughter to weeping and back, or without apparent cause into sudden fury) should be evaluated for mania, dementia, and the somatizing disorders. Unheralded outbursts of temper occasionally indicate medical conditions such as brain infections or tumors. Affect that hardly budges (decreased lability) can suggest Parkinson's disease, severe depression, schizophrenia, or dementia.

The third quality of mood is its appropriateness to the person's content of thought. When I interviewed Joan, she giggled as she talked about the recent death of her mother. Such incongruence of affect with content brings to mind two possibilities: mania and the form of schizophrenia that used to be called *disorganized* (before the DSMs did away with the subtypes). Joan had had episodes of psychosis followed by depression, then long stretches when she was completely normal—clearly suggesting bipolar I disorder. You'll also encounter inappropriate mood when someone with somatic symptom disorder discusses a current physical problem, such as paralysis or blindness, with none of the apprehension you'd expect for such a serious condition.

Depression is the mood symptom most often noted during the MSE. Because of its ubiquity, potential for harm, and response to treatment, I look for depression in every new patient—and a lot of continuing ones. This is important enough to rate its own diagnostic principle. Of course, *always* is always a bit over the top, but depression is so common, so important, and so often missed that I've included the intensifier.

> *Diagnostic Principle:* **Because of their ubiquity, potential for harm, and ready response to treatment,** *always* **consider mood disorders.**

Flow of Speech

Although flow of speech can reveal several possible clues to diagnosis, let's first acknowledge that most of us have speech quirks that aren't usually pathological at all. Examples include verbal tics (such as "you know," "whatever," "awesome," and "like, no way"), *circumstantial speech* (where a person relates a lot of irrelevant detail before coming to the point), and speech so distractible that trying to communicate nearly drives you nuts.

Probably the best-known type of actual speech pathology is what's called *loose associations,* or sometimes *derailment*. Loose associations occur when thought coherence breaks down, so that one idea skids off into another that isn't clearly related. Although you can understand the sequence of words, the direction they take is nowhere on the compass. The result is illogical speech or writing that must mean something to the patient, but that doesn't communicate meaning to others. Here, from my personal archives, is an extreme example:

> "I found out that the English tea which the British drink. And that clam chowder isn't different, like Indian corn is American food. But England has a king, queen, and a prince. Princess Anne is married to an Englishman. Now medication is for help of accidents, sickness, burned people, and blackouts and dizzy spells like me. The truth of Europe, in fact Japan has tea, too. And America. Thanks."

Loose associations and other, less common speech patterns such as *incoherence, neologisms* (made up words), *perseveration,* and *echolalia* (repeating the words of the other person) are usually said to be characteristic of schizophrenia, though they can also occur in mania and dementia.

The interval before someone responds to a question is called *latency of response;* marked deviations often point to a mood disorder. Very long latency is characteristic of severe depression, whereas reduced latency, in which the patient answers almost before you arrive at the question mark, is sometimes encountered in mania. In *poverty of speech,* a patient will spontaneously speak little or not at all; it can suggest depression, schizophrenia, or dementia.

Content of Thought

In the history of the present illness, you will have already encountered most of the material usually described as content of thought. The implications of this information are pretty straightforward.

No matter how you frame them, delusions and hallucinations almost always mean psychosis. However, the sort of delusion you encounter can help define the type of psychosis. Delusions of influence, persecution, passivity (a patient is being acted upon by some outside influence), reference (comments are being made about the patient), thought control, or thought broadcasting (patients feel their thoughts are being transmitted, perhaps by radio waves) often suggest schizophrenia, especially what we used to call paranoid schizophrenia. Delusions of ill health (having a terrible disease) or even of being dead can indicate either schizophrenia or severe depression. Delusions of grandeur, in which patients believe they have great powers or are famous beings such as God or either of the Madonnas, are classic for mania but can also be encountered in schizophrenia. Delusions of guilt suggest either depression or delusional disorder, whereas a delusion that one has become impoverished usually indicates profound depression.

Also note mood *congruence,* which refers to how well mood matches the content of the person's delusion. When I asked a woman I once treated for a postpartum manic psychosis why she seemed so happy and contented, she said it was because she knew she had "the little baby Jesus at home in his crib." Such mood-congruent delusions usually indicate a mood disorder. On the other hand, the delusions of schizophrenia are often mood incongruent, as with the young man who believed that he was the son of Jay Leno and that he could change the weather. Despite these grandiose delusions, he knew that his mental condition had prevented him from maintaining a job and having a normal social life, and he felt severely depressed as a result.

You might encounter hallucinations of any of the senses in a psychosis caused by a medical or substance use disorder, such as delirium tremens, dementia, brain tumor, toxicity, or seizures. In schizophrenia, whereas most hallucinations are auditory, some are visual, and infrequently you will encounter hallucinations of the other senses. The vivid, dreamlike states that we have when awakening or falling asleep are respectively called *hypnopompic* and *hypnagogic* hallucinations, but they are completely normal. Also normal are illusions, *déjà vu,* overvalued ideas (such as a belief in the superiority of one's religion or ethnic background), and depersonalization that is neither protracted nor extreme.

Although phobias or obsessions and compulsions often signal a specific anxiety disorder or OCD, keep in mind two general issues. One is that, as with anxiety in general, a mild degree of these symptoms is common and not at all abnormal. The second, which we'll discuss further in Chapter 12, is the clinical tendency to focus on dramatic phobias and compulsions while ignoring the quiet little depression that sometimes lurks underneath.

Finally, we must mention thoughts about suicide, homicide, and other forms of violence. Suicidal ideas most often point to depression, though they can also indicate a personality disorder, substance use, or schizophrenia. If ideas concerning violence indicate any mental disorder at all, it will usually be one of these three conditions. But violence and homicide are more typical of plain old criminal activity. Remember the Godfather.

Cognition and Intellectual Resources

Reasoning, mathematical ability, and abstract thinking (such as recognizing similarities and differences) largely depend on the person's education and native intelligence; these abilities will therefore be prominently deficient in intellectual disability and other developmental disorders, such as autism spectrum disorder. They can also be clouded by serious mental illnesses such as dementia, schizophrenia, and mood disorders. Problems with comprehension, fluency, naming, repetition, reading, and writing, other than those you might expect from non-native speakers, suggest the need for neurological evaluation.

Orientation is only occasionally deficient, and then almost always it indicates a cognitive disorder—either delirium or dementia. Occasionally a psychotic patient may claim to be Zog from Mars who lives in the Fifth

Dimension, but we would say that such a person is delusional, not disoriented. Impairment of short-term memory can point to dementia, delirium, a psychosis, a mood disorder, or just plain anxiety.

Insight and Judgment

The amount of specific diagnostic information you can gather from the patient's insight may be less than overwhelming. Poor insight into the fact of having a mental disorder often indicates psychosis, but it is also common in patients with dementia or delirium; it can even occur in people who misuse alcohol or other substances. You'll also encounter deficient insight in disorders we don't automatically associate with psychosis, such as severe mood disorders, dissociative identity disorder, anorexia nervosa, body dysmorphic disorder, and instances of OCD so severe that the individual may not identify the compulsive behaviors as irrational.

Both insight and judgment heavily depend on factors that we don't consider abnormal. One is the person's age: Children lack perspective on their own behavior and emotions up to the early teen years, and even for the next few years they still may lack a fully developed ability to comprehend the consequences of their own actions. Hence the 2005 U.S. Supreme Court ruling against capital punishment for minors. To a degree, the insight and judgment of adults are also affected by native intelligence, education, and cultural issues such as superstition and prejudice.

Like insight, judgment may be affected by psychosis and delirium. Any personality disorder can also affect insight (who among us readily admits to having character flaws?), but judgment is especially vulnerable to the more severe forms of personality disorder, such as borderline and antisocial.

With the conclusion of Part II, *you* now have insight into the full range of information you'll need to make accurate diagnoses in your patients. This is the raw material we use during the diagnostic levels already described in Part I. Always keep mentally prepared, however, for new information that could necessitate a reassessment of the facts—as you thought you knew them.

Part III

Applying
the Diagnostic Techniques

11 Diagnosing Depression and Mania

For several reasons, I've chosen to begin Part III with what I continue to call the *mood disorders,* even though DSM-5-TR separates them into the *depressive disorders* and the *bipolar disorders.* Perhaps most important, mood disorders are among the major ills that affect mental health patients. They also rank near the top of the safety hierarchy (Table 3.1), and they present the most complicated challenges to every diagnostician, regardless of discipline or level of experience. I like to begin lectures on diagnosis by explaining that, once you understand the mood disorders, the rest of diagnosis is a relative breeze.

Mood disorders present a variety of challenges:

1. Clinicians must consider numerous depressive syndromes, including major depressive disorder (with its various subtypes and specifiers, such as atypical, melancholic, and seasonal), dysthymia, and the depressive episodes of bipolar disorders.
2. The opposite of depressed mood is a spectrum that includes mania and its variants—hypomania, mixed states, and the high phases of cyclothymic disorder.
3. Once we make a diagnosis of a mood disorder, we must consider the possibility that there may be other, comorbid conditions.
4. Depression shares features with prolonged grief disorder and other losses, problems of living, and adjustment disorders. There is also the vexed question of suicide as rational behavior versus treatable illness (see the sidebar "Can Suicide Ever Be Rational?" at the end of this chapter).

Syndromes of Depression

Mental disorders are somewhat like onions: You can peel away layer after layer until you arrive at the core. Syndromes of clinical depression are like onions in a different sense: There are many different kinds of onions—red, yellow, white, pearl, Bermuda, Walla Walla (which are popular here in the Northwest), scallions, and many others. Each type may be used somewhat differently, depending on its unique characteristics, which you must first identify. So it is with types of depression. Table 11.1 lists the forms we'll consider in this chapter, along with some brief definitions. In addition to the examples given here, you'll find others involving depression in later chapters. By the time you've finished reading, you'll really know your onions.

Kent

Let's start with this relatively uncomplicated example of a patient who seems classically depressed.

> Kent is referred for evaluation by his family doctor, who notes that, though physically healthy, he is "sagging in the mental department." By education and training an electronics engineer, Kent had worked in California's Silicon Valley for 7 successful years. To poise himself for further moves up the corporate ladder, he had enrolled in an MBA program at a local university and was just one class short of graduation when the bursting dot-com bubble downsized him out of a job. With thousands of his colleagues also looking for work, he spent a dispiriting 8 months pounding the pavement before he finally found another job— selling cars for a brother-in-law who "had never even finished college," as he tells the interviewer.
>
> Kent complains of months of depression, which he blames on his loss of status and the struggle to pay the mortgage on his expensive house in San Jose. However, during the first interview, his wife points out that he had been having problems with both insomnia and a diminished appetite for weeks before he'd been laid off. She remarks that "He didn't even show much enthusiasm for the fly-fishing outfit I got him for his birthday." Now he expresses guilt that he cannot provide adequately for his family and distress at the low energy and concentration that hamper his efforts at work. He denies having suicidal ideas, but his wife says that the previous week, he told her that he didn't much care whether he lived or died.
>
> Kent has had no psychotic symptoms or prior episodes of mental illness, and his family history is negative for mental disorder. Although he had used alcohol, sometimes to excess, when he was in college a decade earlier, he hasn't touched it since. He denies feeling worried or anxious; according to him, he is "just plain depressed."

TABLE 11.1. Differential Diagnosis with Brief Definitions for Depression

- *Depressive disorder due to another medical condition.* Physical illness can cause depression, which need not meet criteria for a major depressive episode.

- *Substance-related depressive disorder.* Alcohol, street drugs, or medications cause depressive symptoms, which also need not conform to the definition of major depression.

- *Major depressive disorder, (either) single episode or recurrent.* For weeks or longer, the patient feels depressed or cannot enjoy life and may have problems with eating and sleeping, guilt feelings, loss of energy, trouble concentrating, and thoughts about death. There can be no episodes of mania or hypomania.

- *Bipolar (I or II) disorder, most recent episode depressed.* Currently depressed, the patient has a history of mania or hypomania.

- *Major depressive disorder with melancholic features.* This special type of major depression is characterized by early morning awakening, appetite and weight loss, guilt feelings, and failure to feel better when something happens that would ordinarily be enjoyable.

- *Major depressive disorder with atypical features.* Certain symptoms are the opposite of those usually experienced in major depression—increased appetite, weight gain, and excessive sleeping.

- *Major depressive disorder with seasonal pattern.* In this condition, also known as *seasonal affective disorder,* patients regularly become depressed at a certain time of the year, especially fall or winter.

- *Major depressive disorder with peripartum onset.* A woman develops major depression during pregnancy or within a month of having a baby.

- *Dysthymia (persistent depressive disorder).* These patients typically remain ill for years, with symptoms typically less severe than those of major depressive disorder; they don't have psychosis or suicidal ideas.

- *Bereavement.* For weeks or months, a person whose relative or friend has died experiences feelings of loss and hollowness that typically well up when thinking of the deceased but diminish within days to weeks. If symptoms meet DSM-5-TR criteria for depression, it should also be diagnosed.

- *Prolonged grief disorder.* Someone whose loved one has died grieves for a year or longer, exhibiting multiple symptoms of depression and stress.

- *Adjustment disorder with depressed mood.* Some people respond to life stresses by developing depressive symptoms.

- *Somatic symptom disorder with mood disorder.* Patients who have an extensive history of many bodily complaints for which no physical explanation can be found often also have depression, and sometimes even symptoms of mania. Note my comments on pages 111 and 160.

Analysis

Using the numbered steps in our decision tree for depression (Figure 11.1), here's how I think about Kent. He has no history of mania or hypomania that would suggest a bipolar disorder (step 1). Although his mood is terrible, his family practitioner has given him a clean bill of physical health (step 2). He doesn't drink or use drugs (step 3), has no history of multiple somatic symptoms (step 4), and isn't female so couldn't have premenstrual dysphoric disorder (step 5). At step 6 we note that he has not had prolonged grief, moving us to step 7: Yes, he had had quite a few of the typical major depression symptoms. Lack of psychotic symptoms (step 11) should lead us first to consider major depressive disorder. The asterisk directs us to step 13, which reminds us of the variety of specifiers we can diagnose. Kent did not have symptoms of the melancholic or atypical forms (see Table 11.1), and he was obviously neither catatonic nor postpartum, so we would say he had a single episode of major depressive disorder—the term most often used now for *clinical depression*.

Let's also mention a few of the diagnostic principles that, by either their presence or their absence, have helped us arrive at this conclusion. We have relied heavily on the collateral information from Kent's wife, which proves more accurate than Kent's own estimation of when the depression began. His ancient history of drinking is trumped by 10 recent years of sober living. The social setting of an intact marriage assures us that personality disorder is unlikely to play much of a role in his diagnosis, and anyway, we would want to avoid any personality disorder diagnosis in the face of a major mental disorder. There were no unusual symptoms that would draw us away from a diagnosis of major depression, which is a common diagnosis (a horse, not a zebra).

Comment

In my opinion, the diagnosis of major depression has a major shortcoming: Although it offers the illusion of precision, it obscures the fact that in reality, depression can stem from a variety of causes. Because they are encompassed by one name, we are tempted to view patients who are very different as having the same illness, and *that* can tempt us to prescribe similar treatments (often antidepressant medications) for all. Of course, many patients respond well to the standard regimens, but throughout this book—indeed, throughout your career—you'll find patients with major depression occurring in contexts that should suggest treatments other than pharmacological.

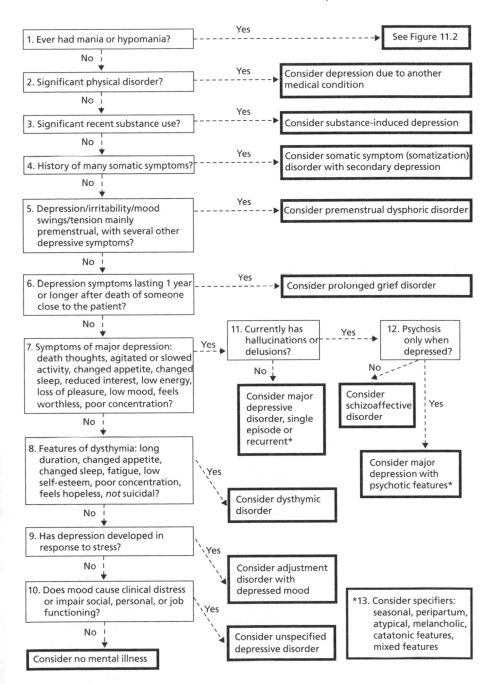

FIGURE 11.1. Decision tree for a patient who experiences depression or loss of pleasure.

Marilyn

Once you have in mind the appropriate differential diagnosis and decision tree, the process of diagnosis is relatively straightforward.

> A 23-year-old graduate student in cultural anthropology, Marilyn has signed up to spend 4 months in Guinea observing and recording the pronunciation of native forest dwellers' fast-vanishing language. Three weeks before she, two other students, and their instructor are scheduled to leave for western Africa, she requests an appointment with the dean of her professional school. "I thought that the thrill and activity of this trip would help me ditch the depression I've had for several years," she confesses. She still has trouble with loss of sleep and appetite, and her mood is low "most of the time." Later, consulting with a clinician friend, the dean repeats this information and asks for an opinion. The answer is unexpected. "Right now, I just can't say," replies the clinician. "We don't have nearly enough information." Here's what an interview revealed later.
>
> Marilyn's depression had first come to light when she was just 15. Pretty and intelligent, she was competitive in volleyball and earned nearly all A's, but still she hadn't adjusted well to high school. By her sophomore year, she felt that she didn't have what it took to make it as either a scholar or an athlete. Though she had a few close friends, she often worried that she wouldn't make the grade socially, either.
>
> Born to a Korean woman who wasn't married to Marilyn's biological father, Marilyn had been adopted when she was just a week old. Her adoptive parents are both college graduates; her mother writes for a biweekly newspaper, and for many years her father worked as a news anchor for a local television channel in a large East Coast city. Two older siblings, who are not adopted, excelled in school and are now entering into professional careers.
>
> Marilyn admits that she feels sad and lonely "most of the time, even when I'm with other people." Although she readily agrees that she is "seriously deficient in self-esteem," her interest and concentration in her studies are good; she has never had suicidal ideas. She strongly denies any substance use (including prescribed or over-the-counter medications); her mother, during a Zoom call with Marilyn and the therapist, agrees. She volunteers that Marilyn has never had a significant medical disorder, "not even the flu."

Analysis

Based on Marilyn's history, we can quickly pass through steps 1–6 of the decision tree in Figure 11.1. Marilyn has just a few symptoms of major depression (step 7), certainly not enough to justify that diagnosis. Her long duration of generally mild symptoms sounds much more like dysthymia (aka persistent depressive disorder, step 8), which is the main diagnosis we should consider.

It is important to recognize, as did the clinician consulted by Marilyn's dean, the need for a comprehensive assessment; without longitudinal information, Marilyn's presentation isn't very specific for any diagnosis. Information about her biological parents might have helped, as suggested by the family history diagnostic principle, but family history is more useful in starting the train of diagnostic thought than in pinpointing its final destination. Although her mother's belief that Marilyn has not used substances is reassuring, of course it is not proof; when a substance use disorder is suspected, objective tests (urine or blood) should be considered. You might think that Marilyn's depression worsened in response to the anticipation of an extended assignment overseas, which would suggest an adjustment disorder with depressed mood. However, that conclusion would contradict the safety diagnostic principle: We should first consider more treatable, more specific disorders.

Although I have said that we could quickly eliminate substance use and medical disorders in discussing Marilyn's disorder, I do not mean—and I will *never* mean—that we can be cavalier about these perilous diagnoses. The trouble is that they are often not at the root of a given patient's problem, so you could blithely ignore them 50 times without incident and reap tragedy on the 51st. Throughout the rest of this book, if I say, "We can safely eliminate . . . ," I mean only that we'll accept it as proven for the purposes of discussion. Whenever evaluating a new patient, I always carefully consider physical and chemical causes.

Comment

Dysthymia, more formally termed *persistent depressive disorder,* can be traced back at least to Emil Kraepelin in the early 1900s. Yet, for all we have learned in its long history, we still relive the old arguments about just where this mild yet prevalent type of depression fits into the family of mood disorders. Of course, the difference in symptoms between dysthymia and major depression is obvious, and other terms have been used over the years to describe types of depression similar to dysthymia. Clinicians have long noted that the chronic low mood and poor self-esteem of patients with dysthymia can seem almost a part of their character structure. However, DSM-5-TR no longer even includes *depressive personality disorder* in its appendix "for further study." Today we seldom encounter *neurotic depres-*

sion, a term once used for depressions that were supposedly reactive to an intense disappointment or some other external stimulus. In counterpoint to this older thinking, some studies have found family histories of bipolar disorders in patients with dysthymia.

Whether we call it dysthymia or persistent depressive disorder, this condition is pretty common, affecting perhaps 6% of the general adult population; you'll also find it in children and adolescents. Although people with dysthymia are less impaired overall than those with major depression, they and their families nonetheless bear a heavy burden; some writers note that these patients tend to channel whatever energy they possess into work, with little left over for personal relationships. The good news is that, like many other types of depression, dysthymia can be effectively addressed with standard antidepressant treatments—provided we diagnose it correctly.

Timothy

The disorders we've encountered so far entail more or less typical depressive symptoms of varying severity. However, it would endanger both the diagnostic process and the patient to rely wholly on symptoms. The following example shows how important it is to seek the diagnosis in the patient's history, as well as in cross-sectional symptoms.

> Timothy, a journalist now in his late 30s, covered the war in Sudan for a major news organization. Shortly after receiving an emergency blood transfusion when injured abroad, he contracted hepatitis C and was started on interferon. "Within a few days I began to feel like I had the flu—achy muscles, tired all the time, stomach pain—and I couldn't sleep more than a couple of hours before I woke up exhausted." However, he had no problems with appetite, and he never felt suicidal; even his sex interest remained good.
>
> Reassigned to the United States, Timothy chafed at the relatively dull stories on his new beat. He complained of trouble focusing on his reporting and began brooding about his health. Noting his insomnia and loss of concentration, his internist concluded that he was depressed and started him on Prozac. "For all the good it did, I might as well have been swallowing Tic Tacs," Timothy says later. "Twelve weeks on, I wasn't any worse, but I sure wasn't any better, either." In answer to a question, he points out that he follows his religion, which forbids the use of alcohol or tobacco in any form.
>
> Timothy and his wife previously saw a therapist to deal with the marital problems surrounding their infertility, so his doctor next

referred him for counseling. It was during "that fruitless 8 weeks" that Timothy, surfing the internet one day when he should have been working, downloaded a podcast that described the mental effects of interferon treatment. He learned that about a third of patients treated with interferon develop serious depression. "I felt outraged and relieved at the same time," he later says, "seriously ticked off that I hadn't been warned about side effects of the drug, but delighted to find a treatable cause."

With his hepatitis in remission, he stops the interferon. Within days, his depressive symptoms remit completely.

Analysis

The absence of a history of mania or hypomania gets us past step 1 of Figure 11.1, but we need to consider whether the hepatitis itself could have caused Timothy's depression (step 2). Typically, patients with hepatitis C complain of poor appetite, weight loss, and fatigue, but not depression. The fact that his depression began at about the time he started on interferon helps move us along to step 3, which is where we stop. The important diagnostic principle—that we should always consider a substance use etiology—is about all we need: Timothy was taking a medication known to produce depression. Here we see a benefit of the decision tree approach, which leads us straightaway to the safest—and correct—diagnosis. A less wary clinician might have settled for an adjustment disorder or for the "wastebasket" diagnosis of unspecified depressive disorder.

Comment

It is easy to assume that "significant recent substance use" refers exclusively to *misuse* of alcohol or street drugs. Timothy's experience demonstrates otherwise: Medications, both prescription and over-the-counter, can also cause mental symptoms. The fact that his depression responded within days of discontinuing interferon is powerful evidence, though not conclusive; only its resumption would confirm the diagnosis, and Timothy was understandably cool to the idea of taking the interferon challenge test. Nonetheless, we can feel pretty confident that we've found the cause of his depression. A medication used for conditions as varied and serious as multiple sclerosis, leukemia, lymphoma, and melanoma, interferon can also produce symptoms of anxiety, delirium, and psychosis. Of course, it is only one of the many types of drugs mentioned in Table 9.2 that can produce mood disorders.

Why does it take interferon and other medications so long to produce emotional symptoms? To arrive at the final common path of depression requires that a drug first reach an effective blood level, which must then cause enzymatic or physiological changes in the brain. Similarly, it may take days or weeks of using a corticosteroid to produce psychotic symptoms. The bottom line is this: Just because a patient on medication for weeks has only recently developed symptoms, don't shrug off this possible cause of mental disorder.

Annette

The following vignette underscores the value of examining a wide-ranging differential diagnosis before accepting the facile explanation for a set of symptoms.

> During 19 years with her airline, Annette has always maintained her weight at 117, svelte for her height of 5 feet 5 inches. Now she is in distress as she speaks with her family physician.
>
> "I've gained nearly 15 pounds in just 6 months—15! I'm huge! I'm so depressed, I feel like crying all the time." Annette wipes her eyes. "And my face, it's all puffy."
>
> Her family practitioner learns that she has been having trouble getting to sleep, and that her interest in her hobbies (she plays the piano and collects dolls) has dwindled to "nearly nothing." So far, she has had no death wishes.
>
> Though she's never had "the opposite sort of mood, like a mania," Annette had been depressed once before, a few years after she started flying for a living. She thinks that her symptoms then were even a little worse than her current misery. She was working short hours during one of the cyclical downturns in air travel, and she had just been dumped by the man she had lived with for nearly 4 years. Her doctor then had diagnosed a "situational depression" and had given her an antidepressant (she couldn't remember which one); within a couple of months, she'd recovered.
>
> Annette has no relatives with mental disorder, and she has never drunk alcohol to excess or used drugs. Her doctor notices that she has hair on her upper lip that seemed heavy for a woman and a few wispy hairs on her chin. "Those have started just recently, too," Annette volunteers. "As if I needed anything else wrong with me. I've tried to pluck them out, but mostly I just don't care."
>
> After the analysis of a 24-hour urine specimen reveals an elevated corticosteroid content, her doctor tells her she has Cushing's syndrome, probably caused by a benign tumor on her adrenal gland.

Analysis

The path to Annette's diagnosis is direct and short. Racing through step 1 of Figure 11.1 with her denial that she'd ever had highs of mood, we come to the question of a significant physical condition (step 2), and immediately we are rewarded. From the physical examination her physician suspected Cushing's syndrome, which typically includes weight gain (especially of the body, but not the limbs), a rounded "moon" face, physical weakness, and an increase in body hair. Testing then revealed that Annette's adrenal glands were overproducing steroids. Steroid medications prescribed for diseases such as asthma or rheumatoid arthritis can also cause Cushing's, but it is more usually associated with tumors of the adrenal glands or of the pituitary gland—the so-called "master gland" located in the brain. Depression often results, as can anxiety, delirium, and even psychosis. Of course, once we reach this step in our decision tree, we'll put on hold the search for other causes of depression and treat the underlying medical condition.

Using the diagnostic principles can be tricky, because some of them conflict. Annette's earlier history of depression that resolved with treatment might have led us down the garden path to a current diagnosis of major depressive disorder; happily, recent history trumps past history to put us right. Then again, tame horses (not zebras) might have dragged us to the common illness of a recurrent mood disorder, but the principle of looking first for a physical disorder keeps us on course as we navigate the decision tree.

Comment

Table 9.1 presents a long list of physical illnesses and other conditions that can cause depression. To be sure, some of these are pretty rare, but overall you could reasonably expect to encounter a good double handful of them in the course of a professional career. It will repay learning these, if only to reassure yourself that you're on the lookout for something another clinician could have missed.

Robert

Of course, we prefer to make do with a single diagnosis, but that isn't always possible. Some depressed patients require at least two.

As a teenager, Robert was intensely interested in math. His first year in high school, he used his babysitting money to purchase one of the early electronic calculators. It could only do basic arithmetic, but he used it to work out his own method for figuring square roots. Forever after, the kids at school called him "Square Root."

Square Root Robert was quiet, but not a loner. He had friends in the science club and on the newspaper, for which he wrote a science column. Based on his science fair participation, he won a scholarship to what he called a "second-class" university. After sailing through college with high marks and earning a degree in math in just 3 years, he worked as an actuary for an insurance company. He used to smile ruefully and say, "I dreamed of being an accountant, but I didn't have the personality."

As long as Robert can remember, he has felt "mostly a little sad, and always a little hurt." His sleep and appetite are about average, and he can focus well enough on his work; however, he frequently complains of low energy, and he claims that he never expects much from the future. He brings doughnuts to work every Friday, but even that gesture never seems to win him any real friendships. He believes that his chronic low self-esteem and lack of drive are why he's remained single. He's had only fleeting relationships with women, though whenever he's has a girlfriend, his sex interest and ability are "adequate for the job."

At 56, Robert is successful in his career, but his personal life has become so miserable that he's sought care. As he tells the mental health clinician who interviews him, "I can scrape together the oomph to get me through the day at work, but once I get home, I collapse. I don't fix dinner; I don't really care if I eat. Living or dying isn't that important anymore. I just want to go to sleep. I can't even do that very well, just lie awake half the night. For weeks now, I just wish it would all end—or that I would."

His clinician notes that Robert had never misused alcohol or street drugs; he was recently given a clean bill of health from his family practitioner. Robert denies the suggestion that he has ever had a mood swing in the opposite direction. "Don't I wish!" he scoffs.

Analysis

To diagnose Robert's condition will require two trips through the Fig. 11.1 decision tree. After paying obeisance at the shrines of steps 1–6, we note that his long-standing history of low mood and self-criticism does not include symptoms severe or numerous enough (extra credit: identify the diagnostic principle here) to answer "yes" at step 7. However, throughout his adult life he would seem to qualify for a diagnosis of persistent depressive disorder (aka dysthymia, step 8).

Now let's heat up our leftovers. Robert's recent, more acute episode adds some yet unexplained symptoms that force us to start over on the decision tree. This time, the introduction of insomnia, death wishes, and reduced interest earn a step 7 "yes" answer. With no psychotic symptoms (step 11) to account for, we arrive at our second diagnosis: major depressive disorder.

How do we list them? Before DSM-5, a diagnostic principle encouraged us to list first the disorder that most requires treatment. In Robert's case, that would be his major depression. Now, however, DSM-5-TR has actually simplified the process just a bit: The criteria for persistent depressive disorder (dysthymia) list a specifier, clumsily named "with intermittent major depressive episodes, with current episode." It allows us to have one diagnosis with a specifier that says: Here's a patient with both a chronically depressed mood and a more intense exacerbation that requires treatment.

Comment

Clinicians have at times termed the combination of these two depressive disorders *double depression*. Despite the fact that it can go undiagnosed, this combination occurs more often than you might imagine—no principle says that having one mental disorder protects against others. Once the major depression is treated, the patient may settle back into the symptoms of uncomplicated dysthymia, though some patients experience lasting improvement in both disorders.

Patients with multiple diagnoses typically have two or more disorders from different chapters of the diagnostic manual—schizophrenia and alcohol use disorder, for example. The symptoms of double depression, however, can look like one big illness, and that's probably the way we should view it. A 2003 study by McCullough et al. found few differences among patients with several types of long-standing depression: chronic major depression, double depression, recurring major depression without full interepisode recovery, and chronic major depression grafted onto an existing dysthymia. Perhaps each of these terms is just a proxy for severity, and chronic depression is really only one disorder—a spectrum disease that sometimes worsens, sometimes improves, but never resolves completely. In any event, with DSM-5-TR we can think of our patients who have long-term depression with acute exacerbations in terms of a single diagnosis.

Of course, regardless of what we call it, what we really want to know is this: How should we treat double depression, and what is the prognosis? A number of studies suggest that patients with double depression (for convenience, let's continue to use the term) may be less likely to recover, as well as more likely to have continuing symptoms, impaired social lives, greater comorbidity with still other disorders, and hypomanic episodes. Double depression may also be more likely to require cognitive-behavioral therapy in addition to antidepressant medication.

Carson (Again)

One last time, let's revisit Carson, our graduate student whose depressions regularly occurred each fall or winter and remitted each spring. I had interviewed him at the point when he was again acutely distressed, apparently due to the prospect of moving his family across the country to a strange town, away from family and friends. We have met him at the beginning of Chapter 1 and discussed his differential diagnosis in Chapter 3.

Analysis

Let us consider first Carson's very recent distress around the issue of moving. Carson lacked mania or hypomania, current substance use, and physical disorders, earning a pass at steps 1–6; the fact that he currently has relatively few symptoms leads us past step 7, and the brevity of his low mood earns a "no" for dysthymia (step 8). The obvious stress-related nature of his condition (step 9) brings us to adjustment disorder with depressed mood. We'd have to go through the decision tree again, with a step 13 specifier, to arrive at his other diagnosis of a seasonal variant of major depressive disorder. Because it was currently summer, only the adjustment disorder required immediate attention, so we'll list it first.

Comment

I would guess that people have been blaming events for their moods ever since we first learned to observe cause and effect. That said, in the wake of the DSMs the type of depression formerly known as *reactive* has sunk nearly out of sight—a victim of our inability to agree on what constitutes a legitimate stressor. One clinician's precipitating stress might be another's irrelevant anecdote. When I was in training, we marveled at the published report of a patient who had become depressed upon learning that his dog had fleas. The concept of reactive depression lives on officially only in the mood specifier *with peripartum onset,* which is in all likelihood biologically based, and in the sort of adjustment disorder that afflicted Carson.

For two reasons, I've put adjustment disorder far down on the differential diagnosis for depression (see Table 11.1): It is much less well defined than most of the other diagnoses, and it is supported with far fewer scientific follow-up studies. Nonetheless, 10% of adults in some mental health populations are diagnosed with adjustment disorder. Is this an error? The relevant data are too scanty, but I believe that adjustment disorder ought to be a category of exclusion, for use only if no other possible diagnosis is appropriate. So if someone's symptoms qualify for major depressive disorder, you shouldn't call it an adjustment disorder. And note that major depression can be diagnosed in someone who is bereaved.

An adjustment disorder diagnosis might be appropriate for acutely developing responses to a severe stressor, such as a threatening physical illness, parental breakup, or upheaval in the workplace. Even when the diagnosis is warranted, it comes with some risk: Although the label carries relatively less stigma for the patient, it may be associated with suicidal behaviors and even with completed suicide. And, perhaps the greatest risk of all, it implies that it is the situation itself that must change. There isn't much practical you can do, after all, to address the root causes of, say, a heart attack or a fire that just burned down the patient's house.

Carson did not at that time qualify for major depressive disorder, and his treating clinician and I therefore agree that this newest episode was most likely in response to multiple stresses: a new program of study, impending fatherhood, and a new and unfamiliar home in some far-off and unknown part of the world. We communicated this to Carson, and the next day he had recovered his spirits as he and his wife drove off to meet their new life adventure. The episode underscores the diagnostic principle that we should be chary of symptoms that develop in response to a crisis; they may well turn out to be transient and not indicative of the patient's overall condition.

Andrea

Perhaps you will recall Andrea Yates, the Texas mother who, one June morning after her husband left for work, fed breakfast to her five children and then one by one, drowned them in a tub of bathwater. Andrea herself provided information for Suzanne O'Malley's book *"Are You There Alone?"*, which meticulously documents the details of her illness and its aftermath. All of the information I've reported here, then, is in the public record.

By the time she was pregnant with her fifth child (and only daughter), several clinicians had already identified Andrea as one of the sickest patients in their experience. Her symptoms read like a textbook summary of grave psychopathology: markedly reduced speech (sometimes referred to as *poverty of thought*), poor attention span, low mood, and delusional guilt about being a bad mother. At one time or another, she cried and had constricted range of affect, feelings of worthlessness, and hopelessness. During her second psychiatric hospitalization, 4 months after the birth of her fourth child, she became nearly mute; a month after release, she tried to cut her own throat.

During her fifth and final pregnancy, Andrea improved, but after childbirth—coping with a new baby and trying to continue the home-schooling of her other children—she once again became severely ill. She stopped eating and speaking, and her insomnia worsened; for long periods, she would just stare into space. She developed the belief that the "mark of the beast" (the number 666) had been written on the top of her head, and she rubbed her scalp raw attempting to remove it.

Andrea's upbringing had been conventional and unremarkable; she had never misused alcohol or drugs, and her physical health was good. An older brother carried the diagnosis of a bipolar disorder.

After her arrest, she told a jail psychiatrist, "I am Satan," and she explained that a camera had been installed in her home to monitor her performance as a mother. She believed that her children were "not righteous, because I am evil." She could hear a variety of hallucinated sounds: the voice of Satan coming to her over the jail intercom; the voice of a character from the Coen Brothers movie *O Brother, Where Art Thou?*; and the sounds of ducks, teddy bears, and a man on horseback, all pouring forth from the cinder blocks of her cell.

Under Texas law, and with conflicting psychiatric testimony, Andrea was judged able to tell right from wrong (never mind that she didn't know which was which) and found guilty of murder. That conviction was ultimately overturned, and a subsequent trial found her not guilty by reason of insanity. She remains in a state mental facility, each year waiving the right to review her competence for release.

Analysis

Which of our two mood disorder decision trees, Figure 11.1 or Figure 11.2 (later, on p. 151) to use for Andrea presents a bit of a problem, for it isn't exactly clear now (it certainly wasn't then) whether she ever had a bipolar disorder. At least one clinician who saw her in jail believed that she did, and this judgment was partly supported by her brother's diagnosis of a bipolar disorder (the family history diagnostic principle). However, at the time of her trial, there was no clear evidence of previous mania or hypomania, so we'll stick with Figure 11.1. Our information brings us quickly to step 7, where all of us will agree that she had many, many symptoms of severe depression. At step 11 we can shout "yes" to the presence of current hallucinations and delusions. Nowhere do we find information that she'd had symptoms of psychosis other than when depressed (step 12), so we have a diagnosis: major depression with psychotic features. Now, step 13 asks about any additional specifiers, one of which is *with peripartum onset,* and the final diagnosis is a postpartum psychotic depression. (This is also where we'd arrive had we used Figure 11.2.)

Focusing on her psychosis, several psychiatrists diagnosed Andrea as having some form of schizophrenia or schizoaffective disorder. They'd have done better using the psychosis decision tree provided in Chapter 13: Figure 13.1 leads us to severe depression with psychosis. In other words, if those clinicians had used a systematic approach, she might at least have had the benefit of a competent diagnosis at trial.

Andrea's depression was foreshadowed by her previous history of postpartum depression and by a superabundance of symptoms that are absolutely typical for major depression—three diagnostic principles in one sentence. The quality of Andrea's delusions also helps guide us: (1) They were not bizarre (each was something that was possible—cameras could have been planted in her house, she could have had a mark written somewhere on her); and (2) they were mood congruent (in keeping with severe depressive disease). Each feature is both typical of psychotic mood disorder and less consistent with schizophrenia than with a mood disorder. In a differential list, I'd put schizophrenia dead last as the least safe diagnosis, which would force us to ignore it until the possibilities of a mood disorder diagnosis had been adequately explored.

In the story of Andrea Yates, we can discern another common diagnostic dilemma. Prior to the ultimate tragedy, she had been treated successfully with an antipsychotic medication (Haldol). The fact that she appeared to respond well to this treatment may have persuaded some of her clinicians that her main diagnosis was schizophrenia, not a mood disorder. However, this conclusion conflicts with her history and the symptoms she presented. Once again, this case illustrates the importance of the decision tree and of a safety-oriented differential diagnosis.

Comment

The peripartum period is one of those special circumstances that can modify the diagnosis of major depression. Various studies suggest that many postpartum women, up to perhaps 15%, will have enough symptoms to warrant a diagnosis of major depressive disorder. This is quite different from the so-called "baby blues," a far milder (and less well defined) syndrome that many women experience and shrug off by the 10th day after delivering a baby. Still not clear is whether women are at any greater risk for depression in the peripartum period than during other periods of their lives.

No one knows just why these emotional states occur, or why they sometimes progress to an actual mental disorder. The many hormonal changes that take place in a woman's body around the time of childbirth must play a major role, but no specific mechanism has yet been identified. We do know that mental difficulties in the peripartum period are by no means limited to depression. Postpartum events can trigger bipolar disorders that in about 1 in 1,000 patients reach psychotic proportions, as was Andrea's tragic experience. The reoccurrence rate for those who have had such a psychosis (about 25% of subsequent pregnancies) is daunting—or should be. The tragedy could have been averted if Andrea's clinicians had only recognized and forcefully pointed out that those who have once experienced postpartum depression are highly likely to have it again. (Charles Dickens's wife reportedly experienced it 12 times!) The good news is that this devastating experience can be prevented, but only if it is recognized and correctly diagnosed.

Increasingly, childbirth is found to precede other mental disorders, including OCD (in which the content of the obsessions is harming the infant) and PTSD (sometimes to the point that a woman will refuse to bear more children). Some women develop panic disorder, though others actually experience reduced anxiety following childbirth.

Mania and Its Variants

A patient once told me, "Mania is worse than depression. At least for depression, there's a floor, and you know it can't get any worse. But with mania, the sky's *no* limit; you just keep going up and up—until you lose propulsion and crash." Some might argue about the floor, but there's no denying the absence of any ceiling for mania.

A pathological upswing of mood signals a whole new spectrum of diagnoses, requiring a new decision tree and several changes in the differential diagnosis. The implications of these diagnoses for treatment and prognosis are huge. When considering any of them, we must look for hints not just in the patient's recent history, but in the past and in family histories as well. Although a type of psychosis called *schizoaffective disorder* can form a part of the differential for the mood disorders, we'll defer that discussion until Chapter 13. Table 11.2 presents the differential diagnosis for mania and its variants.

Herbert

The typical symptoms of mania are classic and well known, and the typical bipolar pattern of illness followed by complete recovery borders on a dead giveaway. Yet still, clinicians will sometimes miss the diagnosis, treating some patients for unipolar major depression, others for schizophrenia or another psychotic disorder.

> After 6 years working as a pharmacist, Herbert had an affair with a woman he met when he sold her a bottle of body lotion. His wife never learned of his infidelity, but the guilty memory stuck with him. It

---

TABLE 11.2. Differential Diagnosis with Brief Definitions for Mania and Its Variants

- *Bipolar disorder due to another medical condition.* Physical illness can cause mania or hypomania.

- *Substance-induced bipolar disorder.* Alcohol, street drugs, or medications can cause symptoms of mania or hypomania.

- *Mania.* For a week or longer, the patient feels elation or irritability; is grandiose; and is unusually talkative, hyperactive, and distractible. Poor judgment leads to problems with social life and work, and often results in hospitalization. Patients with an episode of mania are said to have bipolar I disorder; most of them will also have episodes of major depression.

- *Hypomania.* A patient has symptoms much like mania, but less severe (no psychosis, no need for hospitalization). Patients who also have an episode of major depression and no full-blown mania are said to have bipolar II disorder.

- *Mixed states.* Some patients have episodes with mixed features, in which they have symptoms of both mania and major depression.

- *Cyclothymic disorder.* Patients experience repeated mood swings that are not severe enough to qualify as mania or major depression.

reminded him of his own father, who had suffered from what we would now call bipolar I disorder. When manic, he would drink heavily, then physically abuse both his wife and little Herbert.

Just when Herbert turns 30, that guilt boils over. At the birthday party his wife organized, he bursts into tears when she gives him his present—an antique mortar and pestle he has admired for months but felt they could not afford. Days later, he calls in sick to work. For days, he spends nearly all of his time in bed, much of it sleeping; when awake, he ruminates about the "trick" he played on his wife. He worries that he has infected her with herpes. Though his physician explains that the chances of that are negligible, still he cannot shake his concern. He also worries about the size of his penis: Several times a day he measures it with a carpenter's folding rule, and more than once he clicks on email spam that offers to "Grow your p*nis." Additional symptoms pile up—anorexia, weight loss (10 pounds in just 3 weeks), frequent tearfulness, and finally, thoughts of shooting himself with the pistol he'd smuggled home from service in Iraq. At last, he agrees to start taking medication. Within a week he has improved, and in a month he is back at work.

Although from time to time he still worries about herpes, Herbert remains well for the next 2 years. Then, once again on his birthday, he begins to think about sex. He talks rapidly; within days he develops grandiose thoughts. He becomes convinced that he is the reincarnation of William Faulkner, and he starts writing several "first chapters" dealing with the further doings of the people in Yoknapatawpha County. A couple of nights, he even works late writing a Pulitzer Prize acceptance speech. However, the two policemen who come to remove him forcibly to the hospital turn out to be buddies from his high school graduating class. They all have a wonderful time reminiscing and catching up on their recent lives. His friends depart, still chuckling and exchanging witticisms, leaving Herbert behind. When his wife finally kicks him out, he moves into his camper.

Analysis

Note that *any* history (not just current symptoms) of mania or hypomania starts us off in bipolar territory, even if the patient's current mood is depressed. The lack of any history of medical problems or substance misuse gets us past steps 1, 2, and 3 of the decision tree (Figure 11.2) for a patient with elevated, expansive, or irritable mood. Then step 4 leads us through steps 9 ("yes") and 11 ("yes") to step 12 and the diagnosis of bipolar I disorder.

Had we learned of Herbert when he was 30, rather than years later, there'd have been no history of mania, and his diagnosis could well have been major depression rather than bipolar I disorder—applause for the diagnostic principle that recent history beats ancient history! However, the depressive episodes of patients with bipolar disorders differ in some respects from those of patients who will never have mania or hypomania. Patients with bipolar depression are more likely to have hypersomnia, mood lability, and psychomotor retardation. Bipolar depression also may begin quite suddenly and at a relatively early age. Of course, only in retrospect do these elements stand out, though an earlier clinician could have been alerted to the bipolar possibility by the history of mania in Herbert's father. And, because a patient with first-episode depression may show none of these features, we must forever remain alert for evidence of ensuing symptoms of mania or hypomania.

Comment

In the years after the discovery that lithium proved effective in treating and preventing mania, the tendency of U.S. clinicians to diagnose what is now called bipolar I disorder soared. Yet in 1980 a study by Garvey and Tuason reported that 56% of patients with this disorder had at one time been diagnosed with schizophrenia. And even today, we often *still* don't get it right, or when we do we don't get it early—on average, it takes several years from the onset of first symptoms to make the correct diagnosis of bipolar disorder.

Another common error is the misdiagnosis of *unipolar* major depression in a patient who really has bipolar I disorder. That was the fate of 40% of the patients in a 1999 study by Ghaemi and colleagues. Although this mistake can sometimes be avoided by strictly applying current diagnostic criteria, the first episode of many patients with bipolar I disorder is one of depression. Then the ultimate correct diagnosis can be suspected initially in patients who have a bipolar family history, or who respond with manic symptoms to antidepressant drugs or bright light therapy. Other hints at an eventual bipolar I diagnosis include a rapid onset of depressive symptoms, onset in the teens or early 20s, and unstable mood before or after the depression. Because patients often don't recognize that their own symptoms imply illness, it's important to ask relatives or friends about prior manic or hypomanic episodes, and to report mood lability if it occurs down the road.

Erma

Mental health diagnosis often depends on degree—consider the importance of how much a person drinks, gambles, or eats. The symptoms of mania or hypomania are no exception. When intense, as in the case of Herbert, they can lead to hospitalization, disrupted relationships, or even financial ruin. When milder, if they are noticed at all, they can imply a couple of different diagnoses.

> A news reader for a local radio station, Erma complains that her listeners can tell what kind of a mood she is in. "Every once in a while I get emails from people who say, 'What's wrong? Your voice doesn't have its usual sparkle.'"
>
> Erma used to believe that she was responding to pressures at home; now she realizes that her moods are causing her on-air vocal changes. "Once I got divorced, I went right on having ups and downs of mood. Only now, I fight with the people at work."
>
> Quizzed closely, she describes her moods this way: "They last a few weeks at a time, never longer. When I'm down, I feel as though I'm running on about half-power. I'm still me; I just don't scintillate." During these down phases, she is grumpy and sometimes rude, but her sleep and appetite are about as usual. "And I know what you're going to ask—I never have suicidal ideas. I've worked too hard to get where I am to throw it away." When she is up, on the other hand, "I'm a 50-megawatt powerhouse. I feel like talking and dancing, both at once."
>
> Erma speaks clearly and distinctly, her inflections reflecting years of training and experience behind a microphone. She says she doesn't think her mood swings follow the seasons, and they definitely don't react to her life experiences. "I was up for several weeks after my husband left me for our babysitter, and down the month after I got a raise."
>
> At a recent checkup, Erma's family practitioner pronounced her physically healthy. A Chinese American, she flushes easily if ever she drinks alcohol, so she avoids it almost completely. She has never used street drugs and takes no medications.

Analysis

Erma's up periods earn her a ride on Figure 11.2. The history makes it clear that Erma has no known step 1 (or 3) medical complaints that could

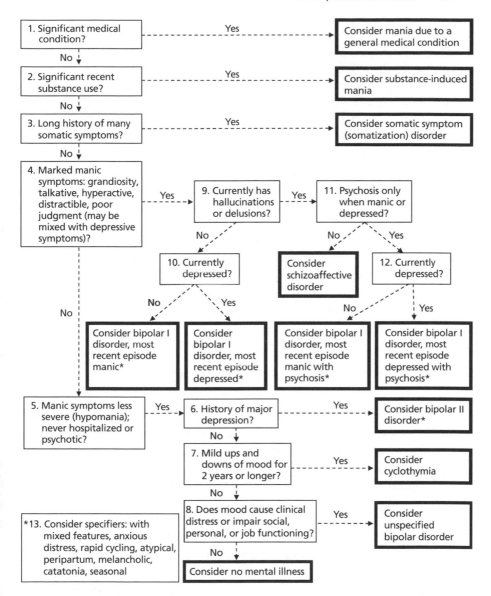

FIGURE 11.2. Decision tree for a patient who has had elevated, expansive, or irritable mood.

explain her symptoms. The fact that, like many people of Asian descent, she becomes acutely uncomfortable with even modest amounts of alcohol would rule out a step 2 alcohol-related illness; we'll take her word that she doesn't use street drugs, either. When feeling "up," she doesn't present the far-out picture of mega-grandiosity that characterizes step 4 "true mania." This moves us on through step 5 to step 6, where her relatively minor depressive symptoms speak against bipolar II disorder. Her ups and downs have persisted for several years (a step 7 "yes"), leading to cyclothymic disorder as our final diagnosis.

The lilt (rather, its absence) in Erma's voice is one of those signs which, as the diagnostic principle says, often beats symptoms in identifying a mental disorder. Her listeners don't have to know her personally—don't even have to *see* her—to know when something is amiss. She herself identifies another principle that can lead patients and clinicians astray: For years she thought her moodiness was due to marital problems, but she discovered that after her divorce she was still moody. The mere fact that one event follows another doesn't mean there is a causal connection; it's a terrific example of the fallacy of *post hoc ergo propter hoc,* a Latin maxim that translates to "after this, therefore because of this." Remember, it's a fallacy.

Comment

Had Erma experienced even one episode of major depression, we could say that she suffered from bipolar II disorder. But with only minor degrees of depression, cyclothymia is the warranted diagnosis. The diagnoses of bipolar I, bipolar II, and cyclothymic disorders are closely related, in that they have similar symptoms and treatment.

Indeed, there may be yet other bipolar conditions that have still not been adequately described. Some clinicians use the labels *bipolar III* for those situations where treatment for major depressive disorder causes the patient to switch briefly into hypomania, and *bipolar IV* for major depressive disorder without a discrete hypomanic episode (just a sunny temperament that is sometimes called *hyperthymic*). However, neither of these two has as yet been given any official stamp of approval. It may be only custom that has averted the use of something on the order of *bipolar V* for cyclothymia—which was, after all, regarded as a personality disorder as recently as the 1970s. And who knows where it will stop? The Romans have lots more numerals.

Rosa

I've mentioned several times that you should always take a complete history, no matter how obvious the symptoms appear. I'll repeat this yet again here, and Rosa's history demonstrates why.

> When she is 46, Rosa notices that she stumbles when she walks. It happens inconsistently—maybe it's worse when she's tired—and at first she tries to ignore it. She is too excitable anyway, her husband has always said, and for once she doesn't want to seem alarmist.
>
> "It's not like I lurch from side to side or anything," she finally tells her family doctor. "It's more of a limp, like I just can't quite get my legs to play nicely together." The doctor can't find much wrong, diagnoses conversion disorder, and remands her to a therapist—for her mood.
>
> Rosa feels fatigued and rather depressed. She has been a homemaker for 25 years; with both children off at college, she hasn't enough to do. With the encouragement of her counselor, she becomes active in her church women's fellowship. Her limp nearly disappears; perhaps the therapy is working, she thinks. Over the next couple of months her mood first brightens, then moves through sunny to a blistering ecstasy.
>
> Now Rosa becomes agitated. She will grip the coat sleeves of strangers on the street to tell them how faith has cured her. She sells her living room furniture and donates the proceeds to a television evangelist. When her husband objects, she calls 911 to report that he has struck her; a policeman escorts him from the house.
>
> Meanwhile, the limp is back, and a peculiar, rapid-fire stuttering makes her speech increasingly hard to understand. Recognizing that something is terribly amiss, her therapist persuades her to return to her family practitioner. Another physical exam leads to a neurological consultation and then to the eventual diagnosis of multiple sclerosis. Treatment with glatiramer acetate, specific for her disease, reduces her physical symptoms, and her mood gradually returns to normal.

Analysis

In Rosa's case, negotiating the decision tree in Figure 11.2 is a pretty quick climb—we've a hit at step 1. However, this apparent success shouldn't tempt us to rest on our laurels with the feeling that our job is done. Although we try to follow the Occam's razor principle and simplify diagnosis whenever we can, it is still possible that Rosa's manic symptoms are unrelated to her physical disease; as we've learned, chronology doesn't always equal causation. However, the remission of her mood disorder once the physical symptoms were under control limits our enthusiasm for having two independent conditions.

Comment

Well into the 21st century, the symptoms of mania (and hypomania) have pretty much become common knowledge, even to laypeople. That which we know well tends to be uppermost in our minds, so it should come as no surprise that every once in a while, someone with a physical condition that is associated with euphoria and the other symptoms of mania/hypomania goes misdiagnosed. It's a shame that Rosa's first diagnosis wasn't based on the differential diagnosis/decision tree model; doing so might have saved a lot of time and anguish.

The number of physical disorders that can underlie manic or hypomanic symptoms is modest (you'll find a list in Table 9.1). However, from time to time I read reports of such symptoms newly associated with another medical condition. These conditions include low blood sodium, uremia (kidney failure), blood vessel malformations in the head, and open-heart surgery. Without a doubt, some of these represent true cause-and-effect situations; but others may be pure coincidence. The trick is to know which is which (see the sidebar "Recognizing Physical Causes of Mania or Hypomania"). As I've noted—well, harped on—previously, the only safe approach is initially to consider an organic cause for *every* patient.

Comorbidity

The patients we've met so far in this chapter have had only mood disorders. However, depressive or bipolar disorders commonly occur with other mental disorders; in fact, a lot of research suggests that this is the rule. Sometimes this co-occurrence is referred to as *dual diagnosis,* but some clinicians reserve this term for a substance use problem combined with a non-substance-related disorder. For the sake of clarity, I'll try to avoid using it.

You will encounter mood disorders combined with nearly every other

Recognizing Physical Causes of Mania or Hypomania

Some useful indicators can actually help differentiate physically caused mania or hypomania from bipolar disorders. (A sidebar on p. 161 informs us that we aren't so lucky with physically caused depression.) Suspicion of physical causes should increase for patients who have some of the following characteristics:

- Late onset (35 or older) of first manic or hypomanic episode
- Clear history of potential physical cause, such as AIDS or recent closed head injury
- Lack of depressive episodes
- No prior mental hospitalizations
- No family history of bipolar disorders
- Mood irritable or dysphoric
- Threatening or assaultive behavior while manic
- Grandiose delusions of worth, power, or special relationships (as with a deity)
- Cognitive dysfunctions, such as defects of orientation and concentration
- Poor response to standard treatment for mania or hypomania
- Rapid resolution of symptoms once a physical cause has been addressed

mental health diagnosis in several possible relationships, which are by no means mutually exclusive:

- Two disorders can begin together; or one (we'll call it primary) precedes the other (secondary).
- Two disorders are present at the same time; or they alternate.
- One disorder induces the other; or they are completely independent. (The former isn't technically comorbidity, but it happens often enough to rate mentioning.)
- The symptoms of one disorder conceal another, such as when a person's heavy drinking masks the fact of depression.

The case histories that follow draw our attention to another issue: Which diagnosis in any pair should you list first, and which later? This issue has more than academic interest. A vast body of research has shown that, for example, secondary depressions respond differently to somatic treatments such as electroconvulsive therapy and antidepressant medication.

Arnold

When he was just 15, Arnold became depressed. He was foundering in several classes in his sophomore year of high school; and he saw "no future in life" and had begun to lose weight. He also couldn't sleep without a couple of pulls at the port wine his mother for years had generously employed as an antidepressant and painkiller; his father had recently died of acute alcohol poisoning. When his grades sank even further, Arnold left school and "just hung out, doing about as much as I wanted to, which was nothing at all." After several months, without any intervention, his depression lifted. He lied about his age and enlisted in the Army.

Arnold was posted to Vietnam, where he served nearly 2 years of his 3-year enlistment. During this time, because he was bright and competent, he was promoted three times; because he had a talent for getting crosswise with his staff sergeant, he was busted twice. He returned to civilian life as a former private first class with a heroin addiction. "There was a lot of it available over there," he tells the VA clinician who interviews him after he is discharged.

Maintained on methadone for the next 15 years, Arnold does reasonably well, using heroin only occasionally and working steadily as a printer. As he gains experience, he moves into desktop publishing and is ultimately offered a partnership in the small firm where he works. After several years, he marries a woman whose first husband had periodically misused alcohol, so she knows the drill. "Use just once," Beth tells Arnold, "and I'm out of here—no, *you're* out of here!" The methadone and Beth's promise keep him clean and sober for the next decade.

But in the late 1990s, Arnold's methadone maintenance program falls victim to VA cost cutting. As he tapers off the drug, his mood darkens and he grows more irritable than he has felt in many years. Although he goes to work faithfully, his interest flags. In his Narcotics Anonymous support group, which he still attends regularly, he hears similar stories from others. One Friday evening, a speaker describes the emotional symptoms of methadone withdrawal—depression, irritability, and sometimes a sense of expansiveness—which can sometimes last for months.

Although this description prepares Arnold for discomfort, it seems that his friends are weathering withdrawal better than he is. As the weeks wear on and he remains methadone-free, the muscle aches and restlessness diminish, but his mood dips lower. He barks at Beth, he growls at his boss, and his work output gradually slows to a trickle. For the first time in years, he begins to think about scoring some heroin—and taking a massive, lethal overdose.

Analysis

With substance use and depression, we have the ingredients for a classic example of comorbidity. A degree of depression can be expected when a person is withdrawing from heavy use of any opioid; methadone is no exception (see Table 9.3). But if Arnold's diagnosis were a simple coast through Figure 11.1 to step 3, we would expect that his depression would improve with time off the drug. In fact, quite the opposite occurred: As time passed, both the number and intensity of his symptoms increased (there's a diagnostic principle here concerning the likelihood of major depression), and we end up with a "no" at step 11 and the diagnosis of major depressive disorder. Arnold's history shows how important it is to consider not just the symptoms themselves but their time course, too.

As to arranging these two diagnoses, I like to list diagnoses chronologically. But, because we believe that Arnold's mood disorder is of major proportions and independent of the substance misuse, it requires our immediate attention; we'll put it first—the safety principle. Besides, his substance use is currently in check.

Comment

In Chapter 4 we met Jakob, whose drinking produced both psychosis and depression. As I've already noted, we wouldn't refer to that relationship, where one illness directly causes another, as *comorbidity*. Patients like Arnold, however, have two (or sometimes more) mental disorders that have no obvious causal relationship. It can take some detective work to sort out the symptoms of each independent disorder to arrive at a diagnosis of true comorbidity.

The work of that detection can be distressingly difficult. It is so easy to encounter evidence of one diagnosis and misconstrue it as support for another. Just think of the symptoms of major depression you can find during the course of intoxication or withdrawal from various substances—they include sleeplessness, social withdrawal, apathy, low mood, and weight loss (see Table 9.3). You can also find symptoms reminiscent of mania—such as rambling speech, periods of tirelessness, heightened psychomotor activity, poor judgment, euphoria, belligerence, and impulsiveness. Alcohol and other drugs can also release inhibitions and induce anxiety states or psychosis, sometimes leading to the morbid thinking that results in suicidal behavior. Table 6.1 lists mental disorders you might encounter in a substance-using patient.

Another deterrent to easy identification is the fact that shame can make patients reluctant to volunteer symptoms of substance use. Fortunately, most people will tell the truth if you question them directly about how much they drink or whether they use drugs. All in all, is it any wonder that a study of inpatients by Lin and colleagues found that nearly 20% of patients with mood disorders also had substance use disorders? And that fewer than one in four had been diagnosed by the physician in charge?

Connie

The depressions we have read about up to now have all been of the sort that respond to standard treatment with antidepressant medications or structured psychotherapy. However, the effective treatment of many other depressed patients depends heavily on an exact diagnosis that may be quite different from the ever-popular major depression.

> Through 2 years of severe depression, Connie has been treated with psychotherapy and 12 different medications for low mood and anxiety, and then a long series of electroconvulsive treatments—none with lasting benefit. Her physician has mentioned the possibility of psychosurgery, but suggests that first she consult another clinician, to see whether there is any other possibility before taking such a drastic step.
>
> There can be no questioning the gravity of Connie's depressive symptoms. At their worst, which is most of the time, she complains of loss of appetite and weight, trouble sleeping, poor concentration, fatigue, and death wishes. She has made three suicide attempts of increasing severity, and she thinks about suicide daily. Because she cannot cope with her three children, she has lost custody of them to her former husband. (She lost *him* due to her chronic pain with intercourse and lack of interest in sex.) Her job has disappeared in the morass of six lengthy hospitalizations. "I'm totally desperate," she says. "I wish they'd just go ahead and cut."
>
> Something about the way Connie brightens after talking for a while makes the consultant reach back for some additional history. With Connie's permission, her mother is interviewed by telephone. She recalls some difficulties that Connie hasn't mentioned. Connie has been chronically ill from the time she was 13. Besides severe headaches, she has had a number of strange complaints, including fainting spells, an attack of paralysis, and even a brief episode of blindness for which no cause could ever be determined. In fact, each of the doctors they consulted during her adolescence and early adult years pronounced her remarkably fit, yet she also consulted doctors or taken

medication for difficulty breathing, heart palpitations, chest pain, dizziness, nausea, abdominal bloating, menstrual irregularity, and pain in her back and extremities.

Connie describes herself as being a sickly child and "always ailing" as an adult, right up to the time that her depression commenced. Recently, however, the physical disorders have bothered her less. Although she experimented with marijuana when she was in high school, it only made her feel sick. She has avoided drugs and alcohol since. "More sickness, I didn't need at all," she remarks with a wry smile.

Analysis

The differential diagnosis we would construct for Connie is very similar to Table 11.1, though we'd need more information to determine whether we should diagnose some form of anxiety disorder. Let's analyze Connie's depressive symptoms with Figure 11.1. For the sake of simplicity, we'll assume that she hasn't had symptoms of mania or hypomania in the past (step 1). At step 2, she has certainly had numerous medical complaints that could suggest a medical disorder underlying her mental symptoms. However, through the years she has been seen by several specialist physicians as well as her family practitioner, and each of them has ultimately pronounced her physically sound. That bounces the ball squarely back into our court. No recent step 3 substance use moves us along to step 4, where we agree that she has had many somatic symptoms in the past. Note that its placement early in our decision tree calls our attention to somatic symptom disorder, regardless of how severe the depressive, manic, or other symptoms may have been.

Here's a problem: How do we list the two disorders? If we slavishly (uh-oh, the word's a dead giveaway, isn't it?) follow the same rules we used for Arnold, we'd mention the depression first. But from all that is written about the somatizing disorders, we know that directly addressing a co-occurring mood disorder (which occurs in about 80% of the cases) is fraught with hazard: A depressed patient with a somatizing disorder often won't respond to standard treatments that help most other depressed patients. Listing the somatizing disorder first puts the disorders into chronological order, which suggests in turn that the depression might need special handling. Similar calculations would apply to other conditions that occur with somatizing disorders, including anxiety disorders, anorexia nervosa, and bulimia nervosa.

Incidentally, the tip-off to Connie's diagnosis is the observation that in the face of a very severe depression, she brightens up after conversing for a while—another example of the diagnostic principle that signs beat symptoms. It may not be invoked very often, but it carries power. Keep it in mind.

Comment

In my opinion, differentiating primary clinical depression from secondary depression that occurs with a somatizing disorder is one of the most difficult problems mental health clinicians face. (Of course, diagnosing secondary depression that accompanies any primary disorder is a challenge; see the sidebar "Recognizing Secondary Depression.") To understand why this problem exists, we'll need to explore a little history.

Somatization disorder has been recognized for more than 150 years. Known for millennia by the ancient term *hysteria,* it was well described in 1859 by the French clinician Paul Briquet. In the 1960s, Robins, Guze, and other clinicians formalized Briquet's findings and co-opted his name for the syndrome they identified. They included more symptoms than are used in the DSM-IV diagnostic criteria for somatization disorder, and *way* more than in the vastly reduced DSM-5-TR criteria for somatic symptom disorder. Of course, there were such physical complaints as various body pains, sexual dysfunction, chest and abdominal complaints, and complaints like an attack of paralysis (see the Chapter 9 discussion, p. 111). They also found that these patients typically had symptoms of depression, anxiety, or even psychosis. In the intervening years, follow-up studies repeatedly demonstrated the predictive value of their work. However, when DSM-III was adopted in 1980, all of the emotional symptoms of Briquet's syndrome were removed from the description, leaving only the physical symptoms. This left clinicians free to make a comorbid diagnosis of any additional mood, anxiety, or psychotic condition for which a patient happened to meet criteria.

One outcome is, I believe, that many clinicians today haven't learned a basic principle of understanding these patients—namely, their almost uncanny ability to sense and conform to the interests of their caregivers. The earliest examples ever described remain the best. On the neurology ward operated by Jean-Martin Charcot in the Salpêtrière hospital in late-19th-century Paris, patients with hysteria (as it was then known) learned to imitate symptoms experienced by epilepsy patients. The interest shown by clinicians from all over Europe encouraged these women to elaborate a ritualized form of pseudoseizure that became known as *grand hysteria.*

Recognizing Secondary Depression

Would that it were simple. About the only easy aspect of secondary depression is its definition: a depression in someone who has a previous serious (that is, it threatens life or the capacity for self-care) medical illness or non-mood-related mental disorder. By some estimations, about 40% of depressions are secondary.

The problem with the diagnosis is this: After years of careful investigations, researchers can only tell us that most secondary depressions are relatively mild (patients like Connie notwithstanding). The symptoms tend to be pretty garden-variety, and there simply aren't any symptoms that clearly differentiate secondary from primary depression. That leaves us with precious few generalizations we can make; however:

- As a group, these patients are more likely to be younger males with a family history of alcoholism.
- Of depressed men with alcoholism, about 95% will have a secondary depression; the figure for women is about 75%. (Yes, this means that among people with alcoholism, primary depression is about five times more common in women than in men. Go to the head of the class.)
- A patient who is psychotically depressed or who has symptoms of melancholy (awakens in early morning, feels worse in the morning, has marked loss of appetite, has unwarranted guilt feelings, loses pleasure in nearly everything, feels no better when something good happens) is unlikely to have a depression that is secondary.
- Depression in patients with a somatizing disorder is almost certain to be of the secondary kind. In all my years of experience, I've known only one somatization disorder patient who I was sure also had an independent, primary depression.
- Depression secondary to medical illness is likely to develop later in life and is unlikely to include the symptoms of suicidal ideas, guilt, or delusions.
- You may not be able to decide definitively whether depression is "real" or is the expected reaction to medical illness, but don't automatically pass it off as the latter. Rather, look for such telltale indicators as previous episodes, history of mania or hypomania, family history of mood disorder, and duration (longer duration is more likely to be found in major depressive disorder).

Thus commenced a worldwide pandemic, which collapsed after Charcot died in 1893.

I don't mean to imply that such patients aim to deceive their clinicians, either in Charcot's time or in our own. Rather, their symptoms seem to evolve almost as an unconscious collaboration between clinician and patient. We can understand why a gastroenterologist who encounters abdominal pain and vomiting, or a mental health clinician who finds depression and anxiety, might well diagnose conditions common in their respective fields. When following up positive responses, the clinician asks about other symptoms typical of the diagnosis. The patient notices the clinician's interest and supplies any number of other symptoms, and the syndrome seems to be confirmed.

Today's patients with somatizing disorders discern and mirror their clinicians' interests in mood, anxiety, and even psychotic disorders. That's why I refer to this disorder as *iatroplastic* (my very own neologism): Clinicians don't cause it, but by their interests they influence its form. Whereas physical and laboratory examinations yield a lack of demonstrable pathology in the case of physical complaints, we still have no such tests for emotional symptoms. Although someone could have two independent disorders—say, a somatizing disorder and major depression—our Occam's razor diagnostic principle suggests that just one is far more likely. The bottom line: A direct assault on such a mood disorder seldom provides the relief these patients seek.

Borderlands

The boundaries of the mood disorders have been sharpened considerably, but a number of fuzzy lines still snake between various forms of pathology or between the normal and the pathological. In this section, we'll explore a few of them.

Bereavement and Loss

Long ago, depressions were commonly divided into two types: those that occur in reaction to some external event (such as loss of a job or a death in the family), and those that have no apparent external cause. The second type was called *endogenous* (coming from within the individual); the first type was termed *exogenous* or *reactive*. Once the DSMs began to spell out diagnostic criteria, the term *reactive depression* fell out of favor; perhaps it was too hard to define what constituted an adequate precipitant for depression. The principal remnant of this simple, logical, but ultimately flawed division of depression into two parts is bereavement—a diagnosis that until DSM-5 served to exclude from consideration for major depressive disorder those who have very recently (within 2 months) suffered the loss of a loved one.

Of course, when someone you deeply care for dies, you naturally feel grief-stricken. What we as clinicians and we as bereaved persons struggle with is to etch the boundary between a clinical depression that requires treatment and the natural grieving process that must be soothed and endured. The diagnostic manuals used to define the difference only as a matter of time: Mood symptoms that lasted longer than 2 months couldn't qualify as only a natural reaction to loss. But so simplistic a distinction contradicts the experience of many patients and clinicians, and finally the manual writers have given up: It no longer makes scientific sense to forego a diagnosis of major depression solely because a loved one died a few weeks earlier.

Still, solid research suggests that bereavement is different from depression. Besides its brevity, it is usually less severe than melancholia and unresponsive to antidepressant medication. A bereaved person's low mood is triggered by memories of the departed individual, whereas those with non-bereavement-related depression feel bad regardless. And it is unusual for bereaved people to have severe feelings of guilt, worthlessness, suicidal ideas, or the slowing of speech and action called *psychomotor retardation*. Bereavement, then, tends to seem rather normal, unaccompanied by seriously impaired activities of living.

Over the past few years has arisen the concept of *complicated bereavement* or *traumatic grief,* which is associated with impaired functioning and relatively poor outcomes. Somewhat similar to PTSD, it is meant to comprise some of the following symptoms: preoccupation with the dead person; longing or yearning; disbelief and inability to accept the death; anger or resentment over the death; and avoidance of reminders of this loss. Now this view has been reified in the diagnosis of prolonged grief disorder, which DSM-5-TR lists not with the other mood disorders but in the chapter devoted to conditions induced by stress or trauma. But from the depressive symptoms it entails, it earns its legitimate place in the Figure 11.1 decision tree.

As a disqualifier for major depressive disorder, bereavement was unique—other losses, such as that of a career or a marriage, didn't count. However, researchers have found that a person who feels devalued by a humiliating event (such as a public put-down by a boss, a divorce brought about by the infidelity of a spouse, or rape) can develop depression similar to grief. And that, of course, lands us right back at the concept of reactive depression. Confusing, isn't it?

For me, here is the bottom line. We expect to encounter feelings of grief and sadness after a major loss, and we should be careful not to join the stampede to diagnose mental disorder. However, a grieving person who develops enough symptoms to qualify for a major depressive episode should be carefully considered for possible treatment, regardless of time intervals or the "logic" of the despair. This is especially true in the presence of despondency unmitigated by happy reminiscences of the dead or unrelieved by visits from friends or other loved ones. And, always, such serious symptoms as suicidal ideas, psychosis, or psychomotor retardation must prompt immediate, effective action.

Minor Degrees of Depression

If there are major depressions, there must be minor ones, right? That thought seems to have struck many researchers, because numerous studies have recently described forms of minor depression that may bear different names, unique criteria, or both. What's resulted so far is a microcosm of the diagnostic chaos that existed before the DSM started getting its—no, our!—act together back in 1980. Most definitions boil down to a relatively brief (2 weeks or more) episode of relatively few depressive symptoms.

Minor depression, however defined, actually nets some pretty interesting findings. Some studies report anatomical changes in the brains of such people, and the diagnosis may predict early death in old men (but not old women). Just like people with major depression, people with the minor variety tend to have difficulty functioning in their everyday lives, and they respond to standard treatments such as the selective serotonin reuptake inhibitors (SSRIs) and maprotiline. Minor depression can also be found as a secondary diagnosis in conditions as varied as Alzheimer's dementia and alcoholism, and it has been identified in patients with bipolar disorders.

Moreover, like patients with major depression, those with minor depression can have both emotional and cognitive symptoms, though vegetative symptoms such as sleep and appetite changes aren't often reported. And though minor depression may be relatively mild, it isn't necessarily brief; just as in the major variety, symptoms tend to persist for weeks or months. Family histories are about the same as for major depression, suggesting that the two forms may spring from the same ground. One problem with the concept is this: Because prevalence data variously put the number of such patients as high as 20% of the general population, it dangerously blurs the line between normal and abnormal. And that—the delimitation from normal—is one area where any useful diagnosis ought to excel.

At least one authority has suggested that the greatest value of minor depression may be in helping to predict major depression later on. However, others who look at the various lines of evidence suggest that differing degrees of depression overlap: A person who develops a mild depression may progress in stages through moderate to severe symptoms later on. In effect, depression of various degrees may best be viewed as existing on a continuum.

Suicide as Rational Behavior versus Treatable Illness

The question of whether suicide can ever be considered reasonable behavior is a complex one. See the sidebar "Can Suicide Ever Be Rational?" for a brief summary of this age-old debate.

Can Suicide Ever Be Rational?

The existence of rational suicide has been hotly debated for many years. Favoring the concept are moral philosophers who regard humans as free agents whose choices should include how and when they will die. Arguing against it are those who cite numerous scientific studies reporting that the overwhelming majority of people who commit suicide have some form of a mental disorder. (Overwhelming, perhaps, but not unanimous—nearly every such study includes a few individuals for whom no mental disorder could be demonstrated.)

Western medicine traditionally regards suicide as an irrational response to crushing stress. One consequence of this view is this logical lapse: Because suicide is a symptom of mental illness, we reason that only mentally ill persons commit suicide. We therefore reject the possibility that occasionally a mentally healthy individual, perhaps threatened by the physical pain or disability of a terminal illness, may desire to stop living. An apparent example is the professor and mystery fiction author Carolyn Heilbrun, who killed herself in 2003 after saying for years that she would one day do just that.

In Oregon, where I live, terminally ill patients may obtain from their physicians lethal medication to help them avoid wrenching pain and incapacity at life's end. In any given year, whereas over 300 patients receive prescriptions for such medications, only about two-thirds actually follow through. A number of careful studies have found no evidence of coercion or ulterior motives, such as on the part of relatives.

In 1995, Werth and Cobia surveyed 400 other psychologists in an attempt to define rational suicide. The group's definition boiled down to the following:

1. The individual's condition should show little hope of remission.
2. There must be no coercion.
3. The process should be sound, as shown by these characteristics relevant to the decision maker: mental competence; rejection of other options only after due consideration; values consistent with this decision; consideration of the impact of the suicide on others; and consultation with other professionals, such as therapists, hospice personnel, and spiritual advisors.

I'm as concerned as the next responsible clinician to maximize the value of anyone's life, but I believe that this must be done with due consideration for its value to the individual who must live it. There is no easy answer here.

12 Diagnosing Anxiety, Fear, Obsessions, and Worry

First, let's define some terms. *Fear* is emotional discomfort caused by a sense of approaching danger. A *phobia* is fear that is unreasonable and intense and is associated with some situation or object. What distinguishes the commonplace fear of, say, spiders from the delusional fear of persecution? It is that spiders usually pose no rational threat, and the phobic person knows this, whereas the delusional person doesn't have the benefit of insight. *Anxiety* is also fear, but it isn't caused by something specific the person can identify; we often say that it is free-floating. *Worry* is mental distress relating to concern for something that might happen. Usually, anxious or worried people have unpleasant physical sensations, such as tense muscles, fatigue, insomnia, and restlessness. A *panic attack* is a discrete episode of intense anxiety accompanied by acute physical symptoms, such as chest pain, choking, dizziness, pounding heart, numbness, sweating, shortness of breath, and trembling.

To a degree, fear, anxiety, worry, and even panic in the form of an acute fright are sensations that normal people experience, and we must therefore discriminate them from ordinary uneasiness. Of course, we clinicians aren't usually consulted for ordinary uneasiness, but even so we need to make sure (by asking) that the anxiety a patient presents has caused *marked* distress or has in some way interfered with social, work, or interpersonal functioning. Table 12.1 presents the differential diagnosis for anxiety states. (Note that in DSM-5-TR, OCD and PTSD now occupy their own separate chapters; for convenience I'll consider them here.)

Panic Disorder and Phobias

Many otherwise normal people experience the highly unpleasant sensation of panic attacks. In fact, perhaps a third of adults in the general population have had at least one such episode. It's when they recur often enough to interfere with normal life that they require treatment.

TABLE 12.1. Differential Diagnosis with Brief Definitions for Anxiety States

- *Anxiety due to another medical condition.* Physical illness can cause panic or other anxiety symptoms.

- *Substance-related anxiety.* Alcohol, street drugs of misuse, and prescribed medications can all cause anxiety symptoms.

- *Panic disorder.* Repeated panic attacks (brief, sudden episodes of intense dread, accompanied by a variety of physical and other symptoms) create worry about having additional episodes. They often occur with agoraphobia.

- *Agoraphobia.* Patients fear places or situations (shopping in a store, being away from home) where they might have trouble obtaining help should they become anxious.

- *Specific phobia.* Particular objects or situations—such as animals, storms, heights, flying, being closed in, or blood or needles—cause anxiety and avoidance.

- *Social anxiety disorder.* The prospect of embarrassment when speaking, writing, performing, or eating in public causes anxiety and avoidance.

- *Obsessive–compulsive disorder (OCD).* Although their thoughts or behaviors appear senseless, patients feel compelled to repeat them.

- *Posttraumatic stress disorder (PTSD).* Patients repeatedly relive a traumatic event, along the way experiencing hyperarousal and avoidance or emotional numbing.

- *Generalized anxiety disorder (GAD).* Without experiencing actual panic attacks, patients feel anxious or tense about a variety of different problems.

Ruth

Sitting alone in the waiting room, Ruth breathes heavily into a paper bag. With mounting dread, she has felt the old, too familiar symptoms: Her heart is pounding and her breathing seems strangled, as though her throat might close forever. She had hoped she could get through at least 1 week without an episode, but now on day 5, just as she is at last about to tell a therapist about them, they are upon her again. As she sits, she again fears that she is on the verge of going crazy: Might she scream? Tear off her clothes? At the moment, she notices that she is sweating and shaky.

At age 29, Ruth works in sales at an appliance store. She was married briefly, and now lives with her boyfriend, Sammy, the assistant store manager, and her 7-year-old daughter.

A few weeks earlier, the episodes of anxiety drove Ruth for a rare visit to her family practitioner. She told the doctor that she tried to stay near a doorway when indoors. Because she lives in earthquake country, she always worries how she'd escape in the event of the "big one." Recently this concern has increased; now, if she must enter the stockroom, she'll ask Sammy to accompany her. That makes *him* nervous, since the store's antinepotism policy is strictly enforced.

Ruth tries to shop only when Sammy can accompany her. If ever she must go alone, she will dash in for her gallon of milk, pay at the self-check, and practically run back out before the panic can take hold. The attacks seem to come at odd times. Once, when she was driving home, Ruth had to stop the car because she couldn't focus on the road. Another time it caught her and Sammy both off guard, when they were beginning foreplay while watching a sexy movie on cable.

The electrocardiogram she'd demanded from her GP was, she was informed, "completely normal, just like the rest of your exam." Because she seemed nervous, the doctor had written a prescription for Valium. But Ruth had tried marijuana in college and didn't like the spacey, unrooted feeling drugs gave her. The Rx went into the bin when she'd arrived home.

Now, however, almost as suddenly as it began, the attack in the waiting room begins to fade away. By the time her new clinician calls her name, Ruth is applying fresh lipstick.

Analysis

Ruth has no other health problems and no history of substance use, so we can move quickly through the first three steps of the decision tree for a patient with symptoms of fear, anxiety, panic, or continuing worry (Figure 12.1). Then, moving unrewarded through the tree, we eventually hit pay dirt: Ruth is afraid of being in a place where she could not get help or escape would be difficult, such as her local supermarket or the storeroom at work (step 14). She also (step 15) has unexpected attacks during which she experiences panic accompanied by a number of physical symptoms. In short, we should strongly consider two diagnoses: panic disorder and agoraphobia. Had we focused on the panic attacks and initially overlooked her symptoms of agoraphobia, we would have arrived at the same conclusion. Along the way, we have considered both somatic symptom disorder and PTSD, both commonly associated with anxiety symptoms. And because depression so often accompanies panic attacks, asterisked step 17 reminds us to check for it as a comorbid diagnosis.

Comment

Charles Darwin experienced repeated attacks of shortness of breath, lightheadedness, palpitations, trembling, and faintness, which today would prob-

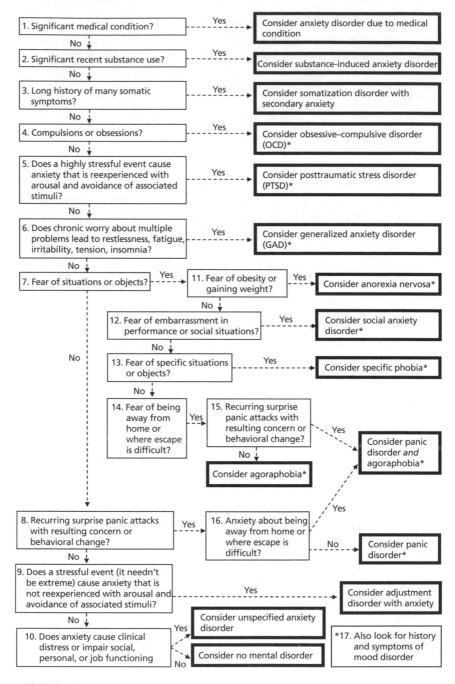

FIGURE 12.1. Decision tree for a patient who has fear, anxiety, panic, obsessions, or continuing worry.

ably qualify for a diagnosis of panic disorder. Various authors have suggested that because he was famously reclusive, he also had agoraphobia. Others believe that his symptoms may have been related to physical conditions such as Ménière's syndrome or Chagas disease (a parasitic infestation found in rural areas of South and Central America). Ultimately, fitness prevailed and Darwin survived. More recently, an adolescent girl was reported by Lee and colleagues to have panic disorder with agoraphobia as the result of a seizure disorder. Additional physical causes of panic and other anxiety symptoms are included in Table 9.1; substance-related anxiety symptoms are covered in Tables 9.2 and 9.3.

Agoraphobia only infrequently occurs by itself, and until recently it wasn't even considered to be a separate disorder. However, DSM-5-TR holds that when panic disorder and agoraphobia occur together, they should be considered two disorders that are comorbid. Other than for coding purposes, however, it doesn't really make much difference: We care less about what we call it than we do about what's wrong and how to combat it. For that, it suffices to recognize whether the patient has panic attacks, agoraphobia, or both. Although a study by Fava and colleagues reported 64% cumulative sustained remission at 10 years after exposure treatment, there is some evidence that agoraphobia symptoms may reduce the likelihood of improvement at follow-up for patients with panic disorder.

Zena

Fear is a word we commonly use to describe negative feelings about the world and our relation to it. When we encounter something we fear— whether it is a specific object, circumstance, or social situation—we immediately imagine that we will be harmed, be embarrassed, or suffer other untoward consequences.

> Though she is an experienced teacher in her mid-30s, Zena has trouble writing on the blackboard in front of her seventh-grade class. A couple of times she has felt panicky, but usually she only experiences trembling, dizziness, and a sinking feeling of dread. When she thinks she hears the kids laughing behind her back, she also feels hot and flustered, and she will shake even harder. When no one is watching, she can write just fine, so she comes to school early every day to post the lesson before the bell. Last year, she requested two extra blackboards, so she could write the material in advance. But it is hard to write everything, because she had a number of different subjects to

teach. Furthermore, she needs to assign readings and other material as she goes along. "Besides the shakes," she tells the clinician, "it always makes me feel that I have to use the toilet, even if I've just gone. I can't be charging out to the loo several times a day."

Analysis

Zena's clinician should first rule out medical and substance use causes for her symptoms (steps 1 and 2 of Figure 12.1). Once that is done, it will be on to a "no" at steps 4 and 5—she hasn't mentioned obsessions or compulsions; we don't think she's suffered a serious trauma. Neither does she seem to worry about multiple problems (step 6); just one was plenty. Rather, Zena's distress takes place in a performance situation ("yes" at step 7 and at step 12)—specifically, writing in public—and her diagnosis will therefore be social anxiety disorder. I hope her clinician will next review the symptoms with her to be sure that they haven't overlooked additional diagnoses, notably mood and other anxiety disorders.

Comment

When diagnosing phobias, clinicians face two problems. The first is failing to recognize that a fear exists; although patients are usually very clear about *what* they fear, they often don't complain of it. It may turn up only when they seek help for another mental health problem, such as depression or a different anxiety disorder. The second problem is to separate abnormal fears from those that are normal. After all, most of us cringe from something—whether it is heights, thunderstorms, or visiting the dentist—yet we aren't about to diagnose the majority of the general population with an anxiety disorder. We only make a diagnosis when symptoms cause enough difficulty to interfere with the person's life in some meaningful way. (Zena came to work early to write on the board, and she suffered distress whenever she had to write in front of the class.) Sometimes we forget to observe the boundary between illness and wellness.

Other types of social anxiety disorder that involve facing strangers include fears of speaking (this is especially common), eating or drinking in public, and performing on a musical instrument. Types of specific phobia include fears of animals; fears of the environment (storms, heights, water); fears of blood/injection/injuries; fears of particular situations (flying, being closed in); and fears of circumstances that could lead to illness, choking, or vomiting. In all types, the person may either avoid the phobic situation or endure it with severe stress or anxiety symptoms. As with other anxiety disorders, the anxiety experienced can take a variety of forms. Many people will have symptoms that fall just short of a classic panic attack, including a sense of impending doom, intense uneasiness, or marked tension.

Rawson

Granted, physical conditions causing anxiety symptoms aren't thick on the ground. Indeed, it is their very rarity that causes them not to stick uppermost in the diagnostic mind. Rawson fell victim to just such a lapse of vigilance.

A British transplant to the United States, Rawson was 25 and worked on the rewrite desk of a daily newspaper. Twice he had become dizzy when eating lunch. The second time, his editor personally walked him down to see the company nurse; she found that his elevated blood pressure rapidly returned to normal as he rested in her office. She recommended that he consult a doctor, but he didn't have one—he'd never been ill, and he didn't smoke, drink, or use drugs—and he didn't feel motivated to find one now.

A few months later, Rawson begins to complain of anxiety attacks. At first, they occur every couple of weeks; later they come more often. At most, they last only 10 or 15 minutes, but they are scary: Rawson feels lightheaded, he has trouble catching his breath, and his heart seems to beat wildly. Perhaps worst of all, they leave him drenched in sweat and dreading the next attack, which always seems to loom just over the horizon.

On the day Rawson finally seeks medical advice, he is actually feeling fine, and his vital signs are all normal. "It's like getting your wireless repaired," he jokes, "it always works fine in the shop." He does acknowledge the occasional headache, feelings of weakness, and shaky hands. His energy is low, and he occasionally feels depressed. His appetite has drifted downward, so that he's lost nearly a stone. "That's 14 pounds," he adds helpfully.

"Your physical health is terrific," the doctor informs him, "but you certainly are anxious. I think you may have an underlying clinical depression." That's how Rawson comes to start antidepressant and antianxiety drugs. When the attacks persist, he is switched from one antidepressant to another—a total of four in the course of 10 months. Yet his symptoms continue; the feeling of dread is marginally better, but the headaches are even worse, and he still has the drenching sweats. Finally, during another visit to his family practitioner, he has an attack right there in the office. His blood pressure, normal when the nurse first checked a few moments earlier, climbs to an astonishing 180/125. A series of tests reveals that he has a pheochromocytoma on one adrenal gland. Surgical removal makes a clean sweep of his panic attacks, his depression, and "the dodgy blood pressure."

Analysis

I'd like to believe that I wouldn't have made the same mistake as Rawson's family practitioner, but I can't swear to it. It is easy to overlook a decidedly uncommon possibility such as a pheochromocytoma, which accounts for only about 1 in 1,000 cases of hypertension. The differential diagnosis/decision tree approach to diagnosis forces us to think every time about substances and physical disorders that can cause mental symptoms. However, the diagnostic principle about atypical symptoms also provides a clue: Headache isn't a symptom usually associated with panic disorder, and though sweating is, it is usually far less prominent than in Rawson's case. And we need only the first step in Figure 12.1.

Comment

Of course, you'll want to know how to tell when anxiety symptoms are medical, not mental. The answer is that you can't—at least, not on the basis of the anxiety attacks themselves. You have to rely on being ever suspicious, looking for symptoms that, like Rawson's headaches and high blood pressure, stand a bit apart from ordinary anxiety symptoms. The most difficult part is always to keep in mind something you infrequently encounter: mental symptoms with physical origins. Quite a few medical conditions can cause panic attacks; you'll find some of them listed in Table 9.1.

Wilson and Harold

Speaking of physical causes, there's another whole class of causes to keep alert for, especially when you're trying to get to the bottom of anxiety symptoms. The next two vignettes present a couple of them that are legal.

When Wilson was younger, he loved coffee. Drinking a lot was fine, as long as he was in college; later, however, he drifted into the arcane world of musical instrument repair, which requires patience and a steady hand. Thus his habits clashed with his livelihood, until he turned to decaffeinated coffee, of which he now drank six cups or more each day.

All was well until a few days ago, when by accident a trainee clerk at Wilson's favorite coffee roastery gives him regular beans. The result is several days of upset stomach, heart palpitations, sleeplessness that was "nearly total," and feeling of restless excitement. Unable to reassemble the silver flute he's been working on, he journeys to his family doctor to try to determine the cause.

The morning his father is diagnosed with lung cancer, Harold quits his 20-year cigarette habit cold turkey. By bedtime, he is pacing the floor and angry, though he hasn't a clue as to the target. Surely not his father? After a sleepless night, feeling "incredibly uptight," he fries up and devours a double helping of bacon and eggs, which for health reasons (!) he usually avoids. At 10 A.M., he can't concentrate at work; he can think only of having a puff—just one deep drag—of a cigarette. Either that, or some more breakfast. At noon he calls his wife and wonders aloud whether he'll be able to stay off tobacco. "Being dead would be better than this," he almost sobs.

"I've already gotten you in to see our doctor, later today," she responds. "I knew this was going to be tough."

Analysis

Because the history sits out in plain sight, there should be no problem in diagnosing either Wilson or Harold, both of whom actually need no referral beyond their respective family practitioners. The use of Figure 12.1 seems trivial, but I would recommend it as an exercise in formulating a complete differential diagnosis. Typical symptoms of intoxication and withdrawal for all major classes of drugs, including caffeine and nicotine, are given in Table 9.3.

Comment

The problem with these examples is this: Beneath what's obvious can lurk other syndromes that are independent of any substance use. I'm referring here especially to mood disorder, though others are possible. When patients are either using substances or withdrawing from substance use, they can develop a variety of anxiety symptoms, including outright panic attacks, phobias, generalized anxiety, or even obsessions and compulsions. Because the anxiety disorders are so often comorbid with other anxiety disorders or with the closely related OCD and PTSD, you often have to make two (or more) trips through the decision tree. Does this mean that the person truly has more than one illness? Perhaps not—the diagnostic science just hasn't advanced far enough yet that we can understand the nuances, as with PTSD and depression.

GAD, PTSD, OCD, and Comorbidity

In his first year with the Boston Red Sox, Jim Piersall was hospitalized for a severe mental problem and treated with electroconvulsive therapy. In 1955 he told his story in the hugely popular book, *Fear Strikes Out,* which included material from his childhood. The following is based on Jim's account in that book.

Jim

From the age of 9 Jim Piersall worried constantly, perhaps triggered when his mother entered a mental hospital for a serious but never specified illness. Treated in an era before the advent of effective medication, she periodically improved enough to be released. However, young Jim never knew when she might be taken away again for a readmission; as a result, he was afraid to go to school and afraid to come home again in the afternoon.

He began to "worry about everything"—about school, about whether his classmates would like him, about what mood his father would be in each evening. In the spring, he worried whether he'd be promoted; in the fall, he worried about who his new teacher would be. As he grew up, it got only worse. In the sixth grade, he worried that the weather would affect his ability to play ball; would he be any good when he was grown? Tense and unable to unwind, he had difficulty sleeping and felt the need to be always on the go. Even when he was grown, physically healthy, and married, with a healthy child and a steady job, Jim worried about the future.

Analysis

Because young Jim was in good physical health and, at the age of 9, hardly a candidate for substance use, we can move right through steps 1, 2, and 3 of Figure 12.1. Nowhere in his narrative did Jim describe obsessions or compulsions (step 4). Did his mother's hospitalization act as a (step 5) stressor?

There's no evidence that he relived the event or that he had physiological symptoms such as marked startle response. These *pertinent negatives,* as clinicians call them, lead us on to step 6, where we can agree that even as a youngster, he chronically worried about many things. Our decision tree urges us to consider the diagnosis of generalized anxiety disorder, or GAD.

However, GAD cannot explain Jim's severe breakdown as a young adult, which resulted in mental hospitalization and subsequent electroconvulsive treatment. The evidence concerning that illness is meager; Jim was always a bit circumspect about divulging details. Although he provides some information in his second book, *The Truth Hurts,* it isn't the whole truth.

> In his first year with the Red Sox, Jim was restless, at times sleepless. He suspected that, by making him a shortstop, the Red Sox were trying to get rid of him. His speech was sometimes logical, sometimes "completely haywire," and he was ejected from games for engaging in fistfights on the field. When admitted to the hospital as violent, he was noted to be talking fast.
>
> After his electroconvulsive treatment, he returned to the Red Sox. He subsequently played 17 seasons in the major leagues, and twice won the Golden Glove award. And after 20 years of good health, when he was no longer playing baseball, Jim suffered an episode of depression, during which he had crying spells. Exhausted and suffering from a loss of self-confidence, he again entered a hospital. With medication, he apparently recovered as completely from his second episode as he did from the first.

Although our information is too skimpy to support a definitive diagnosis, it does provide a pretty good example of how we'd use available information to make our best guess—the way we might evaluate, say, a word-of-mouth history provided by someone's relative. Here's how I'd reason it through: A history of psychosis (paranoid suspicions during his first episode) and of mood disorder (typical symptoms of depression during his second) suggests that Jim might have had a psychotic depression, perhaps in the course of a bipolar disorder. An episodic course would be highly unusual for schizophrenia (we'll cite the diagnostic principle about atypical features). Jim's mother also had a serious mental illness that was episodic, providing yet another possible clue to the nature of her son's difficulty. Here I would assert my favorite diagnostic principle and say that he remains undiagnosed, though in my heart of hearts I suspect that an examination by contemporary standards would confirm a bipolar disorder.

Although Jim's GAD long predated his mood disorder, I would of course list the latter first, because that was the diagnosis in need of immediate attention.

Comment

The worries of GAD go far beyond ordinary "worrywart" status and that, as with any mental disorder, raises the problem: How do you discriminate it from the garden-variety concerns we all have? That's where the issue of impairment or clinically important distress steers us away from the temptation to hang a diagnosis on just about everyone we know. Of course, the clinical relevance criterion isn't perfect; we must still judge what level of distress or disability should serve as our benchmark. But as with so many other mental diagnoses, we can use it to ensure that only people whose lives are truly affected will be considered patients.

There is one more important consideration for GAD: The person's worries must not concern only isolated specific issues that might be typical of a different mental disorder. Here are some examples: Gaining weight would be a source of worry for someone with anorexia nervosa; possible contamination would worry a patient with OCD; and the prospect of having a panic attack would greatly trouble a person with panic disorder.

Although it affects as many as 5% of all adults, GAD is comparatively new, having made its bow only a few decades ago. Before that, such a person would be diagnosed with the old term *anxiety neurosis,* which has since been broken up into a variety of anxiety disorders. GAD affects more women than men and it is more prevalent in midlife than in childhood or adolescence. Although it may fluctuate in intensity, it is a chronic condition that, like major depressive disorder, can be highly disabling. An important feature of GAD is that many patients (perhaps the majority) later develop a mood disorder. Indeed, on follow-up, nearly every patient with GAD has a comorbid diagnosis. No one is quite sure what this means in terms of causal relationships, but it is important to keep in mind for anyone who has GAD symptoms. It's what happened to Jim Piersall.

Wilbur

Fear can be focused on a single entity, as with specific phobia, or on a type of situation, as with social anxiety disorder or agoraphobia. However, clinicians must sometimes link fear with other symptoms and historical features to arrive at the correct diagnosis.

When Wilbur was only 19, the Army drafted him. Lacking any special skills, he trained as a cook and served honorably through two tours in Korea. Because of his job, he never expected to see much combat, so he remained in the Army as a career. "I always figured I could open a restaurant after I finished my 20 years."

That's how Wilbur came to be caught up in Lyndon Johnson's big Vietnam buildup in the middle 1960s. He found himself stationed in the Mekong River Delta, which he later described as "the only place on earth you could stand chest-deep in water and have dust blow in your face." In 1966 his battalion of the 9th Infantry Division participated in a sweep of the countryside northward from Saigon through Tay Ninh province. When the armored personnel carrier a few feet ahead of his rolled over a 2,000-pound bomb buried in the road, men riding on top were thrown dozens of yards. Shrapnel struck his neck and right arm, but it was when the head and spinal cord of his best friend landed on his vehicle that Wilbur threw up and passed out. He remembers little of the next 24 hours, though he was told that he had helped to collect body parts and that he richly deserved his Purple Heart and Bronze Star.

"Since I got back, I've never been the same," he tells the clinician years later at the VA outpatient clinic. "I can't quite accept the fact that I was out of the war zone—I'm always on the alert, always scanning the horizon for threats." Occasionally, as when awakening from a nap, he will momentarily think he is back "in country"; for a split second he might imagine Viet Cong soldiers lurking behind his sofa. Many nights, his wife would awaken to find him screaming in fright and kicking her—hard. Finally, she'd had enough and moved back in with her parents.

"I don't blame her a bit," Wilbur says. "I'm a nervous wreck, always jumping at the slightest sound. I won't watch a movie on TV if there are soldiers, and I'm always tired and grouchy. *I* wouldn't want to live with me!"

The clinician unearths other problems. Ever since he returned from the war, Wilbur's appetite has been off, and his weight has dropped almost 20 pounds. "Everything tastes like C-ration boned chicken," he complains. Although he has found a job as a clerk at his county farm bureau, he is irritable with clients and repeatedly forgets to file the paperwork. He is eventually told, "Get some help, or we'll have to let you go."

The clinical review discloses that Wilbur's tour of duty ended before many soldiers began the heavy use of heroin. "We drank some—you could get a fifth of Jim Beam for three bucks at the commissary—but I never caught the drug habit. I might've smoked a joint or two, but never since returning home. I'm not self-destructive, after all." While admitting to feeling "wired" or "uptight" much of the time, he denies having actual panic symptoms, such as pounding heart or shortness of breath.

Analysis

Mental trauma often goes hand in hand with brain injury, which is therefore all the more important to consider when evaluating a patient for PTSD. Wilbur returned from Vietnam intact though physically scarred, but for others less fortunate, a careful examination might reveal neurological deficits that can help explain their symptoms (step 1). The fact that Wilbur did not use substances is hardly rare, but remarkable in that so many veterans do (step 2). The number of men with somatic symptom disorder is probably vanishingly small (step 3), and Wilbur had no evident phobias or obsessions (step 4). Indeed, as presented, the diagnosis fairly explodes off the page. The dead giveaway is, of course, the severe step 5 emotional trauma that preceded the onset of Wilbur's anxiety and avoidance symptoms. Panic symptoms can accompany the PTSD experience, but they aren't required for diagnosis.

Comment

Wilbur is far from the most deeply troubled patient with PTSD. In my service with the VA, I evaluated returning combat survivors so fearful and suspicious that for years they lived alone in the remote California hills. Elaborate criteria aside, PTSD boils down to five basic concepts: (1) The person experiences or witnesses a seriously traumatic event (death, serious injury, sexual violation), and (2) suffers intrusion symptoms (such as dreams, memories), (3) which the person tries to avoid, but (4) they evoke problems with mood or thinking, and (5) induce arousal symptoms such as irritability, aggression, recklessness, insomnia, hypervigilance, and startle response. The symptoms must last longer than a month. Besides combat, PTSD can develop in civilians who experience civilian trauma (such as hurricanes, earthquakes, and tsunamis), motor vehicle accidents, rape, and other human-caused forms of violence.

Be alert for several confounds in the differential diagnosis of PTSD. Patients with OCD perceive their automatic thoughts as inappropriate, and they won't have experienced a specific traumatic event. Patients with PTSD sometimes behave automatically and later may not remember what they did, setting up a possible confusion with dissociative disorder. Had Wilbur's only stressor been that his wife left him, we might instead consider the residual category of adjustment disorder with anxiety (step 9). Unhappily, at the VA as in civilian venues, financial gain can provide a motive for malingering—which, because it is both pejorative and hard to treat, should be considered as a last resort in any differential diagnosis.

You'll need a careful review to ensure that you aren't missing yet another disorder that must be addressed in treating these patients, for whom anxiety may be only the tip of the mental distress iceberg. Because many patients with PTSD have associated depression, carefully consider the asterisked step 17 at the bottom of Figure 12.1. Nearly always in combat veterans, and often in civilians as well, PTSD and depressive symptoms are tightly entwined. In my opinion, one of the many challenges of evaluating a patient with PTSD is to demonstrate that there *isn't* a history of concomitant major depression. Also frequently comorbid with PTSD is dependence on alcohol, illicit drugs, or prescription drugs, and sometimes on all three.

Peter

Thc drama of anxiety and its cousins can nearly eclipse indicators of other problems. Histories like Peter's demonstrate how important it is to make a full evaluation, even when you are asked for help with a specific issue.

> Because he is so afraid of contamination, Peter resists leaving the house. He lives with his younger sister and his mother, who is an evening shift supervisor at Wendy's. Peter recently dropped out of junior college, where he had planned to major in biology. "I did well for the first semester, but then I just couldn't bear to touch those specimens any longer," he tells the student clinician who is trying to gather the initial history.
>
> For the past 3 months, Peter has also refused to eat raw vegetables ("Can't tell what they've been grown in"), and he has gradually begun to develop odd behaviors—grasping doorknobs with the cuff of his shirtsleeve, for example. He acknowledges that he washes his hands, too hard and too often. An "inner voice" reminds him to wash, even if he's already done so just a few minutes earlier. If he resists and doesn't wash, he'll feel "terribly anxious, as though something truly catastrophic is about to happen." Peter becomes tearful as he says, "I feel totally washed up, quite literally. Who wants to spend his days scrubbing the skin off the backs of his hands?"
>
> The student clinician agrees with Peter's own assessment of

OCD, for which behavior therapy seems an appropriate option. However, during a subsequent interview, the supervising clinician sees something else. Peter gazes almost continually downward, and his eyes redden when he mentions his girlfriend, who has broken off their relationship "because I won't even hold hands with her anymore, let alone make love. I just don't have the interest."

On close questioning, Peter admits to feeling sad most of the time, beginning even before the obsessions started. He's had no suicidal ideas, but he does mention that he dropped out of school after he found that his interest, even in his chosen field of plant physiology, had flagged to the point that he couldn't concentrate well enough to study for exams. Although he denies ever using street drugs, he admits that about the only relief he gets is when he drinks beer; over the past month or two, he has gradually increased his consumption to a 6-pack nearly every evening. "At least it gets me to sleep at night," Peter comments.

Peter's immediate family is well, but the paternal cousin who accompanied him to his first appointment has been treated with a mood stabilizer for a mental breakdown, during which he "went off the deep end" and spent a great deal of money.

Analysis

In discussing Peter's differential diagnosis, we'll need to consider the entirety of Tables 11.1 and 12.1. Although his history contains no evidence of a physical disorder that could explain either his depression or his obsessions and compulsions, for safety's sake we'll recommend a careful medical examination. Alcohol use could not explain the anxiety or depression, both of which began weeks or months before he started drinking beer. That moves us on through the first steps of two decision trees.

You can easily step through the rest of Figure 11.1, arriving at major depressive disorder. Then, following Figure 12.1, you can work your way through to the (not unexpected) diagnosis of OCD. I'd list the depression first, emphasizing its importance as the primary problem. I regard the compulsions as secondary phenomena. Armed with all this information, we'd change our recommendations for Peter's treatment to antidepressant drugs or cognitive-behavioral therapy, which might very well resolve both sets of problems. The vignette also presents a good example of the very last level in our roadmap (Figure 1.1)—reevaluate as new material comes to light—and of the family history diagnostic principle (the cousin who probably has bipolar disorder).

Comment

The benefit of multiple diagnoses is clear: When clinicians learn that patients being treated for one condition actually have several, they often enlarge the treatment program. In contrast to double depression (see the case of Robert in Chapter 11, pp. 139–142), where it can be hard to separate the symptoms of two types of depression, you would think that the presence of symptoms and historical data from diagnostic groups as diverse as anxiety states and mood disorders would make it hard *not* to notice comorbidity. Experience and scientific studies suggest otherwise: We clinicians are sometimes distressingly adept at passing right over comorbid diagnoses.

One solution is more information; you can request previous medical records and talk with relatives and other informants. Another is to use more assiduously the mental health review of systems, which asks questions about emotional and behavioral issues other than the patient's chief complaint—hallucinations, delusions, phobias, obsessions, compulsions, panic attacks, depression, mania, problems with sleeping or eating, the use of drugs or alcohol, and forgetfulness. This plan has been formalized in canned interviews—for example, the Structured Clinical Interview for DSM (SCID), which forces a systematic inquiry about all aspects of a patient's mental health history. Although the value of the SCID and similar interviews has been demonstrated over and again, clinicians may be reluctant to use them. After all, a lengthy questionnaire requires more time than can typically be devoted to a single interview, and its somewhat lockstep format might interfere with other goals, such as forming rapport. However, I've included a semistructured clinical interview as an appendix to my book *The First Interview*.

Linda

No matter how bitter the complaint of anxiety, we need to look beyond the obvious for evidence of other conditions. This requires a breadth of perspective that I feel is too often lacking in our contemporary approach to patients.

At age 61, Linda is one of the older patients I have ever treated for anxiety. Her main complaint was "fear and heart palpitations" that for many months had plagued her—and puzzled the string of clinicians who had prescribed a variety of antidepressant and antianxiety medications. On our first visit, Linda told me that no treatment approach had ever made much difference "except that they all make me feel anxious—even the pills for anxiety!"

No one had ever considered the diagnosis of somatization disorder, which I always include in my differentials for anxiety states and mood disorders. I soon learned that Linda had felt sickly all her life, complaining to her bevy of clinicians about trouble swallowing and walking, blurred vision, weakness, dizziness, nausea, abdominal bloating, food allergies, diarrhea, constipation, menstrual irregularity, and a variety of pains throughout her body. Chronically depressed since age 15, off and on she had felt hopeless, had trouble concentrating, and had suffered loss of interest in her usual activities. She'd had ideas about killing herself but had never made a suicide attempt.

With this information, we agreed to move ahead with a somewhat different plan, one that emphasized behavior modification. Within a few months Linda no longer had panic attacks, and her relentless search for physical cures for her various maladies had, well, relented.

Analysis and Comment

Actually, there isn't a lot to say about somatic symptom (or somatization, if you prefer) disorder that I haven't already written in Chapters 9 and 11. The decision tree search stops at step 3. Technically, you could make multiple diagnoses, including the somatizing disorders, anxiety states, and mood disorders. In my opinion, that really isn't necessary, because anxiety symptoms are so very common in patients with somatizing disorders. Furthermore, with few exceptions, treating the somatization addresses all the problems, and why confuse things with unneeded verbiage? The importance of somatization disorder is signified by its place in Figure 12.1.

Acute Stress Disorder

If you scrutinize Table 12.1 and Figure 12.1, you'll find that I've omitted acute stress disorder (ASD)—the diagnosis DSM-IV created to fill the hole created by PTSD's minimum time requirement of 1 month. The problem with ASD is that it imparts pathological significance to reactions that we might often consider to be normal. Some researchers have reported a strong degree of overlap between PTSD and ASD; others have noted that the diagnosis of ASD isn't especially good at predicting who will recover quickly and who will need health care services down the road. All in all, you probably won't spend a lot of time thinking about ASD. But keep it in mind—one of these days, it just might prove key in someone's differential diagnosis.

13 Diagnosing Psychosis

The psychoses aren't so terribly common. Historically, however, they were of signal importance in helping to establish the mental health healing professions. Many of the great names of 19th-century mental health—Kraepelin, Bleuler, Alzheimer—cut their diagnostic teeth on schizophrenia, bipolar psychoses, and cognitive psychoses. Today the economic impact of schizophrenia alone is huge: For the United States in 2020, the total of direct and indirect costs was over $280 *billion*. And in nonmonetary terms, schizophrenia and its close relatives are responsible for a mountain of human effort, recrimination, and misery, preoccupying patients, their families, and their caregivers. For all these reasons, diagnosing schizophrenia is one of the more important skills of any mental health clinician. Of course, the ability to determine that a psychotic patient does *not* have schizophrenia is also hugely important.

To have a *psychosis* means being in some way out of contact with reality. In a practical sense, this loss of touch can be manifested by having symptoms in one or more of the five groups mentioned below. By the way, whereas I don't ordinarily favor rote memorization of criteria (we have books for that), I do make an exception in the case of these basic criteria for schizophrenia, which clinicians often need in the pursuit of diagnostic clarity.

Psychosis requires at least one, schizophrenia two (including one of numbers 1, 2, or 3), of these five:

1. *Hallucinations*. In the absence of external stimulation, the person perceives sensory input. The result is a belief that the person hears voices when no one is speaking, or sees people, objects, even whole tableaus that are not really there. Although hallucinations of smell, touch, and taste can also occur, they are far less common than those of hearing or vision.

> The film *A Beautiful Mind* shows us hallucinations as real-life mathematician John Nash experienced them. It brings home to the viewer just how real hallucinated sensations can seem to a psychotic person.

2. *Delusions.* Believing something to be true that is not, the individual cannot be persuaded otherwise. These false ideas often involve persecution, such as by government agencies, but other delusions may be of guilt, poverty, ill health, infidelity by a spouse, and influence or thought control through information media (newspapers, television, radio). Grandiose delusions involve being associated with—or being—a deity or famous person.

Consider, for example, Daniel Paul Schreber, whose memoirs Sigmund Freud famously analyzed. Schreber, a judge in Dresden, developed the notion that he was being transformed into a woman so that, as God's wife, he could become pregnant and thus save humanity.

3. *Disorganized speech.* The person's mental associations are governed not by logic, but by puns, rhymes, or other influences that may not be clear to an observer. This so impairs output that communication becomes difficult or impossible. A passage from the first page of James Joyce's novel *Finnegans Wake* provides an unintended example:

The great fall of the offwall entailed at such short notice the pftjschute of Finnegan, erse solid man, that the humptyhillhead of humself prumptly sends an unquiring one well to the west in quest of his tumptytumtoes: and their upturnpikepointandplace is at the knock out in the park where oranges have been laid to rust upon the green since devlinsfirst loved livvy.

It is noteworthy that though her diagnosis remains in question, Joyce's daughter, Lucia, began to show symptoms of mental illness in her early 20s and lived as a patient in a madhouse for 47 years until she died.

4. *Disorganized behavior.* Actions that don't appear directed toward a goal may suggest psychosis. Examples include making gestures (e.g., repeatedly crossing oneself), assuming postures, maintaining unusual or uncomfortable positions for long periods, and removing one's clothes in public.

I once evaluated a patient who had been admitted years before to a mental hospital. He had spent nearly a decade lying so rigidly in bed that his wrists and ankles had become frozen, and he could neither walk nor feed himself.

5. *Negative symptoms.* Symptoms are called *negative* when they indicate the absence of something that normal people have. Examples of negative symptoms include low range of emotional involvement (often called *blunted affect* or *flattened affect*), poverty of speech, and loss of the will to accomplish things (termed *avolition*). By contrast, positive symptoms such as delusions and hallucinations are conditions that most of us lack. Frustrated relatives sometimes mistakenly interpret negative symptoms as indicating laziness or apathy.

> Medication had already abated the hallucinations and delusions of my patient Eric. At age 34, he spent his days lounging around his apartment, which his mother subsidized. Although Eric hadn't worked in 6 years, he seemed totally unconcerned when we talked about it. "Oh, I guess I'll get a job later on," he'd say, often with a yawn. His voice was a little monotonous, and he always wore the same half-smile that never touched his eyes. When he stopped by my office, he would slouch in the chair and look just about anywhere but at me. As long as I knew him, he never changed much, never found work, and never really smiled.

Table 13.1 lists the differential diagnosis for psychosis, and Figure 13.1 (later, on p. 191) presents the decision tree for a patient with psychotic symptoms. Note in the decision tree that, against my usual practice, I've included no possibility of normality: Even the briefest of psychoses warrants some sort of diagnosis. And note that the last box in Figure 13.1 advises us to consider a nonpsychotic hallucination. Well, what does that mean?

Nonpsychotic hallucinations are hallucinatory experiences where the patient retains insight that the sensation is not real. They aren't all that common, but neither are they rare. One source is a condition known as the Charles Bonnet syndrome, in which a blind (or partly sighted) patient has visual hallucinations that can be particularly vivid or complicated. Another source is the visual hallucinations that accompany epileptic seizures. Still others have been reported: auditory hallucinations with deafness; visual hallucinations with migraine; the peculiar phenomenon of phantom limb that occurs in those who have suffered an amputation. All of these experiences, and more, are described in Oliver Sacks's 2012 book *Hallucinations*. None of them can be classified as psychotic disorder due to another medical condition, because, well, the patient simply isn't psychotic.

TABLE 13.1. Differential Diagnosis with Brief Definitions for Psychosis

- *Psychosis due to another medical condition.* Physical illness can cause psychosis, which may not meet the criteria for schizophrenia.

- *Substance-related psychosis.* Alcohol, street drugs of misuse, and prescribed medications can all cause psychotic symptoms.

- *Neurocognitive disorder with psychosis.* Patients with Alzheimer's disease or some other neurocognitive disorder (NCD) can develop psychotic symptoms—often persecutory delusions. (Peculiarly, the actual DSM-5-TR diagnosis would be "neurocognitive disorder with behavior disturbance." In the context of NCD, all accompanying mental symptoms are considered behavior.)

- *Somatic symptom disorder with pseudopsychosis.* Some somatizing patients report hallucinations or delusions that can superficially resemble those of schizophrenia.

- *Mood disorder with psychosis.* A patient with an episode of severe mania or depression, or a mixed state, has psychotic symptoms that last only during the active phase of the mood episode.

- *Schizophrenia.* These patients have been ill for many months and have at least two of the five types of psychotic symptoms listed in the text (p. 185). Mood disorders, substance use, and medical conditions have been ruled out as causes.

- *Schizophreniform disorder.* These patients have all the other necessary conditions of schizophrenia but have been ill less than 6 months.

- *Schizoaffective disorder.* During the same month-long episode of illness, a patient has had an episode of mood disorder (major depression or mania) with psychosis (two or more types of psychotic symptoms). Although for at least 2 weeks there has been psychosis without mood symptoms, the latter are present for the majority of the illness.

- *Delusional disorder.* For at least a month, a patient has delusions, but none of the other symptoms characteristic of psychosis.

- *Shared psychotic disorder (folie à deux).* Rarely, a patient develops delusions similar to those of a relative or other close associate. DSM-5-TR would now characterize most such patients as having delusional disorder.

Schizophrenia: Its Subtypes and Variants

Patients with chronic psychosis typically develop symptoms when young—usually as teenagers or young adults. The early evidence of illness may be hard to differentiate from normal adolescent rebellion. I've included the following vignette not because it presents a difficult diagnostic challenge, but to illustrate the development and nature of a classic syndrome as a baseline for later examples of chronic psychosis.

Ronnie

As a small child, Ronnie had always seemed different. Preferring to build intricate castles and raceways with his blocks, he'd never played much with other children. He'd had several imaginary friends whose company he kept right through eighth grade. He was often mocked because of his odd expressions, such as referring to himself in the third person, and he liked to wear clothing that was old and unfashionable. Having no playmates, he could spend all his time studying; every year his extraordinary grades skewed the curve for his class. This only further estranged him from his classmates.

Just after Ronnie turned 17, his studies began to slide. His high school counselor mailed home a note that said he seemed lonely; he spent most of every lunch hour in the library reading. He claimed that he was only interested in science and physics and that he wanted to "do math" as an adult. Ronnie denied that he had any problems, and the counselor concluded that he was a sensitive youth who might have a mild depression. Neither Ronnie nor his parents were much interested in medication, and he soon dropped out of counseling.

His first year in college started out well enough. Ronnie lived at home in his old room, whose walls were covered with posters of NFL quarterbacks—his father had put them up years earlier, and Ronnie had never cared enough to remove them. Ignoring the mandatory humanities course and focusing on science, he threw himself into his work. Nearly every day, he came home right after class, then stayed in his room. He didn't eat meals with his parents—he'd adopted a vegan diet—and his room soon began to smell of discarded crusts and long-opened cups of tofu spread. At first his mother tried to clean his room, but he added a dead-bolt lock to his bedroom door and wore the key around his neck on a fraying piece of string. He wouldn't even allow her to change the sheets, which gradually turned a greasy gray.

Ronnie's physics professor showed his midwinter exam to the dean. It consisted almost entirely of carefully executed drawings, pentagrams, and upside-down crosses, with text that seemed to combine classical mechanics with Biblical phrases. Before they could question him, Ronnie stopped attending class. Now he stayed in his room and spent his time creating and revising a website devoted to his study of infinity. His mother, who had taken quite a lot of higher math in college, came across his website one day while surfing the internet. She discovered that what he had written there was a mishmash of geometric symbols and religious verses that seemed total gibberish.

Whenever she managed to have a word with Ronnie, usually as he was on his way to the toilet, he would only mutter something too quietly to understand. He grew his hair long and he started to cultivate a wispy beard. He had always been a gentle, quiet boy, but now he yelled at his mother when she asked him to shave and get a haircut. At night she would sometimes awaken to the sound of Ronnie pacing the floor or talking—to himself? A classmate had introduced him to nonfiltered cigarettes; now he went through a couple of packs a day. That bothered both of his parents, neither of whom smoked. Despite the time he spent studying, his science and math grades were dropping toward failure. Just before spring break, his advisor finally telephoned him to say, "Either get some help, or we'll have to drop you."

In his second session with the clinician, Ronnie tells this story: Early in the fall, he noticed that the professor addressed many of her remarks directly to him. At first he was pleased to be singled out in such a large lecture hall. He'd glance carefully around to see whether the other students noticed, but they were all pounding lecture notes into their laptops. Later he realized that the professor was actually talking about him to the others—giving them messages about Ronnie's private life, even his sexual thoughts. One day while walking in the quad, he heard a voice just behind him that said, "He's a wanker, all right." Though he quickly turned around, he saw no one anywhere nearby. Later that evening in his room, he heard the same voice, again criticizing his sexuality.

Although Ronnie tells the clinician that he has plenty of friends, his mother later notes that he has always been "something of a lone wolf." She also mentions a great-uncle who by family tradition had been termed "senile," but his history was one of a deteriorating illness requiring chronic hospitalization from the age of 38.

Although he denies that he does it, several times during his initial interview Ronnie laughs, even with nothing obviously funny as a stimulus. The interviewer thinks he seems to be responding to internal thoughts. When he isn't laughing, he has no facial expression whatsoever. Twice Ronnie interrupts the interview to go outside and smoke, saying that he feels too nervous to continue without a break.

Analysis

The absence of issues relating to health, substance use, and memory help move us quickly through the first several steps in Figure 13.1. (Any faint possibility of a cognitive disorder should be further assessed with a brief assessment such as the Mini-Mental State Exam [MMSE]. This issue is discussed further in Chapter 14.) We note that Ronnie has several step 6 symptoms, but there is no evidence of either depression or mania, bringing

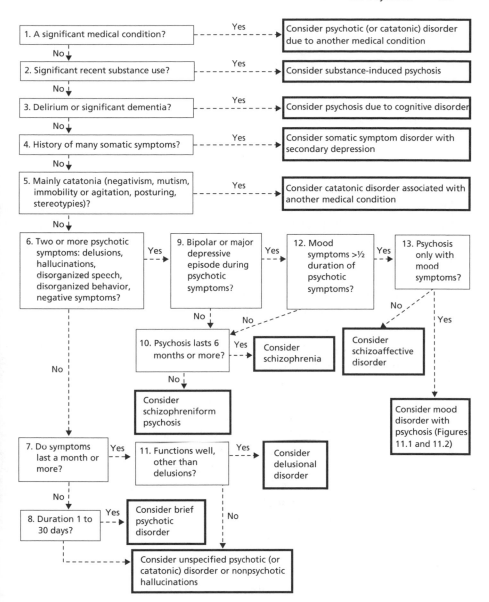

FIGURE 13.1. Decision tree for a patient who has psychotic symptoms such as delusions, hallucinations, disorganized speech, or disorganized behavior.

us to the step 10 question about duration of symptoms. His hallucinations and delusions have lasted for a relatively brief time, but his deteriorating hygiene and negative symptom of loss of the will to pursue his studies in any organized way date back to high school, persuading us that his illness had lasted much longer than 6 months. So, whereas schizophrenia is typically my diagnosis of (almost) last resort, for Ronnie it becomes the most likely to consider.

Along the way, we've used several important diagnostic principles. The collateral history from his mother that he was a loner has more credibility than Ronnie's own claims of friendships, and his laughter during the interview is a sign that trumps his denial of intrusive thoughts. The family lore about his uncle's diagnosis is at odds with the more probable conclusion that he had a chronic psychosis, possibly schizophrenia, which would reinforce our diagnosis for Ronnie. (This shows the value of obtaining what details you can about family history, then forming your own impressions, rather than taking informants' diagnoses at face value.)

Two additional possible diagnoses deserve comment. Ronnie's childhood isolation and discomfort with social relationships suggest a premorbid schizoid or schizotypal personality disorder. These two personality disorders may herald later schizophrenia, but I would follow my own diagnostic principle and decline to diagnose either of them without more information and the opportunity to talk with Ronnie after he had been treated. The other secondary diagnosis might be tobacco use disorder. Although the vignette doesn't provide enough information for a formal diagnosis, can anyone doubt that he is hooked on cigarettes? That's the case in an astonishing 80% or more of patients with schizophrenia, who are about three times more likely than the general population of adults to smoke. The reasons aren't yet clear, though studies have demonstrated that nicotine can enhance cognitive performance.

Comment

In diagnosing schizophrenia, both novice and expert clinicians must struggle—the novices to get it right, the experts to avoid getting it wrong. The latter can happen when experts who come to "feel" the diagnosis of schizophrenia (what's the diagnostic principle lurking here?) forget to consider other possibilities. A couple of generations ago, experts on opposite shores of the Atlantic would have come to very different conclusions when diagnosing psychosis: By a wide margin over their European colleagues, U.S. clinicians tended to use the term *schizophrenia* in questionable cases.

The gulf between the two sides began to narrow in the early 1970s, as the world's clinicians gradually agreed on scientifically validated, conservative criteria for schizophrenia. Even so, errors still occur. As a diagnostic aid, I have put together a list of characteristics that can be used to distinguish schizophrenia from other forms of psychosis described in this chapter (see the sidebar "Differentiating Schizophrenia from Other Psychoses" at the end of the chapter).

Once we've determined that a person does have schizophrenia, are we finished, or should we assign a *subtype?* The traditional subtypes are the terms based on the five classes of psychotic symptoms listed at the start of this chapter. Quite frankly, this step in the diagnostic process is of less than cosmic importance; subtypes don't predict all that much, and some patients change from one subtype to another over the course of time. Furthermore, other than *catatonic,* DSM-5-TR uses none of these terms. Nonetheless, I've mentioned them here, mainly because we'll undoubtedly continue to encounter them for years to come.

- *Paranoid.* Whereas these patients have prominent delusions and auditory hallucinations, their speech and behavior remain well organized and their affect appropriate. Illness often begins later (when patients are in their 30s or older) than for other patients with schizophrenia.

> For many years Kevin has believed that he is being pursued by a secret U.S. government agency—he won't say which one. "They'd find out, and I'd be even more of a marked man." Although he continues to hold down a responsible job and support his family, he spends much of his free time checking his phone and Wi-Fi for bugs.

- *Catatonic.* Patients with this form of the illness, seldom encountered today, typically are markedly slowed down—sometimes to the point of immobility. They may show *negativism* by turning away from you or refusing to follow a command; *posturing* by spontaneously posing or assuming a bizarre posture; *stereotypies* (behaviors that are not goal-directed, such as repeatedly flashing an "OK" sign); *muteness*; and *echolalia* or *echopraxia,* the meaningless repetition of another person's words or actions.

> When I first met Bruno, who had been psychotic for many years, he was lying on his back in bed, rigid and mute. An attendant showed me that when the pillow was carefully removed, Bruno's head didn't budge, hovering in midair, an inch or two above the mattress. He seemed willing to maintain that position for hours.

- *Disorganized*. These patients may have some disturbances of behavior (though less obvious than in catatonia), plus disorganized speech *and* flattened or inappropriate affect. The symptoms of patients with this subtype, which used to be called *hebephrenic,* begin quite early in life. As with all forms of schizophrenia, men develop symptoms at a somewhat younger age than women do.

> With a several-year history of well-diagnosed schizophrenia, Hilda knows the names of all the hospital staff. However, on this admission, she cannot communicate so much as her *own* name. Her brother brought her to the emergency department, because for weeks she has been hiding in her room, refusing even to emerge for meals. When he finally coaxes her to the emergency room, her hair is matted and her nails are ragged. She evidently hasn't bathed for many days; her clothes are mismatched; and one of her shoes is missing its lace. As the interviewer enters, Hilda giggles and hides her face in her hands. Answering the question "Why are you here?", she replies, "I've got jolly sixpence." Then she starts taking off her clothes.

- *Undifferentiated*. This final grouping comprises all those patients who don't fit into any of the previous three categories. Because his psychosis contains both paranoid and disorganized elements, this is how I would categorize Ronnie's illness—were someone to ask.

Although schizophrenia isn't rare, it occurs infrequently enough that early in the course of a young person's illness, we may fail to recognize that something serious is afoot. We also need to continually revisit a schizophrenia diagnosis—patients can change, and even the best diagnosticians make mistakes. The diagnosis of psychosis is a high-risk mental health area, where the stakes are people's lives and families' happiness.

Winona

The typical symptoms of schizophrenia are relatively easy to spot. A greater clinical challenge is to identify issues that are not typical and to recognize what they mean.

> During her first 2 years at an East Coast women's college, Winona earned good grades in a demanding major (physical chemistry) and served as underclass representative to the Student Senate. At least

one of her several boyfriends proposed marriage. Over the summer, she held down two jobs, one of them as lab assistant to her faculty advisor.

In mid-October of the new school year, Winona's roommate drops out of school. The official reason is "fatigue," but everyone knows about Lia's pregnancy; unwilling to have an abortion, she's gone home, and Winona's new roommate has just transferred in as a junior.

Almost immediately, Winona notices that Sherrie is watching her closely, apparently tracking her movements around their small dormitory room. Within days, Winona observes that others on campus have joined the effort to keep tabs on her. By a system of hand waves and nods, one student "can pass me off to another, so the record will be complete," she tells a clinician later. At first, these signals are barely perceptible, but over the next few weeks they become more and more blatant. Soon she detects mocking in the tone of her professors; clearly, the faculty has joined the plot.

Winona makes a trip to her student health service. The faint ringing sounds in her left ear that have bothered her for the past couple of weeks are louder now, and she demands a hearing test. The audiologist is unoccupied at that very hour, so she has her test—which is completely normal. The doctor then asks whether she's been using alcohol or drugs; a little offended, she replies that she has not. "And I haven't been depressed, either, if that's what you're thinking." All in all, the visit is a complete bust—her health appears to be perfect.

A few days later yet, Winona suddenly understands the ringing. It is a way of warning her to be wary of Sherrie, who wants to steal her boyfriend (never mind that Winona doesn't have one currently). In fact, she has begun to hear tinkling laughter with the ringing, which, as she explains later, "gradually morphed into voices. It's embarrassing how simple it all seems now."

Uppermost in Winona's mind is her anger at Sherrie's persecution: "I don't see why I should suffer, just because she can't get a guy."

Analysis

Winona's health overall has been excellent, as attested by her student health visits. This fact gets us past steps 1, 2, and 4. A few minutes' additional interview would confirm that she has no significant cognitive symptoms (step 3). At step 6 we note that she has both delusions and hallucinations. Though for now we can accept her denial as regards depression, her clinician would need more questioning to rule out any hidden depression (step 9). Because she has been ill for only about 6 weeks, far less than the total of

6 months needed for schizophrenia, step 10 recommends that we consider the diagnosis of schizophreniform disorder.

Comment

Schizophrenia usually begins slowly—"insidious" is the word we use to describe the glacial pace at which this disease announces itself. But in 1939 a Norwegian clinician named Gabriel Langfeldt described a psychotic illness that began more rapidly and often resolved entirely. From this concept, through many diagnostic twists and turns, has evolved our current usage of *schizophreniform psychosis* to mean a psychotic disorder resembling schizophrenia that lasts at least 1 month but less than 6 months.

Within a few decades, U.S. clinicians have gone from being distressingly permissive in how we diagnose psychosis to having the strictest set of criteria in the world. Some (such as Schwartz et al., 2000) say that the current criteria may actually be too conservative—that they promote false negatives. A few patients who should receive the diagnosis of schizophrenia do not, or at least they don't in a timely fashion. The time factor may be vital; although the definitive study has yet to be done, some studies suggest that the longer we wait before beginning treatment, the poorer the outcome. As little time as 7 days may make a difference, but the effects of delay may go out to 1 year or more. That's one of the virtues of schizophreniform disorder: It encourages us to proceed with treatment while keeping our options open as regards final diagnosis.

Like schizophrenia, schizophreniform disorder is in all likelihood a group of disorders that we should (but probably won't) refer to in the plural as the *schizophreniform psychoses*. As a group, they are just a parking place we use for some patients until we can figure out a better term to use. After half a year or so, some patients will be rediagnosed as having a psychosis related to substance use or a physical disorder; others will turn out to have a mood disorder. And a substantial minority, those who continue to be ill with their original symptoms, we will have to rediagnose as having schizophrenia.

A few patients, perhaps 20%, will experience complete remission within the 6-month time frame; they are the only ones who can retain the diagnosis of schizophreniform disorder (see the sidebar "Prognosis and Schizophreniform Psychosis"). Be discerning when you read about this condition; I've encountered clinicians who disregard the time requirements and continue to use the diagnosis for patients who have been ill for years.

Prognosis and Schizophreniform Psychosis

Schizophreniform disorder incorporates criteria for predicting which patients are likely to recover completely from their current episode of illness. The outlook is more likely to be favorable if we can identify some features that in follow-up studies have predicted a good prognosis. A patient who has two or more of the following is likely to recover:

- Confusion
- Psychotic symptoms that begin early (within the first month of the illness)
- Good premorbid social and work functioning
- Good preservation of affect

Winona (pp. 194–197) had three of these factors—delusions from the first days she was ill; excellent functioning socially and in her job (school) before becoming ill; and the ability to show anger while ill (therefore, her affect was probably not blunted). However, even when most acutely ill, she did not seem confused. Her clinician told her and her parents that she would probably recover completely, which is in fact what happened.

Organic Psychoses

Numerous physical illnesses can cause psychotic symptoms, which sometimes look remarkably like those of schizophrenia. Table 9.1 lists some of these, four of which are illustrated in the following vignettes.

Edwina

Though she'll tell you she hates the word, Edwina is still spry. She has been a writer all her adult life, and from the retirement home where she's lived for the past 5 years, she continues to pen a weekly column—about retirement. She doesn't smoke or use alcohol, and takes no medications other than vitamin C. Because she has no past history of mental disorder, it surprises staff members at the facility when one Sunday morning she refuses to attend the nondenominational religious services she's always enjoyed. "The specters, they're cursing the Lord," she remarks of phantasms hovering near the ceiling that no one else can see. Edwina claims that the "shade" of a resident who recently died lurks in the chapel, sometimes shaking his finger at her. At Sunday lunch, she refuses to eat her poached salmon; she insists that the cook, a Native American woman who works weekends, has poisoned the fish in retaliation for centuries of mistreatment of her people by the government.

Edwina's doctor recommends an antipsychotic drug, which she refuses to take. But she does consent to magnetic resonance imaging, which shows that she's had a small stroke beneath the surface of the left side of her brain. Other than elevated blood pressure (190/115), her exam is normal. Over the next week she improves, and a month later she's again eating with good appetite. In a column about her experience, she writes that her previous ideas were "peculiar, at best."

Sal

Directly out of high school, Sal had entered the military and served a tour of duty in the first Gulf War. A brave and loyal soldier, he tried to reenlist after his 4-year hitch, but he was forestalled by his history of occasional outbursts of rage, sometimes directed toward his sergeants. These never quite rose to the point of disciplinary action but, coupled with a nagging depression, they caused the Army to reject him for further service. He subsequently worked for a variety of pest extermination companies.

When Sal is 27, his increasingly erratic behavior prompts admission to a VA hospital. He had been found one weekend on the riverfront, running along the levee and screaming about "Star Trekkers" who were threatening to disrupt his visitation with his 4-year-old daughter. He hadn't been hallucinating, exactly. He did say that he might be hearing threatening sounds, though they could be in his head—perhaps put there by the Trekkies. Since his admission, they haven't bothered him, but he keeps trying to alert the FBI to a possible invasion. His doctors first wonder whether he inhaled toxic chemicals from his job, but he patiently explains that his specialty is ridding homes of bats. That involves caulking, not chemicals.

Family mythology holds that when Sal was a baby, his mother had "run off with the gypsies" and hasn't been heard from since. Sal was reared by his father and, later, his stepmother. The only other family history he knows is that a cousin who died in an institution might have had Huntington's disease. A copy of his military mental health evaluation reveals that he had a persistent twitching of his mouth, interpreted as a sign of nervousness that further substantiated his unfitness for duty.

Sal improves with antipsychotic drugs, and his doctors diagnose him as having psychotic disorder not otherwise specified (in DSM-5-TR it would be called unspecified psychotic disorder). Followed in the outpatient clinic, he continues on his medication and does well for 2 years. Then he begins to show distinctive writhing movements of his arms, and problems with his memory are noted. On reevaluation, his diagnosis is changed to psychosis due to Huntington's disease.

Arley

Abandoned by his family when he was 5, Arley had been reared in a succession of foster families. After a disastrous academic career (including repeated fights with students, poor grades, and even altercations with teachers), he left school for good when he was 15. For a time he was homeless and supported himself by petty theft and running drugs for a gang. He began using a variety of street drugs—especially amphetamines, later adding heroin to the mix. By the time he was 20 he was using needles to inject himself; often he was careless about sterility.

When Arley is 25, he is admitted to a hospital with pneumocystis pneumonia. This is the first time he has tested HIV-positive, and it leads to treatment with a cocktail of drugs that at first keep his symptoms under control. Living on the streets, he fears being robbed or molested ("Whatever else, I'm no prostitute," he's told his doctor). Because his medicines make him drowsy, he decreases the dose so that he can stay vigilant, even when sleeping. Gradually he stops taking them altogether. Within 6 months, he is back at the hospital complaining of persistent sore throat, which turns out to be due to candidiasis. He is diagnosed with full-blown AIDS and admitted.

Arley cannot state the current date exactly, but he knows who and where he is. His speech wanders off into descriptions of scenes he claims to see—a valley full of bodies bathed in blood; a crowd of young people waving stumps where their arms should be. During the admission physical exam, he worries that his penis has been cut off; he keeps looking down inside his pants, which appears to reassure him only for a few moments. Within days he becomes mute, staring at the wall next to his bed and threatening to strike out at anyone who approaches. His diagnosis is psychotic disorder due to AIDS.

Trudy

Off and on for years, Trudy has been treated for psychosis. Always rather easily upset, without much provocation she will fly into a rage. Then, at 23, she has her first incident of severe abdominal pain; she carries on so dramatically in the hospital's urgent care center that she is diagnosed as hysterical, despite the fact that she vomited across the shoes of two nurses. She is discharged the following day, but later that afternoon an ambulance returns her to the emergency room.

Curled up on a gurney, Trudy remains completely mute until she is given an injection of Valium. When she gradually begins to speak, she forcefully explains that she is dead already, that her pain signals the onset of her torture in "the spirit world." Days later, her delusions have once again yielded to antipsychotic drugs; her clinician attributes her lingering muscle weakness to a side effect of medication.

Between episodes of her illness, Trudy now faithfully takes the antipsychotic medication—right up to the next attack. These occur every 4 or 5 years, each time resulting in renewed pain, weakness, and hospitalization. But she never experiences hallucinations. When she is 38, a technician notices that her urine specimen has darkened after standing in sunlight on a laboratory bench. This prompts further investigation and the eventual diagnosis of acute intermittent porphyria.

Analysis

Once we know that a medical condition exists, the analysis of each of these patients is trivial. It's the knowing, or rather not knowing, that trips us up. Most such cases will have features that should draw our attention away from schizophrenia and toward a physical cause: a sudden beginning (Sal), onset in advanced age (Edwina), or existence of a prior medical condition (Arley). Trudy was misdiagnosed and treated for schizophrenia for years, but she shouldn't have been, because she didn't have a full enough spectrum of psychotic symptoms—only delusions, with hallucinations completely absent and none of the other five key criteria listed at the beginning of this chapter. Chalk up another plea for the diagnostic principles that urge us to look for more symptoms and typical symptoms of a disorder. And then there's the issue of *atypical* features: Somatic symptoms, such as headache or dark urine, strongly point us toward a physical cause for her disorder. At least two of these patients experienced confusion, which is also atypical for schizophrenia.

Comment

Of course, family history only suggests risk of mental illness; as in the case of Sal, only the Huntington's gene itself can produce the illness. Also, an occasional medically ill patient will have a psychosis that seems typical of schizophrenia, with few if any features that would tip you off to the physical etiology. The only solution is never to be completely comfortable with a diagnosis so fraught with peril as is schizophrenia. With apologies to Thomas Jefferson, the price of accurate diagnosis is eternal vigilance.

Substance-Related Psychoses

You often read that substance use can present as a psychosis that closely resembles schizophrenia, but how many of us have actually encountered such a case? Although the data aren't very clear, it probably happens more often than we realize.

Aileen

Aileen sells major appliances for a discount retail chain. Lately she has noticed something "seriously strange"—the people shown on the television sets displayed throughout the store have begun watching *her*. "They seem almost to follow me around as I move from one aisle to the next," she explains much later to the clinician who eventually admits her to a hospital.

At first, she thought it was funny and mentioned it to a customer, who quickly decamped to shop elsewhere. Later, Aileen was appalled to discover that the characters on TV were also discussing her sex life. She talked it over with another sales rep, who for quite a while stood with her and watched a high-definition monitor. "He said there was nothing going on at all," Aileen scoffs, "but of course, he hadn't a clue." Later that day, her manager discovered Aileen in a back room where there were no televisions, trying to hide inside a side-by-side refrigerator, from which she had removed all the racks. She screamed all the way to the emergency room.

Admitted to a locked ward, she stops talking completely. Several clinicians try to question her, but each time she will only gaze intently at them, then physically turn away until all they can see is the back of her head. Her boyfriend, Geoff, with whom she has lived for 2 years, is away on a business trip, but a coworker supplies the telephone number of Aileen's mother, who drives in from a neighboring county. She states very clearly that Aileen has never had a similar episode, has never used street drugs: "In all her 28 years, she's been a real straight arrow—she doesn't even drink." Her mother does note that at lunch a few days ago, Aileen spoke rapidly and was full of plans for buying a house and renovating it. "I wondered that she had been able to save up the money," Aileen's mother muses. "That big box store where she works isn't a charitable institution."

There is no family history of mental illness or drug misuse, though Aileen's twin brother smoked pot as a teenager. A call to her family practitioner confirms her excellent physical health; she takes no prescribed medications, not even birth control pills. She has fought a weight problem all her life; currently, she's on a low-carbohydrate diet.

When Geoff returns home the following day, at first he says she has been "disgustingly healthy," but later he recalls that for the past week or two she has seemed unusually energetic. Then he mentions that a couple of weeks ago, after her most recent diet had let her down, she tried some tablets from a bottle given to her by a friend. For at least a week, she's been downing several a day. Later he brings in a bottle labeled *"ma huang."*

Analysis

We'll try to determine the cause of Aileen's delusions and other strange behaviors for two time periods: when she was first admitted to the hospital and after her boyfriend provided additional history. First, based solely on the collateral information (from Aileen's mother and her friend at work) of sudden onset and rapid speech, we might entertain a mood disorder diagnosis, though we wouldn't go quite all the way and say that she had a bipolar disorder. Why? Just after admission, she showed some atypical features, such as muteness and negativism—hardly the stuff of mania—not to mention the fact that there were too few symptoms to justify *any* diagnosis. At this point I'd employ the diagnostic principle concerning *undiagnosed,* partly because at age 28 she's had no previous mood episodes, but mainly because there's just too little recent history.

Of course, Geoff's return with further collateral history brings the diagnosis immediately into focus. Although he knows of no physical problems, she has been taking a drug that—a minute spent with Google reveals—contains ephedrine, a stimulant widely known capable of producing manic-like symptoms and psychosis. The Figure 13.1 journey to diagnosis is a short one, requiring just two steps.

Comment

What usually comes to mind when you consider substances that cause mental symptoms? Alcohol and street drugs. However, a wide variety of medications can also precipitate psychosis. The U.S. Food and Drug Administration banned use of ephedrine in 2004, effectively ending an associated series of deaths. However, it can still be found in traditional medicines and imported drugs. The symptoms of toxicity are a lot like those of other stimulant drugs, such as cocaine and amphetamine—which, unfortunately, are still available in abundance.

Vern

One pitfall of a major diagnosis like schizophrenia is that its symptoms are so blatant, so overwhelming that, once we've identified it, we may be tempted to rest on our laurels.

> Vern's emotional symptoms had been accumulating for several years; finally, at age 27, he was diagnosed with schizophrenia. Since then, he has been successfully treated with long-acting intramuscular Haldol, which he tolerates well. He likes his therapist at the mental health clinic. "You're my only friend," he has said more than once.
>
> So 6 years down the road, the therapist notes with some surprise that Vern has once again begun to complain of persecution. Poachers have stolen the flank steaks he purchased for his mother's birthday bash; though he was born in Baltimore, monks from a local commune have collected money to have him deported to Sudan. Within a couple of weeks, he becomes increasingly agitated and belligerent. Finally, howling auditory hallucinations once again precipitate his hospitalization.
>
> There can be no question that Vern is taking his antipsychotic medication: Every 4 weeks the PA plants it right there in his hip. And close questioning cannot dislodge him from his story that he has used neither alcohol nor street drugs. A call to his mother, however, reveals that Vern has finally found a friend—a substance-using patient with a long and checkered history. Sure enough, when directly questioned, Vern admits that he and George have frequently smoked crack together, for about as long as he's been having a recurrence of his psychosis.

Analysis

The use of Figure 13.1 is almost superfluous; you might want to check Table 9.3 to see what other symptoms of cocaine use Vern might be subject to. And Table 15.1 (p. 246) lists the types of substances that can cause psychosis and other mental syndromes during intoxication or withdrawal. I'd arrange Vern's two diagnoses—schizophrenia and cocaine-induced psychosis—in reverse order, to indicate which needs the more immediate (additional) treatment.

Comment

The tip-off here is that Vern's psychosis has returned, despite his continuing use of medication—the effects of which, because it is injected, he cannot escape. Of course, even without street drugs as a stimulus, a patient with schizophrenia could develop renewed symptoms. But the safe course is to suspect that something else has occurred to interfere. Dual diagnosis is far too common a finding to disregard it.

Studies have shown that even excluding tobacco, 40% or more of patients with schizophrenia will misuse substances at some time; most popular is alcohol, then marijuana and cocaine. Substance use is associated with aggression, violence, and relapse of psychosis, and it can persist despite adequate treatment for the underlying major illness. Of course, substance use can lead to homelessness and incarceration, and it increases hospital admissions and costs of treatment. Even marijuana raises these patients' psychopathology scores on standard tests. Although it has often been suggested that patients with schizophrenia use drugs and alcohol to cope with their psychotic symptoms, a 2001 study by Lammertink and colleagues failed to support this "self-medication" hypothesis.

Other Psychotic Disorders and Comorbidity

I have abstracted this description of a patient known only as S. R. from a classic 1933 paper in the *American Journal of Psychiatry*.

S. R.

An active, ambitious young woman who loved to go dancing, S. R. met her policeman husband when she was 18 and married him just 6 months later. Within a year they were the parents of a son. When the child was 5, they moved to a "fixer-upper" house. Some of its features troubled S. R.: The furnace wasn't working well, and she thought she could smell gas. She had trouble sleeping and lost her appetite; several times she vomited. Cross and irritable, she brooded about how coarse her husband seemed and how the 11-year difference in their ages thwarted her desire to mix with other people and go out dancing.

When another policeman in their neighborhood committed suicide early in February, her husband remarked that his line of work could make anyone feel suicidal. S. R. subsequently became depressed, blaming her mood on interference from his parents, who had never taken to her. Feeling oppressed by his sexual demands, she wished that he would leave her alone. She said that she had a bad heart and would soon die.

One night in mid-February, she impulsively requested to go to the home of her parents; there, she accused them of trying to turn her husband against her. Still sleepless the next night, she accused her brother of planning to poison her husband. Then she called the police and asked to be rescued; ultimately she was hospitalized. Five days after admission, her rectal temperature was elevated at 102°F, and her white blood count was 15,200.

S. R. complained of hearing peculiar noises and that other patients were talking about her. She also suspected that her husband had been unfaithful, had begun to use drugs, and would try to steal her son from her. Other patients, using voices that were somehow "rayed" to her from another room, said that her husband was of "mixed blood." When he visited her in the hospital, she thought that his eyes stared and held a glassy look. She complained of physical sensations that she attributed to poison. She lost her appetite, couldn't sleep, and cried a great deal. She smelled many different odors while in the hospital, and she heard her name broadcast over the paging system.

Whereas S. R. had initially been depressed, after several weeks she appeared happy and was once again able to laugh. Now she attributed all her troubles to "radio hypnotism." After 6 weeks of hospitalization, she was discharged home with the diagnosis of dementia praecox. On follow-up 20 months later, she had maintained her recovery and seemed completely her old self.

Analysis

With no evidence of a significant medical condition, substance use problem, catatonia, or delirium, we swiftly advance through steps 1–5 of Figure 13.1 to step 6, which we can answer "yes"—she has at least two symptoms of psychosis. When first hospitalized, S. R.'s psychotic symptoms were associated with serious depressive symptoms (though this account lacks information sufficient to identify a major depressive episode, as DSM-5-TR requires). This leads us through step 9 to step 12, which asks about length of the depressive symptoms. DSM-5-TR states clearly that the mood disorder part of the equation should occupy half (or more) of the total duration of symptoms. S. R. had been depressed for several weeks; this fulfills that criterion and leads us to step 13. To determine that she has schizoaffective disorder would require at least 2 weeks with psychosis but no mood symptoms. And indeed, her psychotic symptoms apparently persisted after her mood reverted to normal, bringing us finally to consider the diagnosis of schizoaffective disorder.

Comment

Whew! This has been about as tortured a trip through a decision tree as we'll encounter in our quest for any diagnosis. Was all that work worth the effort? A diagnosis with ever-changing criteria, schizoaffective disorder was controversial almost from the very first. Of the five patients fully described in Jacob Kasanin's original 1933 article, most would not fully qualify for such a diagnosis according to the criteria in use today. S. R. is the Kasanin patient who most clearly fulfills DSM-5-TR criteria.

Some authors point out that interrater reliability in schizoaffective disorder is unsatisfactory. Other studies use statistical manipulations to suggest that schizoaffective disorder as now described is only a variant of schizophrenia, which it resembles in its prognosis—the direct opposite of Kasanin's conclusion. Indeed, schizoaffective disorder is one whose criteria have changed in each of the three major revisions to the DSM. (In 1980, DSM-III cannily avoided proposing any criteria at all.)

What is the diagnosis of schizoaffective disorder supposed to accomplish? Researchers have long sought a middle ground somewhere between schizophrenia and the mood disorders—a sort of mental health No Man's (sorry, No Person's) Land. If one existed, it would be very much like this disorder. That's why the symptoms have to be so carefully drawn: There must be a substantial period of mood problems accompanied by psychosis, but on the other hand, there must also be a time when there is psychosis without either mania or depression. Otherwise, there would be nothing to differentiate the condition from, say, depression with psychosis.

Let's face it: schizoaffective disorder remains a confused muddle. Its scientific support is weak, and it is too often used as a catch-all for difficult-to-diagnose patients. In 2003, one clinician wrote that because so many of his patients had both mood and psychotic symptoms and gave such poor histories, schizoaffective disorder was one of his most frequent diagnoses. Whereas many studies of psychotic patients lump together schizophrenia and schizoaffective disorder, few publish enough details to determine which diagnosis the clinical features fully support, by any set of criteria. Some authors note that depression is fairly common in patients with schizophrenia, especially those who are older, and that it is correlated with the positive symptoms of hallucinations and delusions. At least one writer (Marneros) suggests that we should distinguish two forms of schizoaffective disorder: *concurrent* and *sequential*. That would require yet another revision of the criteria—a further repositioning of the target while clinicians and researchers alike are still trying to adjust their sights on its present location. All things considered, it's small wonder that William Carpenter, the chair of the DSM-5 task force on psychoses, stated during a 2013 presentation about his committee's work, "We don't even know if it exists in nature."

Camille

The early-20th-century French sculptor Camille Claudel developed a lifelong psychosis that is diagnosable even through the long-distance lens of biography.

> With little formal education, Camille Claudel went far. Though recognized as a talented artist in her own right, her fame largely depends on her position as the longtime mistress, muse, and sometimes collaborator of the great sculptor Auguste Rodin; she contributed entire figures to some of his works. But at around the age of 30, something happened that gradually drew her away from Rodin, her art, and ultimately the world.
>
> Camille had begun to suspect that others, women included, were aligned against her. In fits of anger, she expressed her distrust of Rodin—whom she ultimately accused of deceiving her "by crafty and false character," as she wrote in a letter when she was 38. She became convinced that she knew who was responsible for "depredations committed in the Louvre," and she sent letters containing cat feces to an art inspector. She increasingly withdrew from her friends, and gradually ceased producing works of art at all; she even smashed some of her own works. Poverty-stricken, she was reported to be living in filth, scrounging food from garbage cans. Despite the ample evidence of delusions, nowhere do her biographers ever note evidence of hallucinations or sustained depression.
>
> As the years rolled on, Camille came to the ecumenical conviction that Jews, Protestants, and Freemasons were plotting to poison her. Ultimately, at age 49, she was placed in a mental hospital where she imagined that even the nurses had joined the plot. For the balance of her life, she lived in asylums. Although she would have been provided with art materials, and the income from her work could have

helped her live far more comfortably, she refused to sculpt for fear that, even in institutions, her work would be stolen from her. To avert the poisoning she believed imminent, she would eat only raw eggs and unpeeled potatoes, or whatever cooked food she could prepare herself. By the age of 62 she was still able to compose letters that were completely coherent as long as she avoided the objects of her delusions. At 66 she wrote that, because more than three decades earlier, she had refused to sign a petition at the time of the notorious Dreyfus affair, "the Jewish gang is holding me here."

Although from time to time throughout her life Camille complained of physical illness, there is no record of a physical disorder that could account for her psychosis. She remained lucid until near the end, when she drifted into senility, still convinced that Rodin was the "odious character" who had ruined her life.

Analysis

Our route through the history of Camille Claudel is quite clear: After dashing through steps 1–5, we note that for decades she had delusions but no hallucinations. Therefore, we must answer "no" at step 6 of Figure 13.1. Her ideas, though false, lasted well beyond 6 months (step 7). Outside her delusions, she was able to function well (step 11), bringing us to the consideration of delusional disorder as her diagnosis. Of course, because historical diagnoses rely almost exclusively on collateral information, they can never be more than tentative. (I will also repeat the warning that we must take extra care when trying to diagnose a person we have not personally interviewed.)

Comment

People who have delusions but no hallucinations or other features of psychosis (see the list at the beginning of this chapter) don't meet criteria for schizophrenia; we say that they have delusional disorder. They usually become ill later in life than is the case in schizophrenia, and their functioning is less impaired. The delusions can be of several sorts, but the *persecutory* type, in which the patient is somehow being cheated, followed, slandered, or drugged, is the most common. Other types include *erotomanic* (someone, often of high station, is in love with the patient); *grandiose* (the patient has a special talent, power, or relation to someone famous); *jealous* (a spouse or lover has been unfaithful); and *somatic* (physical sensations, such as insects crawling on the skin or a foul body odor, imply a medical condition or physical defect). Some patients have features of two or more of these types.

Encountered only about 1/30th as often as schizophrenia, delusional disorder's fame far exceeds its numbers. There are a couple of reasons. There is the notoriety that attends instances of stalking, which is sometimes due to the erotomanic form of delusional disorder (the Glenn Close character in the movie *Fatal Attraction* suggests such a case). Then there is our fascination with John Hinckley, Jr., who famously stalked and shot Ronald Reagan in 1981. Hinckley has been described as having delusional disorder, though real doubts linger as to his correct diagnosis. Of course, like those with schizophrenia, the vast majority of patients with delusional disorder do not kill or harm other people. Those few who do so attract an inordinate amount of attention, fear, and rage.

Ted

The symptoms of psychosis are so striking that they can obscure other important aspects of the history and MSE. It's a mistake to allow that to happen, because a second illness can complicate—and a second diagnosis can facilitate—treatment.

> Short and solidly built, Ted vaguely resembles the water heaters and dishwashers he delivers every day for his employer, a major home appliance chain in a West Coast city. He has served honorably in the Army, including a tour in Iraq during the first Gulf War, but after an 8-year enlistment he resigned rather than attend the alcohol rehabilitation program necessitated by a couple of civilian arrests for public intoxication. After that, he bounced from job to job until a divorce finally persuaded him to join AA. He then obtained his present position, which he has held for well over 5 years. Ted settled down, married for a second time, and was engaged in raising his year-old twin daughters.
>
> As Ted is maneuvering an induction cooktop onto his dolly one afternoon, he pauses when he hears something strange—a voice that seems to come from inside the crate. "Ted, drop it," the voice commands. He is so surprised that he does just that, and the box pops open. Looking inside, he sees only a (mute) glass cooktop. After a few moments, he rides it down the lift on the back of his truck and rolls it into the house. Later that afternoon, he hears two voices coming from a carton of microwaves he's picked up at the warehouse. They are discussing him, calling him a failure, a drunk, and an asshole. He tears the carton completely to shreds before bolting from work to gulp his first beer in nearly a decade.

Over the next week, a swelling chorus of crates and boxes have Ted nearly in tears. The following Thursday, he enters his boss's office to try to learn what's going on. The office is empty, but he observes some papers on the desk. "They were carefully lined up with the edge of the desk," as he tells the clinician when he checks himself into urgent care days later, "and suddenly I *knew* it meant that everything was lined up against me." Even his wife "looked funny" at him, proving that she was in cahoots with his boss.

Ted tries his best to avoid further recourse to alcohol, but loses. Even when drinking, he hears the voices, which grow louder and more insistent. After 2 weeks of heavy drinking, he hears a radio announcer say, "Ted's got to learn." At that point, he makes the decision to seek help.

Analysis

Sorting out Ted's psychosis requires some attention to Figure 13.1—and the calendar. It makes a lot of difference that Ted has been psychotic for only a few weeks. This fact, his hallucinations, and his delusions move us to step 10, where a "no" answer brings us to consider the diagnosis of schizophreniform disorder. Although we should always consider prognosis for every patient, schizophreniform psychosis is the only psychotic diagnosis that specifically encourages us to rate how likely the patient is to recover (see the sidebar "Prognosis and Schizophreniform Psychosis" on p. 197). Fortunately for him, recovery from his psychosis is foretold by several of Ted's symptoms: excellent affect, symptoms of psychosis almost from the beginning of his disorder, and very good social and work adjustment prior to the onset of his illness.

We must also discuss his substance use. Ted's alcohol use, quiescent for years, flared up again with psychosis. How should we regard it? Using strict diagnostic criteria (not invariably the best practice, we should note), we might be hard pressed to make a diagnosis of alcohol use disorder. But because it's vital to acknowledge his recent difficulty with alcohol, I'd go right ahead and make the diagnosis anyway, regardless of the number and severity of his current symptoms. We can temper our decision by adding verbiage to indicate that the substance use is recurrent and of short duration. The purpose of diagnoses is to convey as much information as possible, and Ted's clinicians need to know that they must contend with more than just psychosis. Of course, we'll list the alcohol diagnosis second; when psychosis is a factor, it will usually demand our attention first.

Comment

Half or more of psychotic patients will have additional diagnoses. The problem is that psychosis presents a picture so dramatic that we sometimes forget to address any leftover symptoms. Besides substance misuse, we need to keep alert for indications of depression, panic disorder, and several personality disorders.

Jeannie

It's hard to sort out depression in the context of psychosis. There are at least three different constructs to think about—psychotic depression, schizophrenia with depression, and schizoaffective disorder. I've put the information into Table 13.2.

> When I was a medical student, I evaluated a very bright woman who had an MBA and worked in her city's financial district. Always in perfect health, now she had been admitted for her first mental hospitalization ever because of a suicide attempt. After several weeks there, she was still completely miserable.
>
> A little over a year earlier, just after her 26th birthday, Jeannie had begun to suspect that someone at work was spying on her. She had no idea why this would happen, but she had noticed telltale signs—the handset on her desk telephone was replaced pointing the wrong way, and the file folders she maintained on her customers seemed in disarray. Becoming fearful, she drew inward; to keep an eye on her desk, she stopped going out to lunch with her coworkers.
>
> Even so, the signs kept cropping up. Soon Jeannie knew she was being followed: She repeatedly caught sight of the same car in her rearview mirror, and when she was out walking, passersby would wink or wave a folded newspaper to let her pursuers know which way she had gone. For several months she had also been hearing sounds. At first they were only creaking noises—"like a hangman's rope swinging a body," she explained—but lately she had perceived that there were words and now, sentences. "Mad, mad, mad," they mocked her, "Jeannie's gone forever mad."
>
> After her initial diagnosis of schizophrenia, Jeannie had done a great deal of reading about her illness. What she had learned had caused her to become despondent. She knew that she had a chronic illness; that it could be treated, but that it could nonetheless interfere with her work; and that it might even prevent her from marrying and

TABLE 13.2. Mood Symptoms in Psychosis

	Psychotic symptoms	Illness duration	Mood symptoms
Schizophrenia	Two types required	6 months or more	Not significant
Schizophreniform disorder	Two types required	Under 6 months	Not significant
Schizoaffective disorder	Two types required	1 month or more	Duration over half of total, but absent for 2 weeks
Mood disorder with psychosis	One type required	No lower limit	Always present
Delusional disorder	One type required	1 month or more	Not significant
Two disorders: mood and psychosis	Two types required	Depends on diagnosis	Always present

having children. These thoughts had haunted her for weeks; now she had a full-blown depression.

"I'm a chronic schizophrenic," she told me. Tears streamed down her face, which was becoming lined from worry, sleeplessness, and loss of weight. "I'm going to spend my life shut up in a hospital, fouling myself, and talking to phantoms. I'm hopeless. I'll be glad when I'm dead."

Two years later, I recently learned, she was.

Analysis

Confirming Jeannie's principal diagnosis is our first order of business. Once past steps 1–5 of Figure 13.1, we can agree right away that she had delusions *and* hallucinations. Although she had developed significant depressive symptoms, they weren't present when her psychosis began. (If we try hard, we might persuade ourselves that she had schizoaffective disorder, but it would only confirm the tendency of some clinicians to force patients into a favorite diagnosis. To me, her mood symptoms seemed relatively brief compared to the duration of the psychosis.) This analysis takes us through steps 6, 9, and 10, where a "yes" answer yields a consideration of schizophrenia.

Pursuit of her depression sends us through the Figure 11.1 decision tree, where we encounter a problem: It directs us through steps 7, 11, and 12 to consider schizoaffective disorder, which we've already discarded in the previous analysis. What gives? Perhaps we've learned a valuable lesson—that there are limitations to the decision tree method. We can agree that without a doubt, Jeannie had a lengthy psychosis and mood symptoms. But determining how these two concepts are related is problematic; it makes a real difference whether you regard mood symptoms or psychosis as the better point of departure. In Jeannie's case, the dilemma would be best resolved by diagnosing two comorbid disorders, schizophrenia and depression. This would allow a simplified view of her two sets of symptoms, each with its own treatment and prognosis. Jeannie's schizophrenia would be listed first, because its treatment was central: I believed—hoped—that once it was adequately addressed, her perspective on the rest of her life might improve, and her depression might lift. To be sure, this course contravenes the principle of parsimony; Occam would be outraged.

Comment

Depression in schizophrenia is poorly understood and inadequately studied. Postpsychotic depression has often been diagnosed when a bipolar depressive episode might be more appropriate, but even then we are left with many depressions to explain. Some patients with schizophrenia experience anhedonia; others have medication effects (especially from the older antipsychotics) that are experienced as depression. However, still others develop deep depressions that persist even after their psychotic symptoms have resolved. The fact that about 10% of patients with schizophrenia ultimately kill themselves—a rate second only to that found in the mood disorders—should prompt every clinician to watch carefully for developing depression in every such patient.

Brief Psychotic Disorder

For a few patients, psychosis is fleeting—a sort of mini-schizophreniform disorder. Over the decades, such illnesses have received a variety of different names, including *brief reactive psychosis* (discarded because clinicians couldn't agree what constitutes an appropriate precipitant). The category of *brief psychotic disorder* now incorporates postpartum psychosis (but not postpartum mood disorder with psychosis—keep that straight if you can). A single psychotic symptom can qualify a person for brief psychotic disorder, but recovery must occur within 1 month. Because of the requirement for ultimate recovery, this is not a diagnosis you can make prospectively. If the patient has been ill for a month, it is already too late for this diagnosis. You can read a case history in *DSM-5-TR Made Easy,* by an author known to both of us. With both schizophreniform disorder and brief psychotic disorder, what's important is that the patient's prognosis is better than that for schizophrenia.

Shared Psychotic Disorder

Sometimes called *folie à deux,* shared psychotic disorder is a condition so rare that it still elicits case reports in journals. These people are not psychotic in their own right. They only develop delusions in the context of close association with someone else (such as a parent or spouse) who is independently psychotic with, say, schizophrenia or delusional disorder. Then the second person also becomes psychotic, pretty much buying into the first person's delusions. To an extent, the devotees of religious cults occupy this same boat, believing often impossible stories fed them by leaders.

Some of these leaders may themselves be psychotic, as was probably true of Marshall Applewhite, who founded the Heaven's Gate cult. In 1997, seeking to shed their earthly husks and follow the trail of the Hale–Bopp comet, 38 of Applewhite's followers killed themselves with poisoned pudding in tiny, upscale Rancho Santa Fe, California. Other leaders may have personality disorders or other mental issues. Some writers believe that shared psychotic disorder isn't really a specific illness at all, but a phenomenon in some way attached to psychotic illnesses. This was one of the factors (another was rarity) that caused DSM-5 to reclassify *folie à deux* as a delusional disorder.

Whether it's a phenomenon or a mental illness, the belief can only be maintained when the two people involved are relatively isolated from others. Once they are segregated from one another, the independently ill person continues to maintain the psychotic symptoms, whereas the second patient develops insight that the beliefs were untrue all along.

Don't expect to encounter this condition often. If you find an example, look for comorbid intellectual disability, dementia, or depression in the second person. And start writing: Somewhere, a journal editor will probably be interested in publishing it. If not, send it along to me; I'll be fascinated.

Distinguishing Schizophrenia from Other Causes of Psychosis

Schizophrenia is such an important diagnosis, with consequences so devastating for patients and their families, that I want to make sure I've fully impressed on readers the features that set it apart from other causes of psychosis. That's the job of the sidebar "Differentiating Schizophrenia from Other Psychoses."

Differentiating Schizophrenia from Other Psychoses

I thought it would be useful to collect in one place the characteristics that we use to decide when a patient might have schizophrenia, as opposed to other causes of psychosis. Of course, none of the characteristics I have mentioned is absolute. For example, a patient could be young, have a gradual onset, have a positive family history, and *still* turn out to have a psychosis due to the use of cocaine. But on the whole, these are the factors that we should look at in our evaluation of psychosis.

- *Age.* Schizophrenia tends to develop in teenagers and young adults.
- *Marital status.* Patients with schizophrenia are often unmarried.
- *Onset.* Schizophrenia develops slowly; other psychoses are often more rapid.
- *Family history.* As you'd expect, patients with schizophrenia are more likely than average to have relatives with schizophrenia.
- *Drug/alcohol history.* Such a history is less likely in schizophrenia (though these patients may well use drugs and alcohol later on).
- *Confusion.* Perplexity and confusion are associated with eventual recovery in patients with schizophreniform disorder.
- *Premorbid personality.* Some patients with schizophrenia have schizoid or schizotypal personalities before they develop delusions or hallucinations.
- *Affect.* Patients who eventually recover from their psychoses may, while ill, have affect that is neither flat nor blunted.
- *Hallucinations.* Patients with schizophrenia tend to have hallucinations that are auditory; hallucinations of other senses suggest there might be a different diagnosis.
- *Delusions.* Bizarre delusions (things that couldn't really happen, such as being able to direct the world's air traffic by thought waves) suggest schizophrenia; mood-congruent delusions (guilt during depression, grandiosity during mania) suggest mood disorder.

14 Diagnosing Problems of Memory and Thinking

When you think logically about it, there's a lot that's illogical about thinking. We may block out thoughts inconvenient to our line of argument; go off on tangents; allow the intrusion of irrelevancies and rude images; and adhere to prejudices and ill-formed rules rather than to reason. Read the verbatim transcript of, say, a politician speaking off the cuff, and try to count the verbal blind alleys, untangle the twisted syntax, and nail down the indefinite relative pronouns. Yet none of the myriad infelicities of everyday speech indicates much in the way of psychopathology—beyond talking too much while thinking too little.

Cognition refers to the processes we use to involve all of our perceptions and sensations in planning. A person with a cognitive disorder could have problems in several areas, including judgment, memory, orientation, problem solving, language, interpersonal relationships, and *praxis* (doing things). We've already seen how abnormalities in the content of thought—hallucinations, delusions, and phobias, for example—can point to a wide variety of mental illnesses. Although a disturbance in the process of thinking occasionally occurs in schizophrenia or mania, more often it points to a cognitive disorder: delirium, dementia, and their variants. (Newcomers to the sometimes arcane world of mental health nomenclature will have to learn specific definitions of terms that are used in a far more generic sense. For nearly 400 years, *delirium* has meant a state of wild frenzy or excitement; *demented* has been long understood to describe someone who is crazed, mad, or infatuated.) Table 14.1 presents the differential diagnosis for disorders of memory and thinking. It incorporates changes in thinking and nomenclature introduced by DSM-5 in 2013. One of the most noteworthy is the introduction of the term *neurocognitive disorders* to cover the entire waterfront of dementia and delirium. In a bit, we'll talk more about the new terms and update definitions of the old ones.

The term *cognitive* often implies the need for some sort of testing, but we need to be able to recognize a disorder on clinical grounds. Very often, the first symptoms that show up are abrupt changes in personal-

TABLE 14.1. Differential Diagnosis with Brief Definitions for Disorders of Cognition

- *Delirium.* Substance use or physical illness causes a rapidly developing, fluctuating state of reduced awareness.

- *Neurocognitive disorder.* Substance use or medical illness affects functions such as thinking and remembering, interacting socially, using language, organizing and carrying out behavior, perceiving and navigating the environment, and focusing on tasks (attention). Neurocognitive disorder (NCD) can be *major* (it interferes with life in important ways); then it's synonymous with *dementia*. When the patient can compensate, perhaps by keeping lists or using other memory tricks, we say that the NCD is *mild*.

- *Amnestic disorder.* Substances and sickness cause profound memory loss, especially the ability to form new memories. Left intact are general intelligence, ability to focus attention, and ability to learn new tasks (though not new events, ideas, or words). No longer a stand-alone diagnosis, DSM-5-TR calls it major NCD.

- *Major depression with pseudodementia.* A person develops depression so severe as to have apparent (though reversible) problems with memory and thinking.

- *Dissociative disorders.* Profound, though temporary, loss of memory can occur in people who have dissociative amnesia (with or without fugue), or dissociative identity disorder.

- *Posttraumatic stress disorder (PTSD).* Amnesia for important features of a horrific traumatic event can affect these patients, who repeatedly relive the event and experience avoidance and hyperarousal.

- *Postconcussional disorder.* For days or weeks after a head injury that produces loss or alteration of consciousness, a person experiences deficits of memory or attention, plus such symptoms as headache, dizziness, fatigue, mood shifts, personality change, sleep disturbance, and loss of spontaneity. In DSM-5-TR, it would usually be termed a mild NCD due to traumatic brain injury.

- *Blackout.* Heavy alcohol drinking produces subsequent loss of memory for the time the person was intoxicated but awake.

- *Age-related cognitive decline (ARCD).* An older patient worries about trouble remembering things when memory ability, upon testing, is not pathological but perfectly normal for current age. Though it isn't mentioned in DSM-5-TR, it's a useful term for speaking with patients. Sometimes it's called subjective cognitive decline.

ity, interest, or behavior. Circumstances can enhance our recognition: We suspect dementia in hospital or nursing home patients or in those who are older; we look for delirium in postoperative patients and those who drink or use drugs. The *majority* of terminally ill patients will at some time experience delirium! However, we may recognize it less readily in a routine office patient—or the neighbor next door.

Whatever the circumstances, whichever symptoms need evaluating, you should ideally observe the patient on multiple occasions to learn whether the condition fluctuates, as with delirium, or is constant, as with dementia. Your persistence will pay off if you can ameliorate even in some small way the potential havoc wreaked by disorders of cognition, which substitute confusion for clarity and randomness for reason, while reducing what was once personhood to a shell of humanity.

Delirium and Dementia

It is sometimes hard even to identify a cognitive syndrome, let alone to determine its cause. We clinicians must keep in mind a whole range of possible diagnoses, including multiple diagnoses from a differential list.

Bobby

When Bobby is first admitted as an emergency case, no one even knows his name. Two police officers found him wandering on the street, talking to himself and breathing heavily. He didn't seem to know where he was. His face was swollen and he seemed feverish, so they coaxed him into the back seat of their squad car.

At first the emergency room personnel have no history at all; Bobby has apparently lost his wallet, and the envelope they find in his shirt pocket must have belonged to someone else. The doctor doesn't think he's been mugged, because he has no bruises and isn't bleeding, and the physical exam shows no evidence of a blow to the head. His temperature is nearly 104ºF; once in a while he coughs without bringing up much sputum.

Bobby is put into isolation and given some intravenous fluids. Although his gaze wanders as he talks, after a few hours he can speak clearly enough to state where he works; a call established his identity and a home phone number. By the time Clint, his partner, arrives, Bobby is conversing quietly with two women in clown suits whom no one else can see.

Bobby has no history of head injury. In fact, just a couple of days earlier, he seemed a healthy gay man who always takes precautions; he and Clint have both repeatedly tested negative for HIV. The following day, however, microscopic examination of a tracheal washing sample reveals *Pneumocystis carinii*. Bobby has pneumonia, probably due to AIDS.

Once the crisis passes, Bobby is started on a drug cocktail. His T4 cells are low, but his vital signs are normal; he can now walk and exercise without panting. However, Bobby isn't himself. He doesn't return to work, just sits at home watching TV. "He hated it before," Clint observes. Always an attentive and loving friend and partner, now he'll often ignore Clint's attempts at conversation. Once forever busy around the house, he becomes more or less permanently idle, and he doesn't seem to care. He even wears the same socks several days in a row. "He says he's forgotten where he keeps his clean pairs. He's always been so fastidious."

Clint becomes seriously alarmed when he notices that his partner complains of feeling weak and has trouble tying his shoes; this prompts Bobby's final hospitalization.

Analysis

For the first few hours after admission, before the lab results were in and an adequate history could be obtained, Bobby's diagnosis should be "undiagnosed mental disorder." With available data, however, his story suggests two disorders, approximately demarcated by the time of his hospital discharge. During the first, acute episode, he appeared terribly ill and confused. His gaze shifted around the room, and he was alternately alert enough to give vital information and so sick he saw phantom clowns. These symptoms are classic for a delirium (step 1 of Figure 14.1, the decision tree for a patient with cognitive problems). At this point the problem becomes one of determining cause. Because Bobby used neither alcohol nor street drugs, substance use seems unlikely, but the clinician would be right to get blood and urine samples for toxicology. In time, testing would yield the answer.

The testing and hospital stay resolved his immediate difficulties, but Bobby's troubles had only begun. His subsequent history requires a second ascent of the decision tree. Bobby had no history of alcohol use, which gets us past step 3, but wait a minute! What about step 2? Couldn't some of his symptoms, such as reduced interest and activity, be construed as depression? Of course, and at some point his clinician might need to evaluate him for a depressive disorder secondary to a medical condition. But here Occam's razor loses its edge: A mood disorder wouldn't begin to explain the breadth of his cognitive symptoms. And, either of the mood disorder decision trees (Figures 11.1 and 11.2) immediately raises the question of a significant medical condition.

With no history of head injury, we can continue to step 5 of Figure 14.1.

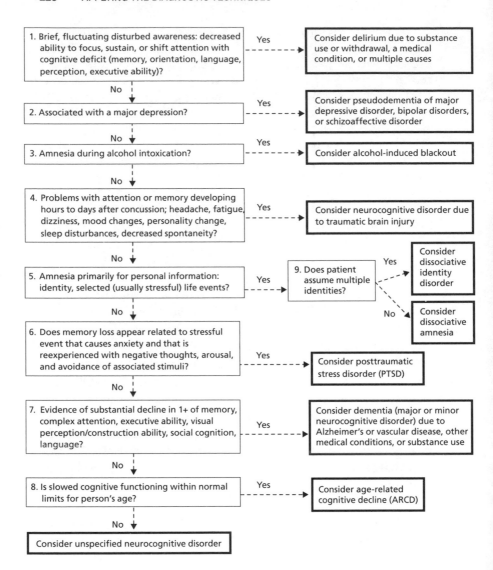

FIGURE 14.1. Decision tree for a patient who has problems with attention or memory loss.

Bobby's memory deficiency wasn't just for personal information, such as his address or stressful events in his life; he even had trouble finding his socks, which carries us past step 6 to step 7. No either/or about it: He clearly had substantial difficulty learning new information as well as recalling previously learned material. In addition, his social awareness had slipped (besides his unchanged socks, he was inattentive to Clint's conversation). All of this moves us to vote "yes" at step 7 to consider dementia, aka major neurocognitive disorder (NCD). The most likely underlying cause would be his HIV. However, before making any final diagnosis, we should obtain a careful neurological evaluation. We'd also want a baseline MMSE or other cognitive test, in order to follow the progress of his condition. (See the sidebar "Do I Need Scales?")

Comment on Delirium

Acute onset (often occurring within a few hours), wandering attention, and fluctuating levels of awareness amply suggest delirium. When they occur,

Do I Need Scales?

Flounders and flutists require scales; for those at other evolutionary stages, the need is relative.

When I was in training, Rorschach inkblots and the Minnesota Multiphasic Personality Inventory were about the extent of tests available, and we used almost no scales at all. Then came the Beck and Hamilton depression inventories, and mental health measurement was off to the races. Now you can find an objective measure for just about any imaginable aberration of thought, behavior, or emotion. If you used them all, you'd spend most of your working life filling out and scoring scales.

Of course, if you're doing clinical research, scales provide the numbers with which you determine change in your patient's symptoms. But most of them don't do much more than formalize the MSE. For many clinical tasks, we can accomplish about the same thing by asking our patients to rate their own discomfort or progress on a 10-point scale from "none" (or "very mild") to "maximum."

However, scales occasionally have great value. For example, many cognitively impaired patients cannot reliably judge how they are feeling or how impaired they are. The Mini-Mental State Exam (MMSE) developed by Folstein and colleagues (and quickly available with an internet search) provides evidence of how these patients are doing, so that we can follow them over time.

hallucinations are usually visual and often quite frightening; however, Bobby's only bemused him. A delirious person's mood may also change rapidly from depressed to anxious, irritable, fearful, or even euphoric. Whereas Bobby's activity level declined and he became quiet, other patients with delirium become loud and hyperactive. Such a patient may be more readily recognized, because their noise and intrusiveness demand attention and motivate caregivers to exert greater diagnostic effort. Of course, some patients will show both states at different points in an illness—another demonstration of the fluctuation that defines delirium. You can see why a single assessment often isn't sufficient to make the diagnosis, and why clinicians often miss it. Delirium can be especially difficult to diagnose when it exists in a context of dementia. Information from relatives or nursing staff may improve the rate of early diagnosis.

Delirium affects 10% or more of medical inpatients, and perhaps three times that many acutely ill geriatric patients. It is a disorder with many causes: brain tumors and trauma; intracranial infections (besides HIV, there's meningitis and encephalitis, which can be caused by numerous infectious agents); infections elsewhere in the body; strokes; nutritional and vitamin deficiencies; and endocrine malfunctions. Besides alcohol and street drug intoxication or withdrawal (remember the classical delirium tremens of alcohol withdrawal), a number of medication types can produce delirium, especially in older patients. See Table 9.2.

Comment on Dementia

Diagnosing dementia is fraught with error, and there are many ways to go wrong. Early on, you can stumble over those everyday *normal* annoyances that affect all of us—forgetting appointments and trouble recalling a familiar name, to name two foremost in my own experience. Many such episodes form a part of what some of us call *age-related cognitive decline* (ARCD, discussed later in this chapter), in which an older person complains of how long it takes to process information. If other cognitive processes—such as attention, verbal fluency and other language functions, memory, and ability to make decisions—remain essentially unaffected, it isn't dementia setting in, but just one more spice in the stew of advancing age.

People with actual dementia don't often spontaneously express feelings of marked unhappiness, but if anyone had asked Bobby whether he felt depressed, he might have agreed—though perhaps he'd only be trying to cooperate. If you learn from caregivers that the main complaints are apathy, reduced energy, and poor concentration, but the person doesn't actually appear sad, the symptoms may well be due solely to dementia. Apathy or depression is fairly common among patients with dementia resulting from Parkinson's, Huntington's, and Wilson's diseases—and AIDS. These disorders are called *subcortical dementias,* because the site of their pathology is far beneath the cerebral cortex. (In Alzheimer's, a *cortical dementia,* depression is less common.)

Although language ability may be intact, the personalities of patients with subcortical dementia may change, especially as apathy, inertia, and decreased spontaneity set in. Often these changes in behavior and personality are what bring patients with dementia to clinical attention. Making a separate diagnosis of personality change in the context of a dementia is a matter of judgment; perhaps it might be justified if the personality change is obvious and clinically important, as when a patient becomes markedly hostile toward people of other ethnicities or loses sexual inhibitions.

In the past decade we've had to cope with more complexity yet, in that we must now consider people whose ability to think has slipped some—a little more than in the ARCD mentioned above—but not so much you'd say they had major neurocognitive disorder (NCD). DSM-5-TR classifies such individuals as having a *mild* NCD; the decline is much less, and although it may inconvenience them, they can muddle through by keeping lists, setting alarms, and using other devices to support functioning. The line between major and mild NCDs is relatively sharp; that between mild NCD and ARCD is fuzzy at best. And we're meant to understand that just because a person can be diagnosed today with mild NCD doesn't necessarily mean that there's a major one coming tomorrow.

Here are a couple of additional points in the differential diagnosis of dementia. Patients with schizophrenia can have difficulty thinking (recall that the old name for schizophrenia was *dementia praecox,* because of its early onset)—either in the acute throes of an episode or after months or years of illness—and many patients with NCD develop delusions or hallucinations. The age of onset, the presence or absence of a medical cause, and the fact that such patients usually don't become psychotic until well along in the course of their disease should clarify the differential. Although the cognitive functioning of people with intellectual disability is subnormal, there should hardly ever be confusion with dementia, which almost always begins far later in life and involves *deterioration* of former cognitive ability rather than a relatively fixed, lifelong incapacity.

Curley

Some patients with serious cognitive difficulties appear quite intact initially. If you speak with them for just a few minutes, you might not even realize that something is wrong.

> The students know that Curley had been a sailor for much of his adult life, and that drink and the devil had at last sought him out. For nearly 5 years, he'd been unable to work or even to care for himself. "I'll give you one more clue," the teacher concludes, just before knocking at Curley's door. "He hasn't hit his head."
>
> "Oh, hi, come on in." With a big smile, the middle-aged man in hospital pajamas welcomes the small group into his room. The teacher and Curley chat for a few minutes. They appear to be on pretty good terms, for they speak about a number of things that touch the lives of each. Just when they seem deep in conversation, the teacher excuses them all and leads the group back out into the hallway. After a few minutes, he knocks at the door again, and all reenter.
>
> "Hello! Come on in!" Curley beams and starts to shake hands all around.
>
> "Do you remember these people?" the instructor asks, gesturing at the class.
>
> "No, I don't think so—wait! It was last night, down in the piano lounge, wasn't it? We all had some drinks, right?" Curley rubs his hands and looks thoughtful. "We were drinking Michelob." He continues to chat for a while, describing the band, the grumpy waitress, the beer that had gone a little flat. Nothing in his tone or facial expression suggests that he is putting them on.
>
> Curley maintains good eye contact, and he seems to focus well on the conversation. When the clinician recites a list of three objects, Curley immediately repeats them all flawlessly. Minutes later, he can recall none of them.

Analysis

Although Curley's ability to retain new memories was at rock bottom, he could maintain his attention on the conversation—and, as he entertained visitors, he seemed perfectly aware of his surroundings and of social conventions. That carries us past step 1 of Figure 14.1. With no hint of depression, no head injury, and no recent alcohol intoxication (he'd been hospitalized for weeks), we can rule out depression, alcohol blackout, and concussion (steps 2, 3, and 4). At step 5 we reject the notion that his difficulty was limited to personal information—indeed, his ability to form any new memories had pretty much disappeared. No suggestion of a major trauma means that we've ducked step 6. Although Curley's other cognitive functions seemed intact, we have enough information to consider (step 7) a major NCD, aka dementia—due, with a high degree of probability, to his past use of alcohol.

A couple of decades ago, Curley's diagnosis would have been amnestic disorder, but DSM-5-TR folds it into the general category of neurocognitive disorder. Along the way, we've vindicated the diagnostic principle that substance use should always be considered.

Comment

Farther back than the DSMs, Curley's condition was known as Korsakoff's psychosis (aka Korsakoff's dementia or Korsakoff's syndrome), named for the Russian psychiatrist who first described it in 1889. It has also been called Wernicke–Korsakoff syndrome. Are there reasons other than historical that it (by whatever name) deserves to be singled out? When you think about it, the relative lack of additional cognitive problems does rather set it apart from other forms of dementia. I say *relative,* because these patients are often apathetic, and their conversation tends to be superficial. Although Curley had no obvious defect of language symbolism or motor behavior, testing might have revealed more subtle difficulties with planning or carrying out the complex behaviors he'd require to prepare his own food, to shop, and to cope with other activities of daily living—activities we must all negotiate every day. In any event, there isn't always a sharp line between amnestic disorder and other forms of dementia.

This form of dementia is caused by damage within the brain's *limbic system*—the structure responsible for new learning that lies curled beneath the cerebral cortex, looking somewhat like a hand clutching a golf ball. The damage is done by thiamine deficiency or by oxygen deprivation (perhaps itself caused by carbon monoxide poisoning or surgical misadventure), or by any of the other usual suspects: traumatic brain injury, strokes, tumors, alcohol, or sedatives/hypnotics such as benzodiazepines and barbiturates. To my way of thinking, Korsakoff's syndrome is worth keeping distinct, if only to remind us of the importance of thiamine in treating some patients with dementia.

When Curley "remembered" that they had all been drinking in the bar the night before, he was trying to compensate for some of the holes in his memory; perhaps they worried him. In any event, such behavior, called *con-*

fabulation, isn't lying (Curley believed what he said), and it isn't delusional (it tends to come and go, evoked by the needs of the moment). Confabulation isn't specific to amnestic disorder. Probably caused by frontal lobe damage, it is just a way that people who cannot remember things sometimes paper over their difficulties with a tissue of desire and habit. With time, it tends to melt away. Indeed, for some patients whose limbic systems are only temporarily out on a limb (so to speak), memory may gradually return if they embrace good nutrition and avoid the drugs or alcohol that have caused the amnesia in the first place.

Other Cognitive Disorders and Comorbidity

Making a diagnosis when there are symptoms of only one disorder can be relatively easy. It is at least as easy to make the wrong diagnosis when a patient has symptoms and signs of more than one illness. Then the differential diagnosis and the decision tree serve an especially vital function, though you need familiarity with the features of both (or all) diagnoses.

Aunt Betty

A few weeks before Betty's 80th birthday, her niece, Gail, brings her to a family practitioner for evaluation. Betty lived with her older brother until his death a month earlier. From almost that day she has been "failing," losing interest in her hobby (she loves to decorate cakes) and complaining that she "just can't do anything anymore." The doctor talks to her for a few minutes; asks her the date (she says she doesn't know) and the name of his long-time nurse (Betty doesn't respond); and prescribes 5 mg/day of donepezil. She is becoming senile, he tells Gail. The medication, specific for people with early dementia, might help to slow its progress, though nothing can alter the eventual outcome. Because Betty also complains bitterly of feeling sad, she is started on amitriptyline (50 mg at bedtime).

Over the next 3 weeks, things rapidly go from bad to worse. Aunt Betty retreats even further into herself; several times her niece finds her lying on her bed, crying. She neglects her appearance and needs help tying the high-top, lace-up shoes she has worn since she was a teenager. Because she is still having trouble getting to sleep, her doctor doubles the antidepressant. Gail learns that the troubles with buttons and shoes are *apraxias,* symptoms of increasing dementia. A fortnight later, Betty is still sleepless, but now she is also agitated—

plucking at her clothing, mumbling something about beetles and wasps, and unable to give coherent answers to questions.

That afternoon, Gail checks Betty into the mental health clinic for a second opinion. There, after 2 hours of assessment and after consultation with her family practitioner, she is taken off all of her medications. Three days later, a calmer Aunt Betty is examined again. At first she has a hard time with the MMSE, several times stating that she can't do the task, but the clinician patiently encourages her to an eventual score of 26 out of 30. When asked whether she can tie her shoe, she again claims at first that she cannot. "Well, just give it a try, anyway," is the response. And with that, she manages just fine.

Analysis

As with several of our other patients, we need to consider Betty's diagnosis at different points in time. "But," you might argue, "with any patient, what we want to know is the diagnosis *now*." Very true, but that often means sifting through information that derives from different time periods and may point to a variety of ills. Nowhere is this process more vital than for someone who has symptoms of both dementia and depression.

When she came to the mental health clinic, Betty's condition had deteriorated. Her loss of concentration and her problems with language (mumbling) and perception (picking bugs off her clothing) strongly suggested a delirium (step 1 of Figure 14.1), which was probably precipitated by the amitriptyline—an older antidepressant notorious for this complication in elderly patients. But what about her diagnosis just before she was treated? For that, we need another quick trip to the tree—where step 2 warns us to give precedence to the depression (of which she had many symptoms) and to consider that her symptoms might indicate a pseudodementia.

Once off medication, Betty's delirium improved—but her depression had worsened. It had lasted longer than you'd expect for uncomplicated bereavement, so she was started on an SSRI antidepressant drug. Within a few weeks, she was once again cheerfully decorating cakes for her neighbors. Her final diagnosis was major depressive disorder.

Comment

Pseudodementia is a slight misnomer: The dementia is real, but it's reversible. It is a diagnosis often made only in retrospect—a great tragedy if some other dementia is erroneously diagnosed first. Because actual dementia resides at or near the bottom of the safety hierarchy, it is vital to defer this diagnosis until all the data are in. And by the way, search the DSMs and you won't find a category for pseudodementia: The DSM-5-TR definition of neurocognitive disorder specifically excludes patients who have a mood disorder that could be causative. The best you can do is diagnose a severe mood disorder and in the summary add—in tall print—verbiage relevant to the symptoms masquerading as dementia.

Depressive pseudodementia is rather common; by one estimate, it occurs in perhaps 10% of older patients suspected of being demented. They may complain of memory loss (not the case for most people with actual dementia) and may even emphasize it, while objective tests show no signs. These people may be distractible, may be slow to respond to stimuli, and may have short attention spans. "I don't know" and "Can't remember" responses are common, though it isn't clear whether such answers are found more often in depressive pseudodementia than in people who have actual major NCD. Risk factors for pseudodementia include a previous history of clinical mood disorder, recent bereavement, and family history of mood disorder. Therefore, getting information from relatives can be enormously helpful in making the correct diagnosis.

Onset is relatively rapid (weeks to a few months), and patients complain of guilt, suicidal ideas, vegetative symptoms—and poor memory. Patients with pseudodementia are especially prone to problems with decreased libido, early morning awakening, and anxiety, whereas patients who have true NCD more often experience disorientation to time, trouble finding their way around the streets, and problems dressing. Table 14.2 lists some of the other features that can help discriminate dementia from depression.

An even more difficult conundrum is the patient who has both an organic ("real") dementia and clinical depression. This will often be the case; perhaps 10–20% of patients with NCD have some degree of depression. You might recognize depression in such a person on the basis of a rapid decline with precipitous loss of general interest, vegetative symptoms (such as insomnia, poor appetite, and weight loss), ideas of worthlessness, and psychomotor slowing that is even greater than in dementia alone.

There's a moral here: Depression and dementia aren't mutually exclusive; we must pursue each one independently. An older patient who has symptoms of either depression or dementia should be considered for both. You need to search for symptoms of depression, even in the face of cognitive disorder.

TABLE 14.2. **Features of Dementia versus Depression with Pseudodementia**

	Dementia	Pseudodementia
Onset	Months–years	Weeks–months
Time of day when illness tends to be worse	Evening	Morning
EEG, brain scans	Abnormal	Normal
Family history of mood disorder	Less likely	More likely
Past personal history of depression	Less often	More often
Social skills intact	No	Yes
Self-blame	No	Yes
Shows concern or distress	No	Yes
Makes good effort at tasks	Yes	No
Cognitive disability	Hides	Emphasizes
Memory improves with coaching	No	Yes
Orientation intact	No	Variable

Wilma

The following vignette illustrates the importance of careful inquiry about each patient's history of medical problems, including illnesses, operations, allergies, and injuries.

> When Wilma finally sees the consultant, she has been suffering for several weeks, and her mother has suffered right along with her. Wilma complains that she cannot sleep; when she gets up in the morning, she is almost unbearably grouchy. "It's a real change for her," says her mother with a sigh. "For her first 17 years, she was the sweetest-tempered thing you could imagine. All my friends with teenage daughters were envious. Now *I'm* the envious one—you'd think she's had a personality transplant."
>
> For Wilma, the main difficulty is headache, which bothers her pretty much the whole day. Combined with the dizziness and persistent tiredness, it is trashing her concentration for schoolwork. She's sure she isn't depressed; they'd studied that in the health class she'd taken the previous semester. However, her memory has been "pretty bum—I couldn't even remember my teacher's name when I went for my piano lesson."

"Have you had any other problems with your health?" the mental health clinician wants to know.

She has had. Several months earlier, against her mother's wishes, Wilma went motorcycle riding with her boyfriend—Frank, that was it. She'd done so before and knew he was a safe driver, but they hadn't reckoned on the patch of black ice at that sharp curve on the mountain road. She'd worn a helmet, but not Frank, an enthusiastic member of the local anti-helmet-law association. He won't be attending meetings for a while, she agrees, not until he emerges from his coma.

After the crash, Wilma was unconscious for nearly an hour. She never could recall riding with Frank that day, and her memory of waking up on the gurney, unsure where she was, is tinged with the sensation of nausea.

Analysis

If her mother's initial impressions had been prime consideration, Wilma might have been subjected to a battery of personality tests. Fortunately, her clinician recognized the need for a complete history. Because we don't think that Wilma had a severe depression and she wasn't currently delirious (though she might have been immediately after the accident), we can quickly bypass steps 1–3. That brings us to the all-important step 4, which encourages us to consider a DSM-5-TR diagnosis of (mild) NCD due to traumatic brain injury. This was formerly called *postconcussional disorder* and was included in DSM-IV as a provisional diagnosis requiring further study. For simplicity's sake, I will continue to use the older term.

Comment

About 5% of adults report a lifetime history of concussion—a blow to the brain that results in unconsciousness or other dysfunction. Mostly, damage is to the frontal lobes, caused when the front of the brain slams against the inside of its hard protective carrying case. Motor vehicle accidents account for a large percentage, but it is also found in football players, shaken babies, and people who fall from ladders. The vast majority of concussions are mild—a brief lapse of awareness or a passing state of altered consciousness when things just don't seem right (the "stars and planets" of the cartoon pratfall).

Concussion almost always produces some degree of amnesia, though it may last only moments. The return to normal is usually rapid and complete. Many people don't need hospitalization; those who do may be off work for a few days, with the vast majority recovered within 3 months. But for weeks or months, a few will continue to have symptoms that constitute postconcussional disorder, which only in the past decade has been given full recognition as neurocognitive disorder.

These patients (their name is legion) have problems with memory or attention, often accompanied by headache, nausea, dizziness, and fatigue. Apathy, insomnia, irritability, anxiety, and (rarely) psychosis can occur. Personality change may be rather mild, like Wilma's, but increased sexuality or other socially inappropriate behavior may also occur. Unlike Wilma, 20% or more experience depression, especially if they use alcohol or drugs, haven't had much education, or have an unstable preinjury work history. If the depression is severe enough to diagnose independently, regard it as you would any other mood disorder.

Postconcussion NCD usually resolves spontaneously. After 3 months of continuing symptoms, we would need to worry about a possible subdural hematoma. Of course, the other cognitive disorder in the differential list is dementia (major NCD) due to traumatic brain injury, which requires the severe injury of motor vehicle accidents or boxing and usually includes neurological abnormalities such as hemiplegia or aphasia.

Cognitive Problems That Are Not Disorders

Usually, differential diagnosis is a matter of deciding among competing illnesses. We sometimes forget to consider another important boundary.

Reggie

In 1994 Ronald Reagan was diagnosed with Alzheimer's disease and announced that he was entering "the journey that will lead me into the sunset of my life." Years later, Reggie goes to see his family practitioner. "I've noticed some things that worry me," he announces. "A lot. I'm afraid I could be getting Alzheimer's."

Just a couple of months earlier, at 63, he'd had a raise and had advanced to a new level of responsibility, even though he secretly plans to retire in a year. Reggie admits that he had begun to slow down a bit. "Well, a lot," he amends.

Reggie has always been a little forgetful of where he's put things. But now it seems to happen distressingly often. When he is deep in thought about his work, any interruption requires moments to shift gears. And it takes forever to dredge up the names of people he's known for years. "My wife says I'm as sharp as ever," he concedes, "but she could be just trying to, um . . . " He breaks off, searching for the word he wants.

"Reassure you?" offers the interviewer.

"That's it. You see, that's what I've been experiencing for months."

Although Reggie feels "pretty anxious" at times about his memory, he's had no panic attacks, and he denies depression or worry related to other issues. Aside from the usual indignities that accompany advancing age, his health has always been good and he's had no injuries. He does drink a glass of wine nearly every day "to help keep up the good cholesterol." A physical exam is completely normal, and he scores a perfect 30 on the MMSE.

Analysis

Experienced mental health professionals might initially suspect a disorder of depression or anxiety, but trips with Reggie through Figures 11.1 and 12.1 don't yield much. And so it would seem at first with Figure 14.1: Reggie showed no evidence of fluctuating levels of consciousness that would suggest a delirium, no depression, and no evidence of either head injury or alcohol misuse. Of course, his clinician should attempt to obtain collateral information on each of these points, but he would seem to be all clear through step 4. His memory lapses didn't rise to the level of amnesia, and they weren't limited to personal information. In fact, we can't say that he had much of any problem learning new information. With no history of mental stressors (absent the aging process itself, I can promise you), we're just about out of options at step 8. The results of the MMSE were comforting if not illuminating, and with his age and history, Reggie's doctor would have the information necessary to offer appropriate reassurance: nothing more than age-related cognitive decline (ARCD), mentioned earlier in this chapter and in Table 14.1. It doesn't imply that there is anything wrong. In other words, we've applied the diagnostic principle encouraging us to consider that a patient might just be normal (see the sidebar "How Many Ways Can We Say *Normal?*").

Comment

ARCD sounds worse than it is. It doesn't even involve, to any important degree, multiple areas of our thinking mechanism. The ability to recognize people and objects, to identify concepts, to perform motor functions, to use language—all these vital areas are preserved. The main difficulty

How Many Ways Can We Say *Normal?*

ARCD (age-related cognitive disorder) is one way of saying *normal,* in the context of a patient's complaint that something seems abnormal. As mental health professionals, we face this sort of situation every day, but how often do we realize it?

Too frequently perhaps, when we evaluate patients for psychological complaints, we feel obliged to "give them their money's worth"—in short, to make a diagnosis. It is better, and far more satisfying, to tell someone straight out, "There's nothing really wrong with you. You have a problem that we can work on together, but your mental health is fundamentally sound." Of course, we can always let it go at "no mental diagnosis," but that wastes information and does an injustice to the myriad people who come to us every day with problems of living. There are better ways.

A number of situations qualify as troubled but normal. Take relational problems, for example, in which members of a unit have trouble getting along with one another. Of course, the cause could be someone's mental illness, but many relational problems exist wholly without any diagnosable mental pathology. The relationships affected are about as varied as you can imagine: child–parent, friend, sibling, spousal, employee–supervisor, workmates. Another normal, if troubled, state is bereavement, a reaction to the death of someone we love. I've discussed it in Chapter 11 (p. 162).

A couple of other terms that indicate normality are less benign. *Borderline intellectual functioning* indicates an IQ somewhere south of the mid-80s, though above the range of patients with intellectual disability and without their problems of living. *Malingering,* a pejorative term I employ only with great care, identifies individuals who intentionally concoct or exaggerate symptoms either to avoid something (work, punishment, or military service) or to obtain something—usually drugs or money, as from lawsuits. Such tangible motives are quite different from those of patients with *factitious disorder,* whose feigned illness may be to obtain medical care. I wouldn't dignify malingering by calling it normal, but neither is it a mental disorder.

For otherwise normal persons with academic, occupational, spiritual, or housing problems, or with difficulty in acclimatizing themselves to a culture different from that of their upbringing, you can use one of those terms (with *problem* tacked on) to give a label that doesn't carry the stigma of an actual mental disorder. For example, someone who's troubled by doubts about the choice of a career might be described as having an *occupational problem.* Finally, there's even a diagnosis for criminals who don't qualify for a personality disorder or other diagnosis: *adult antisocial behavior.* Think Tony Soprano.

is that as we age, and regardless of how smart we are or how educated we have become, the rate at which we process information tends to flag. It's an unhappy fact that DSM-5-TR hasn't seen fit to continue listing ARCD (it had a place in DSM-IV). We can still use the idea of ARCD, however, though it may give fits to the good folks who must apply codes to the stuff we write down.

Regardless of who sanctifies it, ARCD is a statement of normality. Because it isn't a disorder, there can be no criteria; it is a nondiagnosis of exclusion. You must rule out everything else by taking into consideration not just the person's chronological age, but lifelong capacities, educational achievement, general health status, and culture. Here's the good news: It means that nothing is really wrong, and that the person isn't necessarily headed for senescence. Here's the bad news: The situation probably won't improve, and it could get worse.

Jen

Some symptoms point the way to a mental health diagnosis; others do not. In deciding which is which, we must evaluate all symptoms in the context of the total patient. Loss of memory is such a symptom. We must take care not to jump to conclusions about its importance.

> The morning phone call is peremptory: "You've got to fit her in today—she's beside herself." That's Jen's mother. When she'd entered Jen's room this morning, she found her sobbing. "She thinks she's destroyed her mind."
>
> Just 19, Jen is in her second year at an Eastern university that has only recently begun admitting women. She lives at home, but has recently stayed many nights with friends on campus—female friends, her mother hopes. Last night, however, Jen attended an off-campus party thrown by a student she hardly knows. The mob of young people had consumed oceans of alcohol, both beer and hard liquor. Coming off a punishing week of final exams, Jen was ready to party; within minutes of arrival she'd downed several drinks. That was almost the last thing she remembers until this morning, when she awakened, naked and incredibly hung over, in a strange bed with a strange man and an even stranger woman. "I've never done anything like that before," Jen cries when she speaks with the therapist. "I know you can damage your brain with alcohol. I read about it in the psychology class I took last semester."
>
> Before this morning, she hasn't felt depressed or anxious, "but I

sure am now." Jen also doesn't think she hit her head; though it sure hurts like hell, she can't find any lumps or tenderness. She scores a perfect 30 on the MMSE, and apart from the crying, everything else about her seems unremarkable.

Jen admits that she is "pretty upset" by what she might have done while intoxicated: "I've had some experience, but I've been safe. And discriminating, I always thought." After crying some more, she adds, "I'm just so scared I've done something really awful to my brain."

Analysis

Jen's clinician would have to make sure that she hasn't sustained a concussion—common enough during alcohol intoxication, but something to think hard about in anyone who has suffered a period of amnesia. Her MMSE and her focused attention during the interview rule out delirium, and there is no evidence of dementia or a depression so profound as to suggest pseudodementia. In fact, the history points to an alcohol-induced blackout (step 3 of Figure 14.1). Although not an actual mental disorder, blackout is a rather commonplace experience that sometimes requires clinical evaluation.

Before leaving the figure, drop down to step 5. Could Jen's experience have been a dissociative phenomenon that was anxiety-driven? On the surface, this might seem to fit the definition of dissociative amnesia, but we must first rule out more obvious, physical causes before falling back on what some clinicians consider a faith-based diagnosis (see the next section, "Amnesia and Dissociation").

Comment

While blacked out, a person may continue to behave quite normally; it's just that the following day, when the person is sober, little or no memory of behavior remains. During blackouts, people may engage in a wide range of activities, including those as banal as office gossiping, as dangerous as driving, and as intrinsically memorable as having sex. Blackouts result from the effects of alcohol on the region of the limbic system (see p. 225) called the hippocampus. Though established memories remain unaffected, the formation of new memories is blocked. Blackouts can be partial or total; the greater the alcohol consumption, especially if it occurs rapidly, the more severely is memory impaired. However, there is no evidence that an isolated blackout implies anything permanently wrong.

When I was in school, we were told that blackouts were symptomatic of alcoholism, but in recent decades science has determined otherwise. In fact, studies now find that they are common among those who only drink socially—even among first-time drinkers. Perhaps 40% of college students who drink at all have had at least one blackout related to alcohol use. Women may be especially vulnerable to them; a strong minority of young people who drink (especially women) are frightened enough by blackouts that they moderate their drinking behavior. And that's not a bad thing: Despite the belief that they are benign, blackouts can foreshadow later difficulties with alcohol. Jen's experience should serve as a literal wake-up call to reevaluate her recreational choices.

Amnesia and Dissociation

Dissociation is a break in the connection between mental processes that normally occur together. The result is an abrupt, usually temporary change in the person's awareness, behavior, or identity, often with amnesia for the episode after it ends. My dictionary gives *amnesia* as a synonym for forgetfulness or loss of memory. Of course, there is also loss of memory in dementia, but then the defect is global and usually permanent. The amnesia of dissociation implies a gap that, like our hopes for the pothole at the corner, will one day be filled in. Indeed, this is the usual outcome of dissociation—temporary loss of memory that will recover within a period of days or weeks.

Quite frankly, I struggled for days about how to present this topic. Here is my quandary with this set of vexed diagnoses: Dissociation is nearly everywhere, yet it is almost nowhere. It is everywhere, in that it embraces the normal, everyday experiences we all have had, such as daydreaming or becoming so immersed in a magazine article or television program that we lose track of time. Hypnosis is a sort of dissociation often used to assist the treatment of surgical, dental, medical, and psychotherapy patients. Abnormal dissociation, on the other hand, has been identified in the affective blunting of schizophrenia and the numbing of sensation that patients with PTSD develop toward their traumatic experiences. It is also found free-standing, as in *depersonalization* (the sensation of being detached from your body) and *derealization* (the feeling that the world has changed or is not real).

Yet dissociation is also nowhere—almost. In my decades as a psychiatrist, I have rarely encountered someone with an unequivocal dissociative disorder. Some writers question the value of these disorders, which they claim cannot be reliably diagnosed and may be manufactured by credulous enthusiasts. Large series of dissociative patients tend to collect in centers that specialize in their treatment or in the clinics of individual practitioners who have written extensively about them. Like everyone else, clinicians tend to find what they look for.

It can be difficult indeed to resist the allure of the fascinating diagnosis. An interesting patient who wanders into urgent care, suddenly unable to remember vital material from the past, is ready-made for drama. The patient may be highly suggestible; perhaps there is a history of stress-induced pathology. Precipitated by physical, sexual, or other emotional trauma, the amnesia wipes out recall of specific events or time periods, whereas learning going forward is unaffected. The amnesia often departs as suddenly as it began—the happy Hollywood ending.

It is clear to me that, as outlined in Figure 14.1, some patients do lose memory functions temporarily due to dissociative disorders, but many clinicians have only read about them. In 2006 *The New Yorker* profiled such a patient, Doug Bruce, who after 2 years had still not regained his memory. Recent studies have reported that these patients may be underdiagnosed among mental health and general medical patients, so I have mentioned the categories here. But scrutinize your data and your conclusions.

Because few patients spontaneously report dissociative experiences, clinicians must ask: "Have you found yourself someplace and not known how you got there? Have you ever not recognized family or friends? Been unable to recall a span of your childhood or adult life? What about finding unfamiliar items among your belongings, or documents you must have written but cannot remember?" Of course, this sort of questioning risks suggesting symptoms to susceptible people. Carrying the error a step further, clinicians sometimes identify dissociation and then interrogate patients about any possible abuse—a possible cause—that may have occurred during childhood.

As a first diagnostic step, at least one authority advises ensuring that the patient's symptoms are genuine. (Recall Tony [pp. 37–39], the patient known for periodically being at odds with the truth, who claimed to have experienced a fugue state.) Although I hate to diagnose malingering, it is only right to point out that amnesia is the mental illness symptom most often malingered. You might want to review what I've written about it in Chapter 4. Oh, yes, and no one—well, hardly anyone—ever thinks to check the patient for somatizing disorders.

15 Diagnosing Substance Use and Other Addictions

Let me get something off my chest. We are sometimes warned against the term *addiction,* because it doesn't have a scientific definition. While factually true, the same can be said for so much of the mental health nomenclature that if we were to avoid all inexact terms, we'd find ourselves essentially tongue-tied. Depression, paranoia, phobia, anxiety, mania, schizophrenia—on the street and in the popular press—all have meanings rather different from their strict scientific usage.

The word *addiction* comes down from Roman law, where it meant "surrender to a master." How appropriate it is to use such a term for the behaviors we associate today with substance use and other compulsions! This compact term conveys a clear sense of loss of control with harm to the individual and to society. Other than lack of scientific rigor, its principal drawback is a connotation of reproach that we in the mental health field would rather avoid. (*Habit,* a term applied for over 100 years to the use of addictive drugs, has never been much favored by professionals, either.)

Substance Use Disorder

Over the past couple of decades, the terminology has shifted. Whereas from DSM-III on we spoke of *substance dependence* and *substance abuse* as two separate disorders, common sense has at last prevailed, and their criteria have been combined into one grand collation called *substance use disorder.* That term seems a little clumsy to me, however, so I'll probably continue to refer to people who have it as having *substance dependence,* for short. Substance dependence has three principal features:

1. The person will usually be affected physiologically. This means that the drinking or other substance use has been heavy enough and prolonged enough to cause *tolerance,* which is the need for an increased amount to satisfy craving (or a constant amount to avert

withdrawal), or *withdrawal,* in which symptoms develop when the person abruptly decreases its intake. Some people will experience both tolerance and withdrawal.

2. Loss of control is the second constant feature of substance use disorder. It is shown by using more than the person intends, repeated failure to control the use, preferring use to important activities such as family life, and persistent use despite the knowledge that it is either harmful to health or dangerous to the individual or others. I suppose I'd include craving for the substance here—DSM-5 and its successor, DSM-5-TR, are the first manuals to include it as a symptom (and about time!).

3. Finally, several social issues that are the consequence of use affect patients who misuse substances. These include a failure to fulfill important responsibilities, arguments and other interpersonal disputes, and excessive time spent obtaining or using the substance.

I wouldn't get too hung up over the exact number of criteria a person needs for dependence. Two or three symptoms is the range required in DSM-5-TR for a rating of *mild* substance use disorder, but it seems unlikely that many people with substance use problems will stop at 3. Left untreated, those with a few symptoms are highly likely to develop more.

Samuel

How we assess substance dependence is based on two sorts of criteria—the loss of control, and the consequences of use (including social, legal, financial, work, family, and physical/medical). Even though our current diagnostic tools have been forged in comparatively recent times, if we employ them carefully, they can help us mine the past to unearth the perils of the present. As I've noted above, our assessment of substance dependence is based on three sorts of symptom—physiological issues, loss of control, and numerous social and personal consequences of use. See how many of them you can identify in Samuel's history.

Every student of English literature knows that, as a young man, Samuel Taylor Coleridge wrote "The Rime of the Ancient Mariner." Somewhat less well known is how his personal history describes an almost lifelong dependence on opium.

In the waning years of the 18th century, when Samuel's use began, morphine, codeine, and heroin had not yet been derived, and opium was usually swallowed in an alcohol tincture called *laudanum*. Samuel used laudanum intermittently from his mid-20s, to enable sleep and ease both worry and pain. At that time the concept of addiction was little recognized, and anyone with a few shillings could readily purchase narcotics from a pharmacist—no prescription necessary. As an all-purpose remedy for homesickness, exhaustion, and the stress of public performance, Samuel used up to a pint of laudanum per day—a whopping amount by the standards of any era. He also consumed large amounts of alcohol.

Samuel's first serious problems with opium addiction arose in his late 20s. Although he composed his mystical poem "Kubla Khan" largely while under the influence of laudanum, on balance the drug caused him to spend far more time daydreaming of literary glory than working to attain it.

The physical symptoms that result from using opium are numerous and well documented. For Samuel, one of the worst was constipation—"violent stomach pains and humiliating flatulence"—that caused him such agony that for relief, he would resort to enemas and other embarrassments, which he regarded as punishment for his vice. With his mood swinging from elation to despair, he would awaken screaming from terrifying dreams. During a sea voyage, he hallucinated "yellow faces" in the curtain around his bunk, and he had the illusion that the flapping sails were fish flopping about on deck.

In his notebooks, Samuel also noted symptoms that we recognize today as withdrawal: joint pains, sweating brow, "windy sickness at the stomach," diarrhea, fever, and despair. No matter how often he promised himself that he would quit, in the end he always returned to opium's "hideous bondage"—the words of a friend—that left him brooding, lying, and neglecting his work and family. Guilt made him try to conceal the amount he used. In later life he wrote self-pitying letters to friends, whom he accused of misunderstanding him, and he suffered from depression that would suddenly well up and overwhelm him. At one time, he entertained thoughts of suicide.

In later years, Samuel's usage was eventually controlled when a physician put him on a limited prescription, but he sought additional supplies anyway. His druggist allowed him this excess—but in amounts so tiny that he could once again work effectively—and thrive.

Analysis

With a little effort, we can compare the symptoms Samuel showed over 200 years ago to today's criteria for substance use disorder. In Table 9.3, you'll note the symptoms of intoxication Samuel recorded. Next, we'll use the definition of dependence provided at the beginning of this chapter to verify that he was in fact dependent on opium.

From the amount of laudanum Samuel consumed, we know that he tolerated quantities far greater than an individual unaccustomed to its use could have handled, and of course he suffered severely from withdrawal symptoms. His use began when he was a young man and persisted throughout his life; along the way, we can find ample evidence of lack of control. From his own notes and letters, we can see how he craved the drug; he used it despite the evidence of its physical effects, allowed it to displace his work and social responsibilities, and continued using it despite repeated efforts to curtail its use. Even at over two centuries' remove, he fully meets modern criteria for severe opioid use disorder.

The use of multiple substances is common, and today, after a suitable in-depth interview, Samuel would probably be diagnosed as having both opioid and alcohol use disorders. But can we also say that he had a mood disorder? The profound gloom he experienced from time to time was severe enough that he had suicidal ideas; yet, because it seemed entirely consequent to his use of opium, I wouldn't call it an independent mental disorder (shaved by Occam's razor!). Instead, Figure 11.1 points us to a step 3 diagnosis of substance-induced depression.

Comment

One problem in assessing the misuse of substances is the reliability of the informant. In his case, that would be Samuel, who worked hard to hide the true extent of his addiction. I always want to trust my patients, but whenever I know that one may have strong motivation to defer, shade, or otherwise alter the truth, I look for help from trustworthy informants who care about the patient. (For Samuel, we have to read between the lines.) I'll also lean on objective measures such as laboratory tests, which were not available 200 years ago.

Substance misuse is often a story of comorbidity. Various studies have found that a third to a half of those who misuse substances have an additional mental diagnosis, whereas nearly 30% of patients with other mental disorders meet criteria at one time or another for a substance use disorder. Samuel's depression was related to his substance use, which is the usual case. In fact, nearly every class of mental disorder you can think of is more common in persons with substance dependence. Only infrequently, however, is the disorder one that they would have suffered anyway, regardless of their experience with alcohol or drugs. But these secondary disorders can closely mimic independent mental or emotional illnesses. In most cases, with time and abstinence, the secondary symptoms will abate.

Chuck

When evaluating substance use, it can be very difficult to decide whether a person's symptoms are all pursuant to the substance or indicate another, independent disorder. If the former, they should disappear once the misuse has been brought under control.

> At 38, Chuck sought care because of depression. "Life isn't very good, Doc," was his chief complaint. A tradesman who made good money when he worked, often Chuck didn't. June was the financial mainstay of their little household, but she was a bartender who too often sampled her own wares. She had sent along to the clinician a note—when Chuck handed it over, the envelope bore evidence of clumsy steaming and resealing—in which she complained how seldom she and Chuck had sex. He admitted that he had read a lot about alcohol and sexual problems; he'd tried Viagra, but realized it was drinking that had clobbered his sex drive. "Something to do with testosterone levels, Doc," he informed me. "You can read about it on the 'net at . . . " From memory, he recited a URL full of dots and slashes.
>
> Over the years, I've treated a lot of smart patients, but Chuck is the only one who'd actually passed the test and joined Mensa. However, he had never finished high school; after some suspensions (two for theft and one for assault on a teacher), they'd kicked him out. Now he claimed that the Mensa card made him feel that he "had substance."
>
> After leaving school, he kicked around for a time, then washed out of the Army after setting the boot camp record for times AWOL. Next he tried his hand at violent crime. Though he was pretty good at planning, he lacked the drive for effective execution. After he and a partner robbed a 7-Eleven that netted them $84 and several 6-packs, they were nabbed just around the corner as they consumed the liquid proceeds of their evening's work. After his release from prison, he wrote a few bad checks and ripped off several employers for some valuable tools, but for none of this was he ever caught.
>
> By the time Chuck turned 27 his drinking, which had started during his brief Army career, had picked up speed. He was downing nearly a 12-pack of beer each evening, a practice he carried to a series of jobs, none of which lasted longer than a month or two. Then he got married—twice, without bothering about a divorce in between. His first wife's complaints of nonsupport led to information about his other

activities, which landed him "back in the can" for another few months. But with his second marriage came a dowry of sorts—a father-in-law who was a union official in one of the construction trades. After a brief apprenticeship, Chuck seemed set for life with a job that paid well and carried enormous benefits. Currently, however, he was drinking more than he was working—at anything; even June was complaining.

Chuck told me that the feelings of depression had come on gradually, worsening over the past half year or so. Fueled by his drinking, he fought with June "whenever I was sober enough." His appetite was almost nil, his weight had begun to drop, and his sleep had long since gone south.

After an especially hard bender that lasted many weeks, Chuck needed hospitalization. During the admission process, he was unsteady on his feet and even had trouble writing his name. "I'm fine, I'm just terrific," he kept saying, but he slurred his words in a way that said he really wasn't. The next morning on rounds, I was sure of it. After a sleepless night, Chuck's problem with coordination had progressed to a coarse tremor that made him grip his juice glass with both hands.

By the following day, he was in full-blown withdrawal—sweating, pacing (when he wasn't falling down), and vomiting. He also complained about tiny cats "the size of mice" that wore bells that jingled as they danced on his windowsill. He thought that he was in a lockdown at the county jail. While still recovering, he talked about another time he'd been like this, when he was jailed after assaulting an undercover federal narcotics officer who was trying to track a suitcase full of powdered cocaine. "Do I have any regrets? Sure, I'm real sorry I got caught. Or *really* as we say in Mensa. But I don't feel guilty, if that's what you mean. Guilt is for suckers."

Analysis

In addition to his drinking and problems with the law, Chuck had three mental problems we need to discuss—depression, psychosis, and disorientation. Figures 11.1, 13.1, and 14.1 unanimously direct us to consider a disorder induced by substances. That would square with some of what we know about alcohol use disorder. People who drink heavily often have depression, and alcohol-dependent individuals in the throes of withdrawal will sometimes suffer from delirium tremens, during which they become disoriented and have visual hallucinations. In the vast majority of patients, without further treatment the depression disappears once the drinking stops. This was why, though I always give high priority to the diagnosis of depression, I elected to defer treating Chuck's depression.

What about his criminal behavior, and what did it say about his personality structure? Whereas I'd hesitate to offer an early diagnosis for most personality disorders, antisocial personality disorder rests firmly on objective facts that can be obtained from those who know the patient well. Chuck's long history of difficulties with authority and the law (dating to his early teen years, before he commenced to drink heavily), along with his callous lack of guilt, provided a strong basis for this diagnosis.

All things considered, I'd list Chuck's various diagnoses in the order they needed to be treated:

> Delirium due to alcohol withdrawal (delirium tremens)
> Alcohol use disorder
> Depression secondary to alcohol use
> Personality disorder, with antisocial features

Because Chuck was in the middle of his withdrawal symptoms, listing the delirium first underscores the importance of focusing on this potentially life-threatening condition. I believed that his depression had directly resulted from the drinking, so that it should diminish once he got clear of alcohol.

Comment

Close to half of those who misuse alcohol, street drugs, or prescription medications will have at least one additional mental disorder. Some conditions are more or less independent, but often (perhaps usually), the substance use disorder will bring on depression, psychosis, or an anxiety disorder; as such, they are not *truly* comorbid, only co-occurring. (See the sidebar "Independent Mental Disorder or Substance-Related?") We need to know which is which, because we will treat mental disorders that arise only during substance use differently from those that are independent. Outcome for the dependent disorders may be better or worse than for the independent ones, depending on how effectively we deal with the substance use itself.

Disorders Associated with Substance Use

Whether or not they represent independent diagnoses, some other disorders are commonly associated with substance use. Table 15.1 summarizes some of this discussion.

Independent Mental Disorder or Substance-Related?

In deciding whether a patient's mental disorder is substance-related or independent, I consider several issues:

1. If the other mental disorder started first, I would lean heavily toward independence—that is, an illness *not* caused by the substance use. Antisocial personality disorder, bipolar disorders, and schizophrenia are the conditions most likely to begin prior to substance use.
2. If it isn't clear which started first, I'd apply the diagnostic principle concerning *undiagnosed* and use either that label or *unspecified [name of condition]*, then carefully follow to see what happens once the substance use has been dealt with.
3. A substance-related mental disorder should diminish or disappear within a month. If the symptoms persist (perhaps even increase) after detoxification, I'd probably diagnose an independent mental disorder.
4. For an independent mental disorder, I like to see more symptoms rather than fewer, so as to fully meet (or exceed) diagnostic criteria for the illness in question.
5. I search for atypical symptoms. For example, the sudden onset of hallucinations, unusual for schizophrenia, suggests a psychosis cause that is related to other medical disorders or substance use. Visual, tactile, or olfactory hallucinations similarly suggest a nonschizophrenia psychosis.

• *Antisocial personality disorder.* This is one of the few co-occurring conditions that is *not* caused by the substance use. Over three-fourths of patients with antisocial personality disorder also misuse substances, and 10–20% of males and about 5% of females with alcoholism have this personality disorder. Some studies find that an especially heavy history of severe substance use carries a stronger likelihood of comorbidity, especially with antisocial personality disorder.

• *Neurocognitive disorders.* Delirium is found during intoxication with all substance groups except caffeine; alcohol and the sedatives also produce delirium upon withdrawal. A form of dementia can result from heavy and prolonged use of inhalants, and the dementia (it used to be called amnestic disorder) known as *Korsakoff's psychosis* is classic for heavy, prolonged alcohol use with chronic thiamine insufficiency. There's more about this on page 225.

TABLE 15.1. Classes of Mental Disorders That Can Occur during Intoxication (I) or Withdrawal (W)

	Delirium	Dementia[a]	Psychosis	Mood	Anxiety
Alcohol	I/W	Yes	I/W	I/W	I/W
Amphetamines	I		I	I/W	I
Caffeine					I
Marijuana	I		I		I
Cocaine	I		I	I/W	I/W
Hallucinogens	I		I	I	I
Inhalants	I	Yes	I	I	I
Opioids	I		I	I	
Phencyclidine (PCP)	I		I	I	I
Sedatives	I/W	Yes	I/W	I/W	W

[a]Because dementia is associated with long-term, heavy substance use, it scores only a "yes."

- *Psychosis*. You expect the hallucinogens to produce psychosis (sometimes delusional disorder), and they do; occasionally they produce prolonged visual disturbances that don't rise to the level of psychosis. These are flashbacks, during which the person will falsely perceive movement at the periphery of vision, or other visual distortions such as trails, geometric shapes, colors that are too intense ("over-Photoshopped" as one patient expressed it), or objects appearing smaller or bigger than normal. When psychosis occurs with phencyclidine (PCP) use, it usually abates after a few hours; sometimes, however, patients will retain symptoms of catatonia or paranoid psychoses for weeks. Here are two problems that can complicate the diagnostic picture: (1) Some patients may not be aware that they've ingested PCP; and (2) even those who do know may lack insight that their symptoms are caused by the drug. Over half of those who use amphetamines (especially methamphetamine) develop delusions, and some also have hallucinations. Too often, they become violent. Whereas about 3% of those with alcoholism experience psychosis during heavy drinking or withdrawal, marijuana rarely produces psychosis; it creates its mischief by worsening the symptoms of actual schizophrenia.
- *Depression*. Over 75% of individuals with alcoholism develop depression, with symptoms about the same as for other causes of clinical depressions. However, for the vast majority (about 95% of men, perhaps 75% of women) the depression improves rapidly after cessation of alcohol use.

Mood disorder, especially depression, is also associated with most other drugs of misuse, including marijuana (dysthymia tends to predominate), opioids, and the hallucinogens. Depression also develops during withdrawal from amphetamine or cocaine.

• *Anxiety*. About three-fourths of those who use alcohol heavily have panic attacks during withdrawal, and a form of social avoidance similar to agoraphobia is also common during the first few weeks of sobriety. Panic attacks may also occur during withdrawal from sedative/hypnotics and intoxication with amphetamines. Marijuana users, especially novices, commonly experience panic attacks; anxiety disorders are also associated with hallucinogen use.

• *Substance use*. No, I'm not being facetious. Although some individuals who use alcohol disdain other drugs, and vice versa, many patients are equal-opportunity users. Furthermore, we must always take great care to consider all of the "big four" drug sources: alcohol, street, prescription, and over-the-counter.

Other Addictions

We tend to speak loosely and sometimes humorously of many behavioral "addictions," among them eating chocolate, watching TV, and buying things on eBay. However, several disorders that involve difficulty controlling impulses to engage in harmful behavior bear striking similarities to substance use. Because few of them represent much of a diagnostic challenge, I'll discuss them here in less than obsessive detail.

Gambling Disorder

People who gamble to the point of harming themselves and others will have symptoms resembling those of substance use disorder—for example, the need to put increasing amounts of money into play (tolerance) and discomfort when attempting to stop gambling (withdrawal). Other symptoms include illegal acts performed to obtain money for gambling and the disruption of personal relationships. Gambling is also one of the non-substance-related behaviors (another is overeating) that are often effectively managed through 12-step programs similar to AA. These similarities have caused the migration of gambling disorder into a chapter DSM-5-TR now calls "Substance-Related and Addictive Disorders."

Pyromania, Trichotillomania, Kleptomania

For hundreds of years, the Greek word *mania* ("madness") has been used to mean "to have a passion." Although the term is now largely co-opted for the "up" phase of bipolar I disorder, the older usage survives in the names of three contemporary disorders with the general qualities of addictions: pyromania (fire setting), trichotillomania (hair pulling), and kleptomania (stealing), each of which acts as a "master" to which the individual feels compelled to submit. Often beginning in childhood or adolescence, these disorders entail behaviors that can become chronic, lasting well into adulthood. Despite the aspect of surrender, they are *ego-syntonic*. That is, they are carried out in accord with the person's values and conscious wishes—not in response to, for example, hallucinations.

Unlike gambling and substance misuse, these conditions are not defined by lists of behaviors that cause the person to run afoul of society. Instead, each behavior begins with a rising tension or excitement that finds release only as the match is struck, the strand of hair is tweaked, or the unneeded (and unpaid-for) item is swept into a pocket. The tension may be described as "itching" of the scalp in hair pulling, restlessness, or a combination of pleasure and fear (as in kleptomania).

All three disorders entail secrecy—two because they are illegal, the third because it causes the person to look funny and feel ashamed. However, once we've identified the conduct, we're almost home; setting fires and stealing don't require much diagnostic finesse. What they do require is our attention to fistfuls of exceptions. The problem is that these two behaviors are by far most frequently encountered outside the context of mental disorder. In fact, people who steal or set fires with other motives in mind may try to claim falsely that they suffer from the mental disorder. That's why we have to consider the rather long lists of circumstances in which the diagnoses should *not* be made. For pyromania, the fire setting must not be due to poor judgment (as in intellectual disability, substance intoxication, or dementia) or done for profit, revenge, crime concealment, or out of anger or in response to psychosis. For kleptomania, the items must not be stolen in response to anger, delusions, or command hallucinations or for their monetary value. In neither disorder can schizophrenia, mania, or a personality disorder better explain the behavior. For trichotillomania, the restrictions are less severe, though the criterion of clinical distress/impaired functioning would exclude ordinary cosmetic eyebrow tweezing and depilation. DSM-5-TR includes trichotillomania in the "Obsessive–Compulsive and Related Disorders" chapter, which includes a related disorder, excoriation (skin-picking) disorder.

For consistency with the foregoing chapters of Part III, in Figure 15.1 I provide a decision tree for a patient who has problems with addiction. However, you should have no particular trouble making these diagnoses. The greater diagnostic challenges, as I have described throughout this chapter, lie in determining the independent versus dependent status of co-occurring disorders (in the case of substance misuse) and in determining whether particular behaviors may be related to other disorders or motivations altogether (in the case of some of the other addictions).

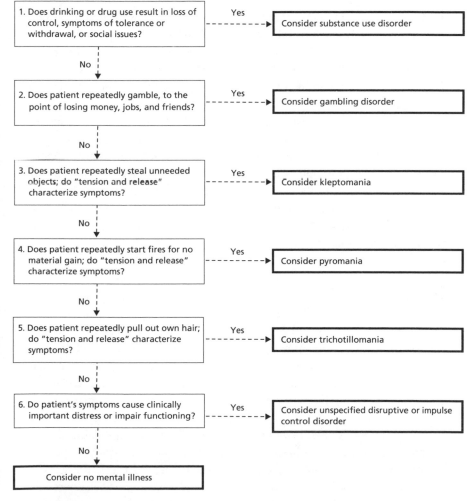

FIGURE 15.1. (Rather boring) decision tree for a patient who has problems with addiction.

16 Diagnosing Eating and Sleeping Disorders

Eating and sleeping are so fundamental to our survival that it's easy to overlook them. We assume that these activities will just happen until, one day, they don't—or don't happen very well. The behaviors included in these two classifications can fly under the diagnostic radar when a patient presents with more dramatic, more pressing problems. But issues related to sleeping and eating can also be the harbingers of other problems far too serious to ignore.

Problems with eating and sleeping occur so frequently in the course of many, many mental and physical disorders that deciding when such an issue is "only" part of an overall picture and when it rises to the status of independent disorder is fraught with difficulty for the clinician. In this chapter we'll take up—though not every possible disorder within these classes of disorder (they are really numerous, especially of the sleeping variety)—problems that mostly affect adults and are likely to be discussed in a mental health clinician's office.

Disorders of Eating

All of the behaviors we mental health professionals encounter are important for the health and happiness of our patients. But only one of them is both subject to conscious decision making and essential for the continuation of life itself. That one is, of course, eating. (OK, sleep is also absolutely necessary to sustain life, but it's pretty hard for a person to control longer than a day or two.)

We must eat to live; if we do not eat, we die. Eating unhealthful stuff can make us sick or even hasten our rendezvous on the coroner's gurney. But what we eat isn't usually the issue for the eating disorders. Rather, the issue is a matter of *how* food is consumed. And a variety of behaviors and attitudes can signal the presence of an eating disorder:

- Eating in binges. The person consumes a larger amount of food at one time than would be required for a normal meal.
- Eating rapidly. Some people gobble their food.
- Fasting and eating too little to sustain good health. Markedly reducing intake is one way patients with either anorexia nervosa (AN) or bulimia nervosa (BN) compensate for their intake, and it can lead to nutritional deficiency. Some patients just flat-out refuse food.
- Fear of excessive weight or of gaining weight.
- Impaired judgment. This can take the form of distorted self-perception (thinking one is fat when objectively gaunt) or it can mean that the person does not perceive just how dangerous the behaviors have become.
- Solitary dining. This is a criterion for binge-eating disorder (BED), but people with other eating disorders do it because of shame or embarrassment.
- Self-induced vomiting or the use of medications to avoid weight gain.
- Extreme exercise. Here is another means of mitigating the effects of too much eating.
- The sense of lack of control over what and when one eats.
- Negative feeling of disgust, embarrassment, or guilt about eating behavior.

Eating isn't just a matter of putting food into our mouths. Apart from the odd sandwich consumed at our desk while we are working through accumulated emails, the social aspect of consumption can be almost as important as taking on fuel. We use the dining experience as a time to exchange experiences and ideas, as a bulwark of family relationships, and as a convenient and recurring excuse to have a good time. None of these important qualities is to be found in the DSM-5-TR criteria for eating disorders, which I've listed with brief definitions in Table 16.1.

Following are some additional issues linked to eating that do *not* constitute symptoms of eating disorders.

- In assessing other mental disorders, we sometimes invoke appetite as a symptom. It may then seem paradoxical that appetite is not mentioned as a criterion for any feeding and eating disorder. Appetite has little to do with feeding and eating disorders—though it does figure in other mental and emotional disorders.

TABLE 16.1. DSM-5-TR Disorders of Eating (with Brief Definitions)

- *Anorexia nervosa.* The distorted self-perception of being fat causes these people such fear of obesity that they eat far less than they need to maintain normal weight and good health. Duration is at least 3 months.

- *Bulimia nervosa.* These folks have lost control of their eating, at least weekly consuming in binges huge amounts of food. They keep their weight down by fasting, vomiting, exercising, or abusing laxatives or other medications. The disorder has lasted at least 3 months.

- *Binge-eating disorder.* These patients eat in binges but, unlike those with bulimia nervosa, do not try to compensate by vomiting, exercising, or using medications. Duration must be a minimum of 3 months.

- *Avoidant/restrictive food intake disorder (ARFID).* Failure to eat enough leads to weight loss or a failure to gain weight, but these patients don't have distorted perception of their own body image. No minimum time is stated.

- *Rumination disorder.* For at least 1 month, these people persistently regurgitate and rechew food already eaten.

- *Pica.* Someone with pica eats material that is nonnutritive—that is, it isn't food. One month is the minimum.

- Obesity is not a criterion for any of the feeding and eating disorders, though fear of gaining weight or being overweight can be.
- The taste of food and our enjoyment of it or of the dining experience similarly do not serve to define these disorders.

Shannon

Each noontime, Shannon avoids the teachers' lunchroom and claims instead a bench at the back edge of the soccer field. Fortunately, where she lives weather during the school year is usually clement. When it rains, she shelters in the privacy of her classroom—with the door firmly closed against intruders.

At age 45, Shannon has taught fifth grade for nearly 20 years. She is well liked by her students and she maintains good relationships with parents, administrators, and fellow teachers. She just doesn't care to eat with them. "I enjoy having my own space, my own private thoughts," she will tell anyone who might ask. She is most keen not to expose her lunchtime habit, which is to consume—no lunch at all. She has pursued this eating behavior for years.

When in her middle 20s, Shannon had been married to the chef at a local luxury hotel. Paolo was always experimenting in their kitchen with variations on main course entrees that he designed for future hotel menus. Of course, Shannon served as principal guinea pig.

"The emphasis was on the pig part," she ruefully explains to her most recent therapist. "I'd nibble bits of whatever was new, hot out of the oven. Later on, I'd scarf down the leftovers from the fridge. It freaked him out, how much I ate, and eventually that helped drive him from the marriage. The day he left I ate an entire New York cheesecake. Homemade."

"Can you describe a typical binge?" The clinician wants a full rundown: What does Shannon eat? In what amount of time? Does she feel out of control? Does it happen when she eats with others? If so, how is it different then? What were the others eating? Suppose someone suggested restraint—would she stop? Whew!

Every few days Shannon will sit down to dinner (by herself), intent upon consuming yesterday's leftover pasta. But after polishing that off, she'll open a can of SpaghettiOs, then another and another. "It's as though someone, or something, has taken over my body—and my can opener," she says. "Whether I'm full or hungry, makes no difference. I just do it."

After the main course ("Three main courses," she corrects herself), it's on to the quart or so of blackberry ice cream—in season—which she also consumes in full. "I hardly even taste it." Afterward, she retreats to her bathroom, where she'll chuck it all up again. "No chemicals needed—a teaspoon touched to the back of my throat works just fine." Sometimes, she puts a towel over the mirror, to cloak her shame for the person she sees there.

Shannon started puberty when she was only 9, and the other girls in her class teased her. Tumbling was all the rage that year and, trying to fit in, she turned out for the squad. But that only led to more teasing—"My body was just too chunky for tumbling; they said I looked like the Pillsbury Doughboy, and they'd try to poke me. Only I didn't giggle." Determined to prove them all wrong, Shannon had begun the series of diets that ultimately spawned a lifetime of fast-and-splurge eating. Of course, tumbling is no concern at all now, but though her BMI is a healthy 21, the shape of her body is "constantly on my mind—I'm alternately appalled and obsessed. Even *I* don't see the sense in it!"

During her second year in college, a friend suggested that she might benefit from weight loss pills. But after a prodigious amount of reading, she decided that pills were, for her, a dead end. "With the emphasis on the dead part," she's happy to add. "Too many people have succumbed to their own amateur pharmacology. I may be obsessed, but I'm not crazy!"

Has anyone else in the family had anything like her disorder? Now that you mention it, Shannon recalls, years ago there was Marty, a cousin who had spent several months in treatment because she refused to eat anything that wasn't white. Food that contained darker colors made her feel nauseous, so she would avoid it completely. She'd eat plain rice and vanilla ice cream and coconut meat, and she would drink milk (not chocolate), but no veggies other than jicama and radishes, if they'd been peeled. And no fruits at all—white peaches and bananas were tinged with color and cherimoyas had dark seeds. "And of course no meat, not even chicken breast—she said its texture was too dry," Shannon finishes up. Marty failed to gain the weight you'd expect for her height. "She was taunted unmercifully, which she said she deserved because she was so scrawny." Shannon thinks that, with therapy, Marty eventually recovered. "Today, she may even be a little overweight. But at least she eats normal stuff."

Analysis

The first branch on the Figure 16.1 decision tree is a decided negative: Shannon is neither underfed nor underweight. That brings us to the decisive node (step 2) where we can agree: She eats in binges and complains of lost control over what she consumes. (I would argue that the control issue is more central to diagnosis than is volume consumed.) Although Shannon doesn't use drugs, she certainly does purge—seemingly, after every humongous meal. That earns another *yes* at step 6 and moves us along to step 9, where we consider our final question: How does she regard her own appearance? Clearly, her self-evaluation is based on her weight and the shape of her body, and she regards her behavior as irrational.

Questions about duration and frequency aren't covered in the tree, but we are up to that task. Her eating behavior has lasted far, far longer than the minimum 3 months, and clearly it occurs more often than the minimum of once a week. And, hey presto! We are fully justified in considering the diagnosis of bulimia nervosa. The behaviors are all current, so we need no statement concerning remission. As for severity, Shannon experiences only a few episodes per week, but the effect on her psyche and her personal and interpersonal life is profound. I'm going to exercise my clinician's privilege and call her degree of BN moderate. (As with AN, the official diagnostic criteria give us permission, as if we needed it, to adjust severity upward depending on the nature of symptoms and their effect on the patient.) If you think it's even more severe than that, I won't argue.

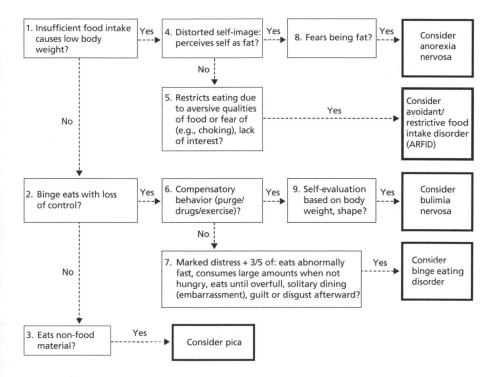

FIGURE 16.1. Decision tree for a person who has a problem with eating or feeding.

Analysis of Marty

We have the briefest description of Cousin Marty's preference for white foods; let's milk it (!) for every drop of information. Right away, step 1 of the decision tree yields a definite positive as we note that the variety of foods in her diet was so limited that she failed to gain weight as expected and was undoubtedly deficient in essential elements such as vitamins and protein. However, at least as Shannon told it, Marty didn't have a step 4 distorted perception of weight or shape (to the contrary, she thought she looked scrawny). At step 5, she clearly refused to eat foods other than those that embodied certain color or other sensory properties (white foods, for example). That lands us at avoidant/restrictive food intake disorder (ARFID) as the explanation to consider. We'd need to know that her physical health was otherwise good and that there was no other medical explanation for her condition (one of our diagnostic principles). Absent any evidence of that nature, we can safely say that her diagnosis at age 10 would be ARFID.

Kenny

In a small restaurant near his home, Kenny sits by himself at a corner table set for two. He eats sparingly of his vegetarian lasagna. Once or twice, as if for reassurance, he touches the toe of his shoe to the large shopping bag parked under the table. The bag bears the logo of that new dessert specialty shop down the street.

The friendly waiter approaches. "From the order, I had assumed you were meeting someone," he says as he scrapes the leftovers into two takeout containers.

"No, I just love this dish and wanted to have it again for a couple of nights." Kenny returns the smile, pays (with generous tip), and departs.

With two bags to manage, he walks carefully. It's several blocks to his apartment, a walkup on the third floor where he's lived all his life. Once inside, he sits down at the single place-setting already laid on his dining table and dumps the first takeout carton onto a platter. With fork in one hand, spoon in the other, he attacks as though the still-warm pasta might try to escape. He gobbles down the last bite and, without missing a beat, dumps and dispatches the second portion. Then he hoists the other carry bag onto the table and says aloud, "Now, for the cake."

Ten minutes later, only crumbs remain. Kenny staggers to the sofa where he collapses, holding his stomach and groaning softly. Following his usual custom, he reaches for the TV remote, in hopes that *The Late Show* will obliterate his gathering remorse.

Now 34, Kenny works as an electronics engineer, designing and building power chips for both military and civilian use. It's a job he can do most anywhere there's an internet connection, so he often works from his home office. Nerdy and somewhat isolated in high school, he continued to live at home while he attended college, from which he graduated, with honors, in electrical engineering.

Kenny's parents were both so heavy that children would point and stare. At one time they had operated a small restaurant; they used to joke, with some truth, that they were their own best customers. Kenny was never very social in school, and he mostly ignored the occasional gibe about his own weight. After his dad died of a stroke, Kenny and his mom carried on with the diner for a time, but eventually they sold out to a developer who paid a king's ransom for the property. Kenny fell back on his engineering training and began his present work. When his mom died, he realized that he was truly alone in the world.

Fully aware of his weight problem and consequences for his health, Kenny spends much of his free time researching diets online.

"Over the years, I've taken most of the popular diet plans for a spin," he admits. "I thought about trying that new drug, Ozempic, but I don't have good insurance, and I found out that, if I pay for the drug, I won't be able to afford food. Maybe that's why it works." But to Kenny's chagrin, nothing has worked longer than a few weeks; he invariably slides back into his old, irresistible habit of binge eating.

Several times a week, but mostly on Fridays and Saturdays, he will cook up one of his mom's favorite recipes; often, it's whole-wheat pasta, which he loads with olive oil and tops with a delicious marinara sauce. There's always enough for three famished adults, and nearly always, he finishes it all in a sitting. He has never purged ("How gross would that be!") and he exercises hardly at all. "The whole thing's unfortunate, and I feel terrible about it," he says, "but there you are."

He once told a therapist he briefly consulted that he thought his eating hides the distress he feels about being lonely, about his fear of a solitary life as he ages. Of course, he admitted, he reinforces these ideas by eating alone—so he can gorge in peace. "And it's not that I'm all that hungry," he admitted then in a burst of self-revelation, "but it just seems nice."

Years ago, when Kenny's doctor told him he was developing hypertension, he agreed to undergo the recommended bariatric surgery. The stomach stapling enabled him to lose over a hundred pounds, a fact he knows courtesy of the baggage scale in the shipping department where he once worked. But with time, he added it all back on "with interest." He's been back to the doctor numerous times, expressing deep concern for his health, which he sees as sliding inexorably downhill. A nutritionist he once consulted advised ("without stinting") about his choice of foods, his eating habits, his feelings about himself. Although he agrees with everything he's told, he cannot seem to translate what he knows into effective action for regaining control.

Analysis

Well, starting in at step 1 of the Figure 16.1 decision tree, Kenny certainly doesn't have low body weight or insufficient caloric intake. Next stop is step 2: Does he binge eat? Of course, that hearty *Yes* is coupled with his own acknowledgment that he has indeed completely lost agency over his eating behavior. However, he emphatically denies any of the step 6 behaviors (exercise, purging, laxatives, or diuretics) some people use to ameliorate the effects of their overeating. And that drops us into step 7.

As is necessary for the diagnosis of BED, Kenny feels distressed about his behaviors (we can infer remorse from his repeated attempts to get his eating behavior under control and from what he expresses directly to his physician). And now it gets a little complicated: Does he have enough of these specific behaviors to qualify at step 7? It is the amount of food that Kenny craves, not its taste or texture, and he rapidly eats large quantities (even when not hungry) to the point of feeling marked discomfort. We've noted that Kenny eats alone (we will presume because of embarrassment) and he dispatches huge amounts when he is already full. Afterward, he feels guilty and irresponsible, as though he's betrayed himself and perhaps even his long-dead parents. Yep, if you're keeping score at home, that's a clean sweep of all five possible qualifiers; we only needed three. And that slides him right over into a consideration of binge-eating disorder.

With the big steps behind us, we must not forget the seemingly picky bits of information, omitted from the decision tree yet needed to nail down a diagnosis. In the case of BED, that would be frequency of bingeing. Kenny does so significantly more than once weekly, which is the rather undemanding DSM-5-TR requirement. And, although we haven't learned it in so many words, it's an easy inference that his problems with overeating have persisted far, far longer than the required 3 months.

No statement concerning remission is possible for someone who is still actively symptomatic, so the only other issue would be severity. Here, I'd tend to take issue with the DSM-5-TR guidelines, inasmuch as Kenny's severity ought not be judged by frequency alone. I would factor in duration, degree of distress, past failed efforts to ameliorate the behavior, *and* the considerable social consequences. Even though Kenny binges less often than daily, I'd say he is severely affected by his disorder. Anyone want to argue that?

Roxanne

Roxanne is eating lunch at her desk. That's been her habit for the past several years, starting even before she began her current job supervising trainees at a multinational corporation. All morning she interacts with coworkers, fielding complaints and questions that resurface every few days, in varying accents and turns of phrase. By noon, she's had it up to here with people. A generous bag of raw veggies at her desk while she skims her text messages suits her to a tee.

Unfortunately, when the fresh group of newbies comes on board every 4 weeks, she must share at least one lunchtime with them. Then, she contends not only with perhaps a dozen new faces but with a lunch menu that is always the same—heavy on processed meat, light on appropriate herbs and spices, with fruits and veggies honored by their dearth. That menu must have been written in stone: She has tried to have it varied, but someone higher up on the organization food chain (!—the punctuation is Roxanne's) seems to love menus rich in foods that Roxanne cannot abide. Each month, the experience calls to her mind the terrifying fear that she is gaining weight.

This fear dates back far too many years. As a young child, she loved her dance lessons, but quit when someone pointed out that she was too pudgy to be a ballerina. (Her mother fixed her a consolation cheeseburger with all the trimmings.) A decade later, when in high school and still a few pounds overweight, she was frequently heckled, especially by her two brothers, both of whom were athletic and svelte. Though only a little heavy for her height of 5 feet 8 inches (she calculates her BMI then was 27), she felt self-conscious enough that she didn't even date until long after she started college.

Roxanne has long since internalized the gibes of her youth: She doesn't just think she looks fat; she *knows* it. When she catches her reflection in a mirror, she is horrified at the chubby upper arms, her "enormous butt." She obsessively monitors her weight on her digital bathroom scales, each day hoping for the miracle of "just a few ounces less."

When her oldest brother eventually moderated his physical conditioning routine, Roxanne requisitioned his elliptical trainer and began religiously logging more than 60 minutes in her spare bedroom every evening. She tightly restricts her intake, but once or twice a week, when she has consumed more than she can tolerate, she will bring it back up with a tidy, almost dainty spew into the toilet.

Even so, she believes she is grotesque and fat beyond words. She won't talk about it—too likely that someone will try to argue with her about what she considers "my body, and that's private." But she admits to weighing herself frequently, sometimes multiple times a day, and wishing she could trim off a few more ounces of disgusting fat.

Roxanne also maintains an extensive collection of recipes on her iPad. Often she will meticulously prepare a main dish (cheesy pasta her specialty). Then she sits down at her dining room table with a plate full of delicious, home-cooked food—and tease it with her fork until it's grown leathery and cold. Any bite she does take will stick in her throat; the idea of death by culinary perfection almost makes her laugh. In the end, she tosses nearly everything into the bin.

Now, whenever she can force herself to look in the mirror, she sees not the manifest concentration camp survivor with vanishing biceps and scrawny chicken neck, but a human balloon that threatens to explode all over her tiny apartment. Recently, when a colleague pointed out that she had begun to look like the stick figures she draws on the whiteboard to illustrate corporate structure, Roxanne gazed stonily ahead for a moment, then turned and stalked off.

Analysis

For Roxanne, our Figure 16.1 decision tree excursion will be brief. At step 1, let's agree that she eats far too little, resulting in a dangerously low body weight. Indeed, the last time she weighed herself, she tipped the scales at a scant 95 pounds; strung out along her 68 inches of height, that yields a BMI of just over 15—alarmingly below the normal, healthful range (see sidebar "What Is BMI?").

At steps 4 and 8, Roxanne views herself as overweight (arms and buttocks especially), which is an evaluation markedly different from the stick-figure perception of anyone who knows her. The vignette makes crystal clear that she doesn't just worry about her appearance; rather, she actively fears being fat. With these three criteria amply fulfilled, we conclude that we should consider her for the diagnosis of anorexia nervosa.

The only explicit duration requirement for AN lies in the 3-month window we use in determining type: restricting or binge-eating/purging. Of course, most every patient will have been ill far longer than this: It takes a lot of time to lose weight (or, for a child, to fail to add weight concurrent with growing taller). Although the vignette does not state the duration of Roxanne's disorder, from her distress over the immutable workplace luncheon menu we can infer that it has gone on for many months, and probably for years.

What Is BMI?

The idea that a person's weight increases proportional to the square of their height dates back nearly 200 years to a Belgian mathematician named Adolphe Quetelet. (Exceptions to the rule occur in the first few months after birth and during puberty, but for the majority of our lifetime, the formula works just fine.) In modern times, we call this quotient the body mass index (BMI) and calculate it by dividing square of the height into weight. By convention, these measurements are expressed in meters and kilograms, yielding a normal range of 18–24.9. Score below that, and you are underweight; above it, you are either overweight or, in extreme cases, obese. Calculators are readily available on the internet, though in 2023 the American Medical Association noted that, because it was derived without including many ethnic groups, BMI should probably be used clinically with other measures.

Along the way we should pay particular attention to other possible explanations for weight loss. We haven't learned anything about a possible mood disorder (one of our diagnostic principles), and her personal physician hasn't released anything that would suggest an underlying physical condition such as an intestinal malabsorption syndrome; it's another diagnostic principle. We should consider these, despite their neglect by the official DSM-5-TR criteria.

When it comes to writing down Roxanne's diagnosis, we can first discard any question of remission. But then we still must determine which subtype best describes her journey toward starvation. The choice is binary, so it should be pretty simple: Did she binge-eat and purge, or did she not? Well, the vignette is pretty clear: It's yes and no. Mainly, she controlled her weight by restricting her eating, but once in a while, she would vomit up what she considered to be excessive consumption. Binge-eating/purging type of AN only requires the purging to be recurrent, and "once or twice a week" fits that description like size 4 sweats.

Putting it together, we can diagnose Roxanne as having AN of the binge-eating/purging type. I confess that I'm a little unhappy with the subtype, inasmuch as she didn't binge but achieved her goal mostly by limiting intake. But rules are rules and binge-eating isn't necessary to qualify for this subtype; purging alone fills the bill, even if it's only twice a week. The purging episodes have been recurrent for far longer than the minimum 3 months specified. And severity? Her current BMI is a shade above 15, dropping her into the severe category. I don't expect any pushback about that.

Comment for the Eating Disorders

Did you notice that each of these vignettes began with the image of eating alone? I didn't really plan it that way, but it does underscore the fact that these disorders bear some remarkable similarities. Of course, for BED solitary dining is sometimes a criterion, whereas for AN and BN (and sometimes rumination disorder), it is only a by-product. With two minor exceptions, these conditions are all about individuals having personal issues around the consumption of food. In only one criterion (for ARFID) do we consider any interference with psychosocial functioning; and one of multiple possible symptoms of BED is eating alone out of embarrassment.

The decision tree begins with low weight and reduced nutrition intake. That's partly because profound loss of weight is dangerous and requires early, certain identification. But even moderate AN carries with it considerable morbidity, and folks with AN can die of their disease—some by suicide, some due to medical complications. Starvation states can induce low mood and further entrench the obsessional thinking that characterizes AN.

Until the DSM-IV, there wasn't even an eating disorders chapter. AN, BN, and the others were lumped in with conditions first encountered in childhood. BED, though more frequently encountered than either AN or BN, didn't enter the pantheon until DSM-5. The three lesser members of this club—ARFID, pica, and rumination disorder—though hardly rare, only infrequently come up in the assessment of adults. Indeed, regardless of ethnicity or other demographic characteristics, eating disorders in general are relatively uncommon, certainly as compared with the prevalence of mood and anxiety disorders in the general population.

But among the eating disorders, BED is actually the most common, with a prevalence of close to 1%; women predominate, but not as much as for AN or BN. BED is especially common in obese people, though being overweight is not necessary to the diagnosis. Fasting or dieting can serve as a precipitant. When people plan their binges, they may purchase special, favorite foods. After a binge, they may have trouble even recalling what it was they consumed.

We tend to think of patients with AN, and perhaps, by extension, of those with other eating disorders as being young and female. Though often true, it's important not to ignore other potential populations: males (who are less likely than females to seek treatment), people of color, and older people.

Pica may have no consequences—similar to rumination disorder. It can be free-standing or coexist with other eating disorders. All the other eating disorders are mutually exclusive. Many people will cross over from AN to BN.

We don't know how ARFID is related to other eating disorders: Is there crossover? Are there family histories in common? We do know that it can be dangerous, even resulting in the need for parenteral feeding (the use of gastric intubation or even IVs).

DSM-5-TR includes one more feeding/eating diagnosis, and that's rumination disorder (RD). It denotes people (not just children, but also some adults, especially those who have a developmental disability) who regurgitate and rechew their food. RD doesn't fit comfortably onto any decision tree that I've been able to devise; because of its rarity in a mental health provider's office, I'll just briefly mention it here. Rumination usually begins within the first few minutes of completing a meal. Sometimes the individual swallows, sometimes spits out the just-chewed glob, and an episode may last as long as 2 hours after eating. Criteria do not require that patients or others suffer harm or other untoward sequelae, so you might think it more of a curious behavior than a disorder—but you'd be wrong. Rumination can lead to malnutrition in infants or older people, to dental disease, to esophageal lesions. It is sometimes confused with gastroesophageal reflux disease; indeed, RD is claimed as home turf by gastroenterologists as well as by mental health clinicians. In any event, RD is not a condition you are likely to encounter in the casual patient who drops by for an evaluation. Some patients with RD may eat alone, so as to prevent others from knowing that they pursue behavior that is frowned upon by others. Does this sound familiar?

We also should mention how to regard a patient with an eating disorder who fails to meet full criteria for any DSM-5-TR condition. For example, suppose Kenny had had too few of the behaviors required for BED? We would have to give him a diagnosis of unspecified eating disorder and reassess when more symptoms developed.

Finally, waiting in the wings for official recognition is yet another eating disorder: orthorexia nervosa (ON). Those with this condition strive so hard to eat a healthful diet that they may eliminate entire food groups or focus on fasting (which they regard as purifying). Should they violate their own, self-imposed dietary rules, they feel shamed, fear they'll become ill, or experience other negative ideas about themselves. They may suffer from weight loss or malnutrition. ON wasn't included in DSM-5-TR's conditions for further study, but who knows? It may yet be served up in a future edition.

Sleep Disorders

Disorders of sleep pose danger for the patient, yet, because sleep is something that everyone does every day (night), when they come up we tend to ignore problems with sleep or pass them off with a cliché: "You'll sleep better tonight"; "Catch up on the weekend"; "People sleep more than they need to, don't you think?"

For some patients, sleep is a symptom; for others, it's a freestanding disorder. So it doesn't always work to focus all your attention on what you think is a primary condition (e.g., depression). How well or ill a patient sleeps may be important enough that it needs to be addressed independently, hence the need for accurate assessment of the sleep itself. How we record a particular person's insomnia depends on knowing the antecedent (if any) medical or mental condition. That's one reason for starting the decision tree in Figure 16.2 as I have done.

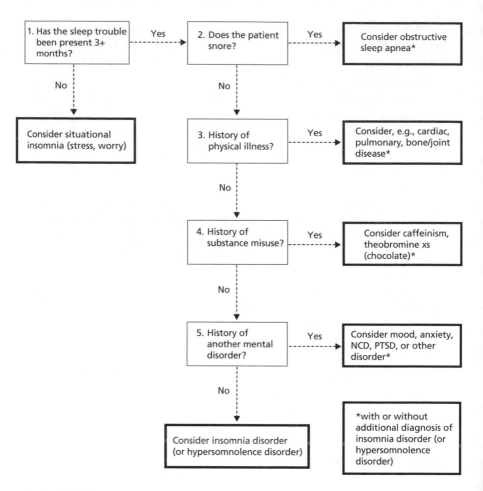

FIGURE 16.2. Decision tree for someone who has a problem with insomnia. You can substitute hypersomnia as the main complaint and still use the tree.

Depending on how you count them, you could find 13 or you could find 30 disorders of sleep defined in DSM-5-TR. Some you'll encounter frequently among mental health and medical patients. Others are uncommon, some even so rare you'll hardly ever see an example. So, I'll try to hit the high spots of those sleep disorders that you can expect to come upon in the course of ordinary clinical care, emphasizing those in which the person doesn't get enough sleep.

We'll explore some of the possibilities through the story of Henry, who over the years experienced a variety of symptoms and evaluations.

Henry, Part A

For his 21st birthday, Henry receives a smart watch that he can pair with his phone. "This watch is *really* smart," he explains, "It even tells me how long I sleep each night." That information has been a comfort for several weeks—until the last couple of nights. "Now, it tells me that I'm getting only about 5 hours of deep sleep." His dad had been a technician for a sleep lab, so Henry knows how important sleep is. "'You are what you sleep,' Dad always said."

Henry has a job and girlfriend. Lorelei works evenings and likes him to be awake when she comes home just before midnight. His own job involves staffing a telephone help line that services the East Coast. "That's a problem for someone who lives in L.A.," Henry points out to the interviewer who is trying to determine what's wrong. Eventually, that determination is: nothing. The clinician sends Henry away with reassurance and a pamphlet that discusses some advice for good sleep hygiene.

Analysis

Creating a broad differential diagnosis is our first rule, so basic that it's not even a diagnostic principle: Rather, it's the umbrella title for my first six diagnostic principles. But wait! There's a question we need to ask early, namely: Does the patient meet the criteria for any disorder, a sleep disorder in this case? And when we think about Henry so far as we have become acquainted, he does not. And why not? Because, like most of the disorders described in DSM-5-TR, the patient's symptoms must be present for a minimum specified duration to gain admission to the particular corner of the diagnostic ballpark. In the case of insomnia, that duration must be at least 3 months—and occur three or more nights per week during that time. Of course, Henry has been troubled for only a couple of weeks. At one time or another, everybody (or nearly) will experience that level of trouble sleeping—the result of stress, worry, or bedroom activities that are more interesting than sleep.

So, we'll choose "no" at the first node of our insomnia decision tree and consider what practical steps we might suggest for dealing with the stress of his situational issue. (Henry's clinician appropriately gives him some tips concerning sleep hygiene.) But we won't burden him with a sleep disorder diagnosis. Not yet.

Henry, Part B

Henry absorbs all the good counsel and reassurance that his sleep is almost certainly normal and that, with healthful good living and positive outlook, his issues will soon clear. And that's exactly what happens. He practices good sleep hygiene and he has the information from his clinician; later he consults Doctor Google and finds the same information everywhere. When he does experience a restless night, he tells himself that it's just a blip, not a calamity.

Fast forward 10 years. Henry now works for a local electronics fabricator. He and Lorrie are married; they have a daughter, Mattie. Several times a year they drive to the mountains for skiing. On their last trip ever, Henry gracefully swoops around a mature stand of conifers. At the bottom of the slope he pauses, turns, and watches in horror as Lorrie disappears into a tree well. He frantically herringbones back up the slope while her personal beacon cries for help. But thick powder snow has collapsed in after her, and though Mountain Rescue rapidly deploys to the scene, by the time they can dig her out, Lorelei isn't breathing. They persist with CPR way past the point of any hope.

The rest of that day and nearly all the next Henry can never recall—how they got her down the mountain, how he broke the news to her parents, to Mattie—what words do you use to tell a 5-year-old that her mother has died, for God's sake! In the aftermath, Henry sells all the ski equipment, except for Lorelei's skis; those he burns. He vows never again to drive to the mountains, and he won't even watch a film that involves the sport.

But the hours leading up to the event he recalls with crystal clarity: how she really hadn't wanted to go, how he had insisted, how it was so clearly his fault she had died. If someone tries to suggest otherwise, he'll argue or groan aloud, then shut down and kick the furniture or punch the walls. "I have the plasterer on speed-dial" is the rueful comment he makes, only partly in jest, to a clinician months later.

In dreams he relives the horror, the helplessness of being able only to watch as they dig, deeper and deeper, with a sense of both urgency and futility. He can do nothing but weep, which he does until—as usual, he awakens halfway through the night, drenched in sweat and panting. Then, for hours he will lie in wakeful misery. As a result, he is drowsy and listless throughout the day, cannot focus on his work and, half a year on, is told to take sick leave—or find another job.

It is the sleeplessness that eventually drives him back to the clinic that had once solved his distress with hope and reassurance.

Analysis

Once bitten, twice shy, so this time we'll check first for duration of the problem, which approaches 6 months, meeting minimum criteria for nearly every disorder in the book. And the frequency? It seemed to happen almost nightly. We need to pay attention to the other qualifiers for seriousness, too: clinically important distress or impairment we can definitely endorse. And Henry had plenty of opportunity for sleeping.

So, let's get down to it. Because something terrible has happened, we turn to the trauma chapter for guidance. Henry directly viewed the horror of Lorelei's death, satisfying the first DSM-5-TR criterion for posttraumatic stress disorder (step 5 of Figure 12.1). Over and over he revisited the event, both in memories of the day and in his horrifying dreams. He burned her skis and refused to return to the mountains, either of which would meet the requirement for avoidance behavior; these are external reminders, though taking steps to avoid thoughts or memories (that is, internal reminders) would also serve.

The diagnosis of PTSD demands that we identify symptoms from a number of different categories. One such is negative changes in thoughts and mood; Henry qualifies with near-amnesia for what happened that day subsequent the event, and with his distorted self-blame for Lorelei's death. And in the months that followed, he also experienced changes in arousal and reactivity, namely his sleep issues and his angry lashing out. He hadn't been using drugs or alcohol, and his distress—the final element needed to qualify for the diagnosis of PTSD—was only too obvious.

The mood symptoms and the circumstances could argue for either PTSD or for the new diagnosis in our toolbox, prolonged grief disorder (PGD). Again, time plays a central role. The operational definition of PGD includes the requirement of a least 1 year of symptoms before the diagnosis can be entertained. Obviously, Henry's symptoms have not yet passed that landmark, so we must put PGD to the side. A full year out, we might need to revise our conclusion—these two disorders can exist together.

And actually, Henry's first symptoms developed within the first few days—perhaps we should say hours—of watching in horror as his precious wife was buried alive. That would set him up for an immediate diagnosis of acute stress disorder (ASD). But as time drags on and his symptoms persist, ASD will morph into a classic case of posttraumatic stress disorder.

So let's review—this is, after all, a complicated disorder: After the traumatic event, Henry fully met the requirements for a stress disorder: intrusion symptoms (those horrid dreams); attempts to avoid stimuli that reminded him of her death (disposing of ski equipment, shunning the mountain); negative beliefs (self-blame, inability to remember parts of that day); and changes in arousal (I'd say that kicking the furniture was irritable behavior, and, oh yes, troubled sleep).

Uh-oh, here's a complication: Although we can diagnose insomnia disorder in the face of another mental, sleep, or physical condition—in fact, DSM-5-TR provides handy specifiers for just such instances—the rules say that the insomnia must be sufficiently serious to require (*warrant* is the term of art) clinical attention on its own. At the same time, however, the insomnia must not be completely explainable on the basis of the other disorder. Clearly, that puts us clinicians into the position of rendering some judgment calls. But we are up to it: Henry's problems with sleep instigated his seeking care and they are serious enough to require special attention. Comorbidity is the rule, not the exception; happily, we don't have to determine that one disorder causes the other.

So, in my clinical judgment, here is where the second part of Henry's story ends. He has plenty of symptoms justifying two disorders, and we would recommend treatment for them both: posttraumatic stress disorder *and* insomnia disorder.

Henry, Part C

With therapy and medication, Henry's insomnia and PTSD symptoms dwindle; at length, they fade away. He takes up the challenge of working from home (finally, he returns to his old job in IT) while single-parenting his only child. All of his free time he spends caring for Mattie, who with love and support comes to terms with horrific death and thrives—as does Henry.

Fast forward another dozen years. Henry has succeeded brilliantly in his dual roles of breadwinner and homemaker. Well, perhaps too well—since Lorelei's death he has gained a lot of weight. "Too much of my own home cooking, too little exercise" he ruefully observes. But he is both grateful and proud that Mattie's weight has tracked perfectly within the normal range for a growing child.

However, a serious issue has come up, something that Henry has negotiated with concern, with care, with grace. Six or seven years ago, perhaps driven by looming puberty, questions about sex and gender began to creep into Mattie's conversations with Henry.

"I wonder that I—this seems so weird!—that I don't really feel like a girl?" In ever-stronger language, the question comes up over and again. It is during the pandemic, and Henry has carefully supervised their homeschooling sessions. Mattie despairs at one day having to fulfill a woman's role, in fact wonders whether the name *Matt* might be a more comfortable fit. One day, she finally articulates it: "I actually feel more like a guy."

"Wow!" Henry responds, "I didn't see that coming." Though on reflection, for years he has noticed that Mattie—Matt?—has never been interested in dolls or other typical girls' fantasy play, preferring baseball and hockey and wrestling to quieter activities. After much thought, Henry cautiously offers this: "More than anything, I want you to be happy, and this is a really big deal. We shouldn't decide anything suddenly. I think we need some help with this—and we should probably start by sleeping on it." The counsel and sleep eventually help them understand the emotions wrought by gender dysphoria. Together they find a way forward with puberty blockers and other gender-affirming care.

Now, mostly, Henry seems to sleep well. But for some months he has found that, even after a full night's sleep, he feels groggy, almost hung over. It has become an enormous struggle to drag himself out of bed. Their family physician calls it "sleep inertia," for which specific medical remedies are thin on the ground. Henry absorbs all that the internet has to offer and doses himself with caffeine when he first awakens. It helps some, but still he's left feeling so fatigued that, in the past few weeks, he has had the experience of nodding off suddenly, unexpectedly, even when he's fully occupied with his work or, once, while eating supper. He certainly doesn't trust himself to drive.

Fortunately, Matt has taken driver training, passing the operator exam on the first try. "Of course!" Henry brags, his too-ample chest swelling with paternal pride. And so, with Henry's daytime alertness too compromised to be ignored any longer, Matt (literally) drives him back to . . . you guessed it: The sleep disorders clinic.

"He's always snored," Matt tells the clinician, who has invited input. "Even when I was little, I'd sometimes awaken in the night to its steady, sawing rhythm. After a couple of minutes, it would stop for a while. The quiet then would last such a long time, I'd sometimes wonder whether he was still alive." Eventually, the silence would be shattered by a profoundly resonant snort, which signaled the return to rhythmic snoring.

"Lately," Matt adds, "it all seems to have worsened, especially since Dad has, um, chunked up a bit. You know those jokes about the neighbors complaining? Well, last week that actually happened. The woman who lives next to us down the hallway came to the door. She was apologetic but she wondered whether something could be done so *she* can sleep."

Analysis

Once again, we'll need our decision tree, which allows us to start out with a complaint of daytime drowsiness. Henry's sleep period is, as far as we know, plenty long enough to get us to step 2, where we hit pay dirt. Of course, this third episode in the saga of Henry leaves "obstructive sleep apnea" dancing on our lips. With onset after marked weight gain, it seems a good fit for Henry's symptoms.

However, right away we do encounter an issue. Sleep apnea is one of those disorders that official criteria state you can diagnose only with a laboratory study. This means that my grandfather, for example, who died before polysomnography was even a thing, could not have received the diagnosis, despite his (and my grandmother's) lifelong experience with window-rattling snores and snorts.

So, for the purposes of our discussion, let's just agree that, in the case of Henry, a sleep study would only underscore our unsurpassed clinical judgment. Then, look at the symptoms required in addition to the lab studies: either of "nocturnal breathing disturbances" or "daytime sleepiness, fatigue, or unrefreshing sleep." Yep, Henry scores on both accounts. I'd say that, clinically, his is at least moderately severe, but the professor in the machine may ultimately rule differently.

Comment

Henry's case is hardly unique: Obstructive apnea affects over 10% of American adults and is especially frequent among those whose weight is too generous. Indeed, problems with sleep overall are extraordinarily common. I'd wager that the number of people reading this who have never had any issue with sleep is small. Sleeping too little—insomnia—is a complaint that perhaps a third of all adults will make at one time or another. However, only about a third of these folks could ever qualify for an official diagnosis. (As with so much else in life, we tend to complain about more than objective data can support.) Of those with verifiable insomnia who consult a sleep disorders clinic, about a third will turn out to have an underlying mental condition; half of these will have a mood disorder. Plenty of other medical disorders will also be diagnosed.

Even aside from insomnia, there's a lot more going on in the sleep disorders clinic than we've dreamed of in our philosophy, Horatio. Narcolepsy isn't so common, affecting fewer than 1 per 1,000 persons, but it can seriously impair those it touches. Circadian rhythm disorders come in a variety of flavors and tend to affect young people especially; these disorders have even crept into our everyday language as we speak of "larks" and "owls."

And sleep apnea? Well over 10% of adults (more men than women) have it, but is it truly a disorder of sleep? The answer, I suppose, depends on whom you ask. The sleep disorders clinician will give you a firm "Yup." Other clinicians (nose and throat specialists, say) may also claim it for their own. Of course, it has the word *sleep* in its name, but then so does sleeping sickness—an infectious disease caused by a parasite that tsetse flies transmit. But sleep apnea does appear prominently in the sleep section of DSM-5-TR, so we mental health clinicians must be prepared to reckon with it.

Then there are all those things that go bump in the night—such as sleep terrors and REM sleep behavior disorder. Up to 5% of adults have nightmares that occur at least weekly; and over 10% have episodes of sleepwalking. Don't forget the substance-related sleep disorders, and if you ever see someone with sleep-related hypoventilation, text me. They all occur, and we all need to have at minimum a nodding acquaintance with them. Each gets taken for a spin in my book, *DSM-5-TR Made Easy*. Highly recommended.

Finally, there's restless legs syndrome, affectionately known to its sufferers as RLS, which doesn't really have all that much to do with sleep at all—except that it can disturb yours if you experience it at night. (Using this standard, that raucous raccoon paying a nocturnal visit to your backyard is also a sleep disorder.) RLS affects between 1 and 2% of adults in the United States, and for them, whether or not it disturbs sleep, it's a real bummer. Trust me.

I haven't heard whether Henry ever did get a sleep study, but he did acquire a continuous positive airway pressure (CPAP) machine; now everyone's sleeping better. And by the way, Matt continues to thrive, his transition now well advanced.

17 Diagnosing Personality and Relationship Problems

Personality disorders (we'll abbreviate them as PDs) primarily involve problems relating to oneself and to other people. They are lasting patterns that can show up in the realms of thought, feelings, behavior, and motivation; they affect interpersonal relationships and the control of impulses. Personalities disordered in some way affect nearly 10% of the general population and about half of all mental patients. In the latter, it will often seem an afterthought when someone's main problem is a major mental disorder of the sort described in the foregoing chapters. Your realization that a given patient has a PD may only develop slowly, after several interviews.

Unhappily, with this chapter we approach the limits of science and certainty as regards our ability to characterize and diagnose mental disorders accurately. Our descriptions of PDs are categorical, which means that we count symptoms until we have enough to cry "Aha!" One result is that there is no theoretical limit to the number of personality types we might declare disordered. (At a lecture some years ago, an expert in the field claimed that there may be as many as 2,000 PDs. I later told him—in jest, of course—that anyone who believed that might have "multiple personality disorder disorder.") Another result is that many patients qualify for two or more PDs; this confuses everyone. Perhaps the biggest problem of all is that categorical systems depend so heavily on interpretation that we are tempted to slip confusing patients into a convenient PD (some would say "wastebasket") category.

Other classification systems rate personality along a handful of dimensions that attempt to quantify how we regard ourselves and adapt to different circumstances. For example, the well-known five-factor model uses the dimensions of neuroticism, extroversion, openness to experience, agreeableness, and conscientiousness. Other systems employ a score or more of dimensions. Dimensional models eliminate the possibility of multiple PDs for an individual, but they also increase the amount of effort needed to determine where anyone belongs on each of these ranges.

Defining a PD Diagnosis

Whereas most diagnoses represent a change in a person's usual thinking and behavior (the few exceptions are early childhood conditions such as autism spectrum disorder, ADHD, and intellectual disability), PDs start early in life and continue more or less forever. This fact requires a big shift in our diagnostic method. With most other disorders, we need to notice what has changed about a person; when discerning the pattern of a PD, however, we must instead pay attention to what has remained the same— the lifelong background of attitudes and behaviors. We must tread carefully the path to diagnosis, scrupulously adhering to the several requirements for assessing PDs. Table 17.1 presents a differential diagnosis for PDs and other personality or relational problems.

Characteristics of PDs

- The symptoms of a PD are present throughout the person's adult life, at least since late adolescence.

> In the half dozen years he'd lived just down the street from the crisis residential house, Bruce's tendency to secrecy seemed to be increasing. His long hair was now unwashed and uncombed; his nails had grown long and ragged. No one liked him, especially the kids he repeatedly chased from his unfenced front yard, which was nearly as scruffy as its owner. "Personality disorder, schizoid type" was the guess of the mental health specialists who encountered him nearly every day, though they admitted they couldn't be sure without an interview. So it was with surprise and, ultimately, sorrow that after he died suddenly one rainy Saturday afternoon, they read his obituary. Years earlier, Bruce had been a rising star in the summer comedy circuit in the Catskills. Then, inexplicably, he'd dropped completely out of sight. He was only 54 when he died of a slow-growing meningioma, which could have been treated if only he'd been appropriately diagnosed.

Already, you can see this isn't going to be easy. *Accurately* defining a PD requires a lot more detective work than some other conditions, where most of the relevant symptoms are low-hanging fruit.

- Can other disorders, physical or mental, better account for the symptoms?

TABLE 17.1. Differential Diagnosis with Brief Definitions for Personality Disorders (PDs) and Other Personality or Relational Problems

- *General description of a PD.* A lasting, inflexible pattern of "inner experience and behavior" different from cultural expectations that presents problems in thinking, emotions, interpersonal relationships, and impulse control. This begins at an early age and manifests itself in a variety of work, social, and interpersonal situations.

- *Antisocial PD.* Egocentric and driven by desire for personal gain, these people lack concern for others and the capacity for intimate relationships. To gain their ends they will lie, deceive, and manipulate others while callously disregarding their personal responsibilities. Their attitudes toward others are often described as hostile or callous. They will impulsively take inordinate risks without considering possible consequences. Antisocial PD cannot be diagnosed before age 18.

- *Avoidant PD.* Low in self-esteem and ultrasensitive to rejection, these patients hesitate to become socially involved unless they can be certain of acceptance. They are reluctant to take risks in the pursuit of their goals, and when they do try to participate, anxiety is likely to preclude enjoyment, especially in social situations.

- *Borderline PD.* Instability characterizes these patients—it defines their self-image and aspirational goals, and it infects their close relationships, which they find fraught with the fear of rejection. Their emotions are labile (often angry or hostile), and they are prone to depression, hopelessness, and intense anxiety. Easily insulted, they cannot recognize the feelings and needs of others. They impulsively take risks without considering possible consequences.

- *Dependent PD.* A need to be taken care of leads to clinging, submissive behavior and fear of separation.

- *Histrionic PD.* Emotional excess and attention-seeking behaviors are typical.

- *Narcissistic PD.* Looking to others for their sense of self-esteem, these self-centered people seek attention and approval, even admiration. Their grandiosity (fantasized or actual) makes it hard to perceive feelings of others as distinct from their own needs. With little genuine interest in others, their lack of empathy renders their relationships with others superficial.

- *Obsessive–compulsive PD.* With their sense of self deriving from work, these people are production-oriented; however, their rigid and unreasonably high standards prevent the achievement of goals. Lacking empathy, their relationships are secondary to productivity. Their demands for perfection apply to themselves as well as to others. Preoccupied with details and organization, they will persevere at a task long after it stops working for them.

- *Paranoid PD.* These patients distrust and suspect others, whose motives they interpret as malevolent.

- *Schizoid PD.* Isolation from social relationships and restricted emotional range in interpersonal settings characterize these patients.

- *Schizotypal PD.* These odd, sometimes bizarre people often have confused ego boundaries and life goals that tend to be unrealistic or ill thought out. Sometimes

TABLE 17.1 (*cont.*)

helped along by perceptual distortions, they misunderstand or misinterpret others' behavior, yielding mistrust that impairs relationship intimacy. Their thinking is vague, and others consider their beliefs to be peculiar or odd (restricted affect can encourage this). Suspicious of the intention or loyalty of others, they prefer solitude.

- *Personality traits.* A person's experience of self and interpersonal functioning is impaired, and there is pathology of at least one personality trait domain: negative affectivity, detachment, antagonism, disinhibition (or compulsivity), and psychoticism. However, these don't add up to a clear diagnosis.

These three can start later in life:

- *Relational problem.* Two or more individuals interact so as to impair functioning or produce clinical symptoms.

- *Personality change due to a medical condition.* There is a lasting change in a patient's established personality after a traumatic brain injury or physical illness.

- *Intermittent explosive disorder.* Without other demonstrable pathology, there are episodes of aggressive acting out, resulting in physical harm or the destruction of property.

For as long as anyone can remember, Max has been the grouchiest postal worker in the history of his branch office. His nasty disposition has featured in many performance reviews, but his work is so meticulous that no supervisor has wanted to fire him. At home, he is "a bear to live with," as attested by three ex-wives and a bevy of angry stepchildren. Since his high school days, Max can never remember feeling anything but "lonely and sad"—feelings he's declined to share with any of the mental health clinicians who have tried to help him over the years. "Borderline personality disorder" is what at least a couple of them have written into his chart.

To the joy of his coworkers, when he turns 55 Max retires and takes a job managing, of all things, the office of a mental health clinic. After a few weeks, one of the clinicians suggests that he try medication for dysthymia. Within weeks, Max's "personality disorder" disappears. In a special ceremony the following year, fellow employees fete him as "Mr. Personality."

Before patients are diagnosed with a PD, they should be scrutinized for a variety of other conditions. For example, dysthymia can create dependency; mania may underlie belligerence; and long-term substance use can set the stage for impulsivity. Also, don't confuse with illness issues such as patients' trouble fitting into cultures or subcultures different from the ones in which they were reared.

- The pattern must be stable. I realize that "stable instability" is a bit of an oxymoron, but you get the idea: It's the pattern that's constant, even if the behavior wobbles a bit. Consider some counterexamples: You wouldn't make a PD diagnosis for a person who displays antisocial behavior only when intoxicated or in the throes of a manic episode. And, you can identify antisocial behavior in lots of adolescents, most of whom will probably straighten out with time. Although official criteria allow you to diagnose a PD in anyone, even (except for antisocial PD) someone quite young, I think it's safer to wait until the person has fully matured. PD is serious stuff; once one is diagnosed, it tends to follow the patient around forever. I wouldn't want to be responsible for such a label unless it's fully deserved.
- PDs affect several of the features that contribute to a person's character: affect, cognition, impulse control, and interpersonal functioning. If, say, only mood is affected, you should focus your diagnostic interest on a bipolar disorder or dysthymia—but probably not a PD. Or if mood is stable and the only trouble is controlling the impulse to steal, you might first consider kleptomania.
- A PD must be more or less consistent across the spectrum of life areas, including work, social, sexual, and family life. For an example, revisit Chuck (we met him in Chapter 15, pp. 242–244), whose antisocial behavior wreaked general havoc.

Table 17.2 presents a brief list of personality-related questions that might help you detect PDs in your patients. Wherever indicated, ask for examples.

Recognizing a PD

Many experienced clinicians claim that they can sense when a patient has a PD. What they are really doing is (1) matching what they observe against the countless patients they have evaluated in the past; (2) noting certain behaviors and items of history that are typically associated with a PD; and (3) identifying discrepancies. I can't help you with the first of these—only time can confer that sort of experience—but I can cast a few pearls from groups 2 and 3. Unhappily, without a reliable history, in some cases there is essentially nothing that will tip you off. For example, it will be nearly impossible to recognize an antisocial person like Ted Bundy, the charming

TABLE 17.2. Assessing Personality Disorder in Mental Health Patients

1. What sort of a person do you think you are?

2. What do you like most about yourself? What do you like least?

3. Do you have many friends, or are you more of a loner?

4. Do you have any problems getting along with members of your family? With friends?

5. Do you tend to be suspicious of other people's motives?

6. Do you like being the center of attention, or are you more comfortable staying in the background?

7. Do you feel that other people would like to deceive or harm you?

8. Do you tend to bear grudges?

9. Are you a superstitious person?

10. Does your mood tend to be pretty stable?

11. What are your dreams for yourself? Do you sometimes fantasize about them?

12. Do you feel you deserve special treatment or consideration?

13. Do you often feel inadequate in new relationships? Do you feel you need a lot of advice and reassurance when making everyday decisions?

14. Do you sometimes get so preoccupied with details that you lose sight of the point of what you were doing?

15. Are you especially stubborn? Are you a perfectionist?

Note. Adapted from *The First Interview* (4th ed.) by James Morrison (The Guilford Press 2014). Copyright © 2014 The Guilford Press. Adapted by permission.

butcher of over a dozen young women in the 1970s. In that sense, the diagnosis of antisocial PD demonstrates the value of third-party informants.

Note that no single behavior is diagnostic of a PD, so you can't take any of these items to the bank; each must be evaluated in the context of all else you can learn about this person. The items are meant as flags, not criteria. What you observe may not be a PD at all, but just personality traits, which we all possess to some degree. Sometimes the clues you spot may mean another diagnosable disorder entirely.

Information from the History

Some items will be obvious from the history, even when the patient is your only informant.

- In particular, problematic behaviors that recur—for example, repeatedly firing one's own clinician (operationally, I'd say three or more times; there are plenty of legitimate reasons to change medical care providers). Other examples include repeated legal difficulties (especially incarcerations), mental hospitalizations (in the absence of a confirmed diagnosis of a bipolar disorder or schizophrenia), or changes of spouses or jobs (neither of which carries quite the stigma it once did). I'd also include behavior patterns such as hoarding, recurring suicide attempts in response to disappointment, and repeatedly running away after fighting with a relative.
- Multiple suicide attempts, though PD should never be your first diagnosis in this instance.
- Exclusive focus on any one aspect of life: workaholism, partying, sex, playing bridge, or other hobbies. For example, I'd worry about a college student who did nothing but study, partaking in no extracurricular activities or social life.
- Obviously false answers (e.g., $2 + 2 = 5$) or a vague story that keeps changing.
- A family history of PD (such as antisocial or borderline).
- A childhood history of sexual abuse, or being reared by parents who are long-time, heavy substance users.
- Certain diagnoses with a strong likelihood of associated PD: eating disorders, dissociative disorders, somatic symptom disorder, social anxiety disorder (often found with avoidant PD), schizophrenia (often linked with antecedent schizotypal PD), and substance misuse.
- Chronic difficulty working with other people.
- Lack of friends and close relationships, especially someone who seems to have no need for any.

The Patient's Affects and Attitudes

Certain affects and attitudes may be evident even during the initial interview. Here are a few from a list you will eventually augment from your own experience:

- Negative attributes of disposition maintained without apparent embarrassment. Examples include expressions of violence, arrogance (often found in narcissistic PD), and conscienceless lack of remorse and empathy (for example, bragging about criminal exploits or indifference to the suffering of others).

- Disregard for one's own suffering, long associated with histrionic PD.
- In the absence of dementia, mania, or schizophrenia, discrepancies or inconsistencies between affect and stated mood, or mood and content of thought.
- Perplexity when asked to describe feelings of others.
- Excessive rigidity, as shown by inability to "get along by going along" in the workplace or family.
- Attitudes of chronic victimization (someone else was at fault, "I didn't do it," "I was framed").

Behaviors Observed over Time

Often, only after you begin working with a patient do you learn enough to diagnose a PD. Some indicative behaviors include the following:

- Glancing toward the window or door in a show of enhanced vigilance.
- Repeated suicide gestures or episodes of self-mutilation such as (perhaps superficial) wrist cutting.
- Excessive dependence—chronically stating, in effect, "I want you to decide."
- Demanding something, then rejecting it. Examples include hospitalization, followed by against-advice discharge; medication that the patient then refuses to use.
- Repeated failure of therapeutic measures that are normally effective for the patient's current major mental diagnosis.
- Paying close attention to clothing and grooming while neglecting relationships.
- Impulsivity, including extravagant gestures such as setting one's hair on fire or other modes of self-injury.
- Extreme reactions to events—perhaps attempting suicide upon learning that a relative has cancer.
- Evidence of consistently faulty judgment: multiple instances of not following medical advice, persistent promiscuity that results in rejection or disease, repeated legal troubles (especially criminality).

The Therapeutic Relationship

Again, some issues in the therapeutic relationship will become apparent quickly; others may take a while to emerge.

- Initial extravagant praise for your clinical abilities, with disparagement of the patient's previous therapist, followed later by complaints and devaluation—of you.
- Negative affects directed toward you, including dysphoria, anxiety, anger, and belligerence. Also there can be overt acts of hostility, such as kicking in an office building wall or letting the air out of your tires. (Ask me about those sometime.)
- Seductive, self-dramatizing, whining approaches to you and others.
- Manipulative behaviors: requesting a hospital pass from one caregiver when another won't allow it; demanding a certain favored hour for therapy; implying disaster if medication isn't forthcoming; repeatedly inquiring about your personal life; asking to be held, massaged, kissed, and more; attempting to smoke in the office; using your first name despite requests to do otherwise; making repeated telephone calls to you on weekends; changing appointments at the last minute.
- Gift giving—even a Danish and coffee can come with strings attached.
- Repeated tardiness for appointments.
- Stalking the clinician, the ultimate clinical nightmare. (Again, you have it from someone who's been there.)
- Neglecting physical symptoms such as sharp abdominal pain or an abscessed tooth—a worry to any clinician.
- Negative feelings on the part of the clinician: annoyance, fear, distrust, anger, or even, despite misbehavior, attraction. Any of these can suggest that one of you may have a PD.

Recognizing a PD can be a challenge in some patients, though in others it may seem obvious.

Robin

"There are some things I won't talk about," Robin declares on her first visit. With her unlighted cigarette, she gestures toward the scars laddering her left arm. "That's one of them. I saw you looking."

It is late November, but Robin has a deep tan. Although she's pulled her burnished auburn hair back in a long ponytail, she looks every day of her 37 years. "I just don't feel happy," she complains. "Some days I'm depressed, but mostly I'm just out of sorts. I hate my life." Sometimes, she says, she feels bad around the time of her periods, but more often it seems related to whatever is going on in her life. "My low-end job sucks, and no one really likes me."

Robin's complaints are legion. Last year at Thanksgiving, she accused her mother of favoring her older sister, Alicia; the three haven't gotten together since. And that is only part of Robin's rupture with her family. She lost one job when she impulsively danced topless at an office party. Over several weeks, she picked up men from the singles bar she frequents after work. More than once, she has brought one home with her to spend the night—causing no little inconvenience for Alicia in their shared apartment. Tempers flare late one evening when Robin walks through the door with yet another "drunken loser," in her sister's words, "though she never drinks more than a beer or two herself." Now they aren't even on speaking terms, compounding Robin's misery.

With Robin's permission, the therapist calls Alicia for some background information. Because they work at the same government office, Alicia has a lot of insight into what she calls her sister's *modus operandi*. "Ever since she was a little kid, she's been a walking focus of discontent," Alicia reports. Over the telephone, you can almost hear her frown. "She's always suspicious that someone else is saying things to make her look bad, to try to get her in trouble." Back when she was a senior in high school, Robin broke off contact with her best friend, who she thought was trying to steal her boyfriend. "I'm certain now that this girl was a lesbian—what would she want with *anyone's* boyfriend?" Alicia asks.

She continues, "During the last election, Robin was wild in support of the president. She was always talking politics and passing out campaign literature, even though it's against office policy. But when the White House issued a presidential order she didn't approve of, she said she felt betrayed, and started campaigning for the other side. That's how she is—always blowing hot and cold. Our boss'd love to get rid of her, but you know the government—that would take an act of Congress."

To a fellow employee, Robin criticized their boss for the decision not to hire a temp when a coworker took paternity leave. Later Alicia overheard her telling their boss that the choice was solid, because the coworker hadn't been pulling his weight. "When I called her on it, Robin blew up and threatened never to speak to me again. Typical of her, also, that she always comes crawling back. I've never known someone who is so afraid of being alone, but so often shoves other people away."

Analysis

First, we would need to know whether Robin has a major mental diagnosis (see step 1 of Figure 17.1, our decision tree for a patient with character/interpersonal difficulties). Although the details reported in this vignette are sketchy, her clinician learned enough to determine that she probably didn't qualify for an anxiety, mood, or psychotic disorder, and that she didn't drink or use drugs. (Had she qualified, we'd want to be doubly careful about also diagnosing a PD, though the figure encourages us to explore that possibility.) More information would be needed about her physical health, but Alicia's historical review argues against any recent change (step 2). Robin's

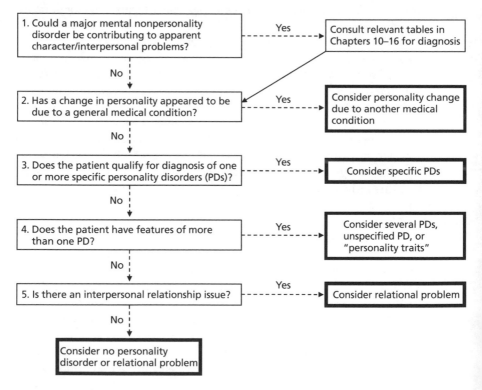

FIGURE 17.1. Decision tree for a patient who experiences character/interpersonal difficulties.

challenge early in the interview alerts us to the possibility of a PD. Robin herself mentioned numerous instances of difficulty getting along with other people, especially those in her own family.

Robin would seem to fit the general description of someone with a PD: She's had lifelong difficulty with her self-image and maintaining her interpersonal relationships; without evident psychosis, her thinking is skewed by ideas that others oppose her; her emotional state is precarious. These characteristics affect all areas of her life. None of the patterns typical of the recognized PDs (see Table 17.1) adequately defines her character, however, so we'd have difficulty giving her a specific PD diagnosis (step 3). She does appear to have several disordered personality traits, including dramatic need for attention (dancing seminude), paranoia (suspicions about her girlfriend), and borderline characteristics (multiple episodes of self-mutilation). At step 4, then, we might well consider her for several personality traits or an unspecified PD. Although we could theoretically continue on through our decision tree and look for a relational problem in addition, in the face of so many personality traits it seems unnecessary.

Comment

The diagnosis of a PD is beset with many problems. Here are just a few of them:

1. Contrary to the impression you might get from a casual reading of diagnostic manuals, most patients with PDs have mixtures of traits and PDs. Yet clinicians tend to diagnose only one PD, even when patients meet criteria for two or more.
2. When more than one PD *is* diagnosed, what does this actually mean? Surely not that the patient has several personalities. And how does this help inform treatment?
3. There is no sharp dividing line between PD and normality.
4. So far, little work has been reported that would pinpoint the cause of PDs.
5. PDs are especially hard to evaluate. Often the patient interview alone doesn't suffice, even when a standardized interview is used; neither does psychological testing. Rather, to demonstrate that the behaviors in question are both enduring and pervasive, we need interviews with relatives and others who have known the patient well, at least from late adolescence.
6. The three DSM-5-TR PD clusters (odd or aloof; dramatic, impul-

sive, or erratic; anxious or fearful) currently in use have little basis in objective research.

Some PDs have special issues. Many researchers place schizotypal PD on a continuum with schizophrenia; in addition to discussing it with the PDs, DSM-5-TR and the *International Classification of Diseases* (10th rev.) even list it in the same chapter with schizophrenia spectrum and other psychotic disorders. Although we list somatic symptom disorder as a major mental disorder, it so often goes hand in glove with histrionic PD that it's hard to determine where one leaves off and the other begins. Avoidant PD is often found with social anxiety disorder. Some clinicians use *borderline* more to express general disapproval than to describe a specific disorder. And fears of abandonment are symptomatic of both borderline and dependent PDs.

We could address some of these issues by describing personality with a hybrid dimensional system of the sort DSM-5-TR offers in its Section III alternative descriptive model; with time, it might be adopted formally as the standard for PD evaluation. It requires us first to identify, as we already did for Robin, moderate or greater problems with self (identity or self-expression) or interpersonal relations (empathy or intimacy). DSM-5-TR provides a table (on p. 884) to facilitate that task. Then, using the Personality Inventory for DSM-5-TR (the long form is available for free download at *https://www.psychiatry.org/File%20Library/Psychiatrists/Practice/DSM/ APA_DSM5_The-Personality-Inventory-For-DSM-5-Full-Version-Adult. pdf*) I entered the answers I thought Robin might give. Note that she was no longer available to do it herself, and besides, clinicians are encouraged to use informants' responses. Here's how she (well, we) scored for the five top-level personality domains: Negative affect, 1.6; Detachment, 1.4; Antagonism, 1.4; Disinhibition, 1.7; Psychoticism, 0.2. Each of these but the last ranked about midway between mild and moderate. I determined that she did not score at a moderate (2.0 or greater) level on enough of the individual facets, as they are called, to qualify for any of the PDs named in this assessment measure. (With elevated scores on the facets of emotional lability, impulsivity, and hostility, she would come very close to qualifying for borderline PD.) For anyone who is interested, I encourage you to play around with the form.

Although clinicians sometimes focus so strongly on the major mental disorders that they ignore the presence of PDs, the opposite problem also arises: An apparent PD drives away consideration of other, more treatable (and even more dangerous) mental conditions.

Consider the case of Elizabeth Shin, an enormously bright and talented MIT sophomore. After many months of care related to anxiety and depression, she burned herself to death in her dormitory room. On several occasions she had cut herself, which prompted speculation that she had borderline PD. Did her clinicians pay too much attention to an apparent PD and thus give short shrift to her repeated statements that she wanted to kill herself?

What can we take away from the discussion of PDs and their confounds?

- Maladaptive traits are present in many people who don't meet criteria for a PD.
- Examine all patients for character issues that influence how they do business with the world, whether or not they meet anyone's formal criteria for a disorder.
- Although I've complained about the criteria, it is *far* better to use any standard than to depend on your subjective impressions—a much-ignored diagnostic principle.
- An important function of the PDs is to remind us to look for associated major mental disorders.

Phineas

In addition to the problem of detecting major mental pathology, we must also keep alert for how long the person has had character pathology and the circumstances in which it was acquired.

One fall day in 1848, Phineas Gage, the foreman of a railway construction gang in Vermont, had just tamped down an explosive charge when all hell broke loose. As reported by a local newspaper, an accidental explosion blasted Gage's tamping iron through his left cheekbone and out through the top of his head. The tapered iron was 43 inches long and over an inch in diameter at its widest; it weighed just over 13 pounds. Although most of the left frontal lobe of his brain was destroyed, Phineas possibly didn't even lose consciousness. The newspaper stated that he was "in full possession of his reason, and free from pain." His recovery was so successful that 10 weeks later, he returned home to New Hampshire.

     Within a few months he sought to return to work, but as his friends sadly noted, "Gage was no longer Gage." Formerly capable, efficient, and possessed of a good business sense, now he was profane, irreverent, obstinate, impatient with others, vacillating, and capricious. Indeed, his personality was so altered that his company would no longer employ him. Able neither to plan for the future nor to hold a job, 13 years later he died penniless. Although his brain was not autopsied, his skull is on display at the Warren Anatomical Museum at Harvard Medical School.

Analysis

At step 1 of Figure 17.1, we can conclude from the history that there does not appear to have been a major mental disorder (we're talking here about mood, psychotic, or substance use disorders). That gets us to step 2, where we can agree that Phineas's change in personality was well explained by the horrific injury he sustained, and he fits neatly into the DSM-5-TR category of personality change due to traumatic brain injury. Although relationship problems might have developed later, they do not form part of this particular exercise.

Comment

The obvious difference between a PD and Phineas's personality change is time: The former must be continuously present from a young age. Personality change can embrace many possible symptoms, including agitation, passivity, irritability, aggression, labile moods, childishness, irresponsibility, apathy, rigidity, and lack of motivation, reduced empathy, disagreeableness, and diminished conscientiousness. As with PDs, informants other than the patient are of critical importance; newspaper accounts are optional.

Personality change is often related to a traumatic brain injury, which when severe is likely to cause symptoms. But it can also result from diseases such as strokes, Alzheimer's disease, benign or malignant tumors, HIV disease, multiple sclerosis, spinocerebellar ataxia, neurosyphilis, Huntington's disease, cerebral malaria, toxicity, and encephalitis—in fact, just about any disorder that affects the metabolism or structure of the brain. If the personality change is prominent, you can diagnose it even in a patient with dementia; in fact, it may be how dementia first announces itself. Some researchers have found that personality change early in the course of Alzheimer's disease predicts that the functional decline may be more rapid than usual. The obvious conclusion is that any patient whose character structure has changed should receive a full medical workup for possible physical causes.

Diagnosing Relational Problems

In every chapter of this book, we have wrestled with boundary issues between different illnesses. Here is a case that explores a different sort of boundary.

Marcie

At age 32, Marcie is the mother of two small children. Although she abandoned a promising career in marketing when she became pregnant, she loves being a stay-at-home mom. However, for the past several weeks she has been distressed, anxious, and somewhat depressed. Actually, she tells the clinician, she feels fine most of the time, but her mood begins to slip toward evening, when Ian arrives home from work. She doesn't know whether that could have anything to do with it, because "we have a great marriage, and he's a terrific dad." She hesitates. "But, well, we have been fighting a lot."

The clinician probes: "Money? Sex? These are the big issues for most couples." Their battleground is her brother's drinking. Ray lives across town, but he spends much of his time with Marcie and her family. From the garage of her home, Marcie and Ray run the small mail-order business they inherited from their mother just a year ago. "On her deathbed Mom begged me to take care of Ray, and I promised I always would. And I never dodge my responsibilities."

Ray had been sheltered by their mother, and lately Ian accuses Marcie of behaving just like her. Marcie acknowledges the truth in this claim, but she can't just let Ray go. "He may be heavy, but he's still my brother," she explains. (Ian has long resented the jokes she uses to slide away from serious discussions.)

However, Ian doesn't dislike Ray. In fact, he rather enjoys his company, when Ray is sober—which, Marcie admits, "any more is mostly never." Now she and Ian fight nearly every night, and much of the weekend, too. She said that she has no problems with sleep or appetite. In addition, she denies actual panic attacks or death wishes, and she remains passionately interested in her children and her business. And her sex interest is excellent, she says, "when Ian and I are on, um, speaking terms."

Analysis

Marcie lacks the symptoms for a step 1 major mental disorder, and there is no evidence of a medical condition or a lifelong PD (steps 2 and 3). Indeed, she doesn't really have enough symptoms to warrant *any* of the usual clinical diagnoses. The fact that she becomes symptomatic only when her husband is home should move us in a different direction.

An adjustment disorder would seem to be a real possibility, but let's think about that diagnosis and its several drawbacks. For openers, the criteria are vague: "Clinical significance" is required; there must be no other disorder that can account for the symptoms; and you as the clinician must judge that the symptoms occur in response to a stressor—even if your crystal ball is in the shop for repairs. Furthermore, any prospective diagnosis must be listed as *provisional:* You can only know that you've made the right diagnosis if the symptoms go away once the stressor lifts. What a stressful set of criteria!

In Marcie's case, both she and Ian were apparently contributing to the difficulty, which would make it seem just about perfect for a relational problem. By the way, this diagnosis also suggests the path necessary to deal with the problem, whereas a diagnosis of adjustment disorder depicts a patient as a passive vessel, filled with anxiety and depression until something happens to take away the strain. If you feel strongly that you would want to give Marcie a personality diagnosis, I'd go with *undiagnosed*—I wouldn't even know what kind of *unspecified* diagnosis to use.

Comment

It's a truism that many people consult us not because they are ill, but because they have problems working, living, or just plain getting along with others—their siblings, children, parents, spouses or partners, and even coworkers:

- For a year, a brother and two sisters have fought over their parents' estate.
- A mother and her teenage daughter quarrel about dating; the daughter stays out late, the mother nags. Both are angry.
- Lovers in a 10-year committed relationship are at odds over whether to adopt a baby.

- A man uses amphetamines and frequently beats his wife, who will never agree to press charges or seek shelter.
- A woman lies in a coma for 15 years while her husband and parents argue about whether she should be allowed to die.

The examples above share several features. The behaviors in question often act as a circle of cause and effect: A mother punishes her daughter for staying out, and the daughter in turn rebels at the perceived overcontrol by staying out later. In other words, the way the individuals respond to one another perpetuates the dispute. The pattern involves anguish and sometimes danger, and it is relatively constant from one situation to another. It usually isn't simply a response to a particular event, and it persists not for days or weeks, but for months or years. It is unresponsive to social or religious suasion, and there is evidence of impact on individuals' health and functioning.

Recognizing Relational Problems

Shelves groan with books that propose to assess couple and family discord, and I promise not to burden them—and you—much further. Instead, here is a brief outline to help you decide whether a relational problem describes your patient's difficulties:

1. You'll probably need collateral input to ascertain that this is an interpersonal issue—that two or more individuals contribute to the conflict. Even if the second person denies it, the behavior you observe may tell another story.
2. The relationship must be important. No matter how heated it becomes, an argument between strangers on a train doesn't qualify.
3. The conflict itself must be relatively enduring. Most relationships have their ups and downs; we mustn't react with alarm to every lurch on the Ferris wheel of family life.
4. Does an individual's mental diagnosis provide background? If so, it must not be the sole source of the conflict. It probably happens often that a given clinical situation entails both an individual diagnosis and a relationship problem. They may be completely separate, or one may flow from the other, in which case the relationship problem is said to be *embedded*.

5. To identify an impairment of social functioning between the parties, you might find some help in the Global Assessment of Relational Functioning (GARF), which guides clinicians to evaluate the relationship in terms of problem solving, organization, and emotional climate. (You can find the GARF on p. 814 of DSM-IV-TR. DSM-5 deep-sixed it, along with the GAF. Too bad.)

The early years of the 21st century have witnessed a huge debate over whether to include relational problems as a regular part of future diagnostic manuals. At this writing, the issue hasn't yet been definitively sorted out—but regardless of the degree to which they are formalized in criteria, the problems still exist and must be identified and treated. They represent part of the enormously important aspect to the overall provision of mental health care called *problems of living,* which can include just about anything that isn't an actual mental disorder. The diagnostic manuals include a lot of this psychosocial and environmental stuff, with code numbers, so you can note it right along with your other diagnoses. The list of potential problems of living includes the following:

Family (death, divorce, neglect, abuse)

Support group (living alone, being a victim of discrimination, emigrating)

School (difficulties with teachers or classmates, illiteracy)

Workplace (stressful schedule or working conditions, discord with supervisor or coworkers)

Housing (homelessness, unsafe conditions, trouble with neighbors)

Finances

Access to health care (through lack of insurance, geographic isolation)

Legal difficulties (being a victim of crime, getting arrested, involvement in litigation)

Other issues, such as problems of acculturation, religion, retirement, and the effects of war or terrorism

Distinguishing Disorder from Normality

And here is yet another sort of boundary to keep in mind.

Horace

After Horace reached his university's mandatory retirement age of 65, he spent his first 20 emeritus years teaching his old subjects as a volunteer. He later tells a clinician, "I eventually got too old to get myself there on a regular basis, so I've spent the last 8 years working in my garden, writing letters to the editor, and reading the classics." What brings him to mental health attention is his response to his general physician's news that there is a small cancerous growth in his left kidney. Horace buttons his shirt and smiles as he says, "Well, good. At 93, I think this is just the right time for me to take my leave. Exit Horace." Subsequently, he refuses even to discuss the operation that, if undertaken right away, will almost surely provide a cure.

The mental health consultant learns that Horace sometimes feels down for a few hours ("And who wouldn't? My wife died years ago, and I've outlived all my old friends"), but he has no other symptoms of a mood disorder. He drinks two glasses of wine each day ("It's good for my cholesterol"), but he denies having any difficulty whatsoever interpersonally, financially, or with the law.

Analysis

Several mental health clinicians review Horace's story with his attending doctor. After half an hour of digging for further symptoms, they determine that they cannot make a case for any major mental disorder (step 1). They agree that he regards his situation with equanimity, speaks dispassionately, and appears to have made a rational choice. There has been no step 2 personality change. In fact, there is no evidence of any problem with his personality (step 3); he has always been a sweet-tempered man, beloved by family, colleagues, and students. Finally, other than the distress felt by Horace's physician, there are no interpersonal issues that might merit a diagnosis of a relational problem (step 5). We are apparently left with a person who, with no mental illness, has every right to make what he regards as a logical, everyday decision about his own health care needs. The consulting committee does encourage the treating physician to discuss again the merits of an operation.

Comment

How often does a clinician wonder, "Could this patient have *no* mental illness?" I suspect it happens rather less often than it should. Indeed, research in this area is apparently entirely lacking—Medline searches for *no mental illness* and similar phrases consistently come up empty. One problem is the absence of a bright line between normality and illness. Extend Horace's momentary "feeling down" to a few days, and would he be ill then? Add sleeplessness; would he be ill then? What if he lost his appetite? At some point, all would agree that he had a clinical illness, but the gray area leaves much room for dispute.

The follow-up: Horace's physician does press the issue of the kidney operation, emphasizing the pain and loss of control if his cancer were to metastasize. Horace ultimately relents and speedily recovers from a successful operation.

18 Beyond Diagnosis
Compliance, Suicide, Violence

All clinicians need to keep in mind three issues that are important for evaluation but transcend the boundaries of diagnosis: compliance, suicide, and violence.

Compliance

When I was a student, *noncompliance* meant that the patient didn't follow the clinician's directions. Now an ethos of cooperation—partnership between patient and care provider—has changed how we view this important subject, which some clinicians now call *adherence*.

Of course, there are degrees of noncompliance/nonadherence. One patient might just disregard a recommended exercise program; another might "forget" many doses of Antabuse, endangering sobriety. In between are myriad opportunities for confusion and error.

Research in this area lags, but we do know a fair amount from controlled studies—though much of it is pretty predictable. For example, nonadherence is greater among outpatients than inpatients. It increases with more time in treatment, with a more complicated treatment regimen, and with more side effects. You can reduce it with careful supervision, education about the nature of the disease and the nature of the treatment, and a supportive environment. Patients who are satisfied with the course of treatment are much more likely to be adherent than are unhappy ones. Indeed, nonadherence per se may not be the only reason—or may not be the reason at all—why treatment is not working; other factors may need to be considered (see the sidebar "Why Doesn't Treatment Work?").

The effects of nonadherence run from major to mundane. Of course, no treatment can be effective if it isn't utilized, and for some patients, not taking the prescribed treatment (say, a course of cognitive-behavioral therapy) may only mean that depression continues without relief. More serious

Why Doesn't Treatment Work?

The question "Why doesn't treatment work?" has a number of answers, each of which is probably right some of the time.

- *Wrong treatment.* Some patients with depression respond to SSRIs, others to cognitive-behavioral therapy. Still others with apparent treatment resistance may require ketamine or a drug combination.
- *Insufficient time.* Often patients despair of treatment that simply hasn't yet had enough time to work. This is famously true of psychotherapy, as well as most medications.
- *Wrong dosage.* Usually this applies to drug treatment, and usually it means that too little of the medication has been prescribed. Some drugs have a "therapeutic window" of effect, which means that either too little *or* too much can prevent optimal response.
- *Interference from other treatments.* Here's another problem with medication: The use of one can decrease the effectiveness of another.
- *Side effects.* Very often, unwanted effects (another medication issue) cause such grief that patients reduce doses or drop out of treatment altogether.
- *Other adherence issues.* The patient doesn't do the exercises, attend day care, practice the homework assignments for cognitive-behavioral therapy, or take medications as prescribed.
- *Use of substances.* In many ways, the effects of street drugs or alcohol can complicate treatment and its assessment.
- *Wrong diagnosis.* This may be the most common, though least heralded, factor of all those that contribute to the apparent lack of treatment effectiveness. It is also one of the easiest to rectify.

consequences could include repeated episodes of illness and multiple hospitalizations.

> When in the depressed phase of her bipolar I disorder, Belinda is a model patient who always recovers quickly. But when manic, she neglects her medication and might end up in a hospital over 1,000 miles away, where she grew up. With her fourth or fifth episode, I was called to her house one evening to find her in her front yard, spraying her living room furniture with the garden hose.

Still other patients may *become* estranged from family and friends.

Maude had been a champion swimmer, who often won medals and one year came close to qualifying for the U.S. Olympics team. But at 23 she developed schizophrenia, and forever afterward she claimed that her antipsychotics made it difficult to perform in the water. Time and again, she would stop taking her medication and become psychotic. With each hospitalization she refused medication, necessitating a court hearing to determine whether she should be medicated against her will. More than once, the judge was sympathetic to her pleas and discharged her from care. When I last spoke with her, she was in a nursing care facility, so psychotic that she couldn't even feed herself. Eventually her husband divorced her and took the children to live with him.

Sometimes the results are dire, as shown in two brief reports:

Severe recurrent depression caused Jolene to retire from her job with the post office when she was 44. About every 2 years, she became severely melancholic, couldn't sleep, lost weight, and refused to answer the telephone when her brother called to ask how she was doing. In her despondence she would develop suicidal ideas, but with every episode, she waited so long before calling for help that she couldn't be managed at home and had to be hospitalized. Each time, she stayed in the hospital only long enough to receive four electroconvulsive treatments, then signed out against advice. "I stopped because I felt better" was her usual rationale. She then failed to follow up with outpatient visits or treatment. This pattern went on for more than 20 years. After my last contact with Jolene, I heard nothing more for about 2 years, until a relative called to say that she had hanged herself.

In December 2005, a distraught Rigoberto Alpizar ran from his plane, which was about to take off from Miami, and onto the jetway. After allegedly yelling something about a bomb, he reached into his carry-on bag as he refused to surrender to the air marshals. They shot him dead. His wife told another passenger that he had bipolar disorder and had not taken his medication. No bomb was found, and no link to terrorism was ever suggested.

Obviously, identifying adherence issues is important for clinicians and patients alike. Here are some clues and resources you can use to assess the risk of nonadherence in your patients.

- *Ask the patient.* At every visit, I routinely ask each patient to describe each medication and its schedule of use. I frequently learn that the regimen is different from what I have recommended. Routine questioning offers a chance to discuss the issue without sounding critical. Differences from my expectations are easily discussed as a misunderstanding or as the patient's response to side effects; the usual solution is a successful compromise. Similar procedures could apply to diet, schedules of exercise, cognitive-behavioral homework, and more.

• *Ask relatives.* Collateral information from those who know the patient well may turn up problems with adherence.

• *Note lack of improvement.* Nonadherence is a likely factor when patients do not experience the expected response to treatment.

• *Are there side effects?* With drug regimens, *lack* of expected side effects can tip you off that your patient may not be getting enough medication—perhaps none at all.

• *Check environmental factors.* Is there a support system? Does this patient's peer group pride itself on refusing drugs or other treatment modalities?

• *Monitor caregiver factors.* How fully have you educated your patient about the need for treatment? How often are appointments scheduled? (Monthly or more often will help ensure adherence.) Does the patient perceive your relationship as strongly positive and helpful? Does the patient understand the theoretical reasons behind the treatment approach?

• *Watch for telltale symptoms.* Nonadherence can result from depression (the patient may have an apathetic response to treatment recommendations), euphoria (the patient may feel "too well to be sick"), delusions (the patient may be suspicious of your motives), poor insight (the patient may be unable to understand that an illness requires treatment), or anger (the patient may be acting out).

• *Observe red flags.* Adherence issues are especially relevant to mania, schizophrenia, dementia, personality disorder, and substance use. Patients with both substance use and another major mental disorder are especially vulnerable.

Suicide

The base rate of suicide (it's infrequent, at about 1% of deaths in the general population) and the inexact nature of the science make it hard to predict which individuals will attempt suicide and who will succeed. We have to rely on the seemingly numberless studies that try to pinpoint characteristics of suicide risk.

Jay retired after 30 years of honorable service in the Marine Corps. For a time he worked in his brother's machine shop, but now he mostly just sits at home. A couple of years ago, his wife died. They'd been childless, and he has never been a particularly social person. Now, in his late 60s, he lives alone on his military pension and Social Security.

No one has heard much from Jay until he is brought to the emergency department after he attempted suicide by carbon monoxide poisoning. He was discovered unconscious in his garage when a neighbor returned home unexpectedly at lunchtime and heard the purring of an engine. After several touch-and-go hours in intensive care, he recovers enough to speak with a mental health consultant, who learns that he has been drinking heavily to combat a severe melancholia.

Jay is sallow and gaunt. His clothes hang on his 6-foot frame—clearly, he has lost 20 pounds or more. He says that when he awakens at about 3 or 4 each morning, he will lie there and brood about the death of a friend with whom he served in Vietnam. "I could have picked up that grenade and heaved it, but I just jumped behind some sandbags." He has lost his interest in hunting, but he still keeps two rifles and a pistol locked in a cabinet. He has smoked all his adult life; a doctor recently told him that a spot on his lung is "suspicious" and he should come in for more tests. Not a religious man, Jay says that if he learned it was malignant, he wouldn't have it treated, though his father had died a horrible, lingering death from lung cancer. Jay would either move to Oregon and request physician-assisted suicide, or "just do the job myself, in the comfort of my own living room."

From the available information, Jay's clinician feels that there is an extremely high risk of further suicide attempts and places him on a one-to-one suicide watch. That evening about 10, Jay goes into the toilet and closes the door. Five minutes later, the aide attending him calls out, and the staff breaks down the door. They find him, hanging nearly lifeless from a loop of bath towel, and cut him down.

There are two basic sets of risk factors for suicide: those that pertain to mental illness, and those of a personal or social nature. I've put them into a couple of lists for reference.

Mental Disorders and Suicide

Like Jay, the vast majority of those who attempt or complete suicide have a diagnosable mental illness. Although suicide and suicide attempts are not tied to any one diagnosis, each is associated with suicide behaviors.

• *Mood disorders.* Major depression and bipolar disorder account for about half of all suicides, mostly when such a patient hasn't been treated adequately for depression. Risk of suicide increases as depression becomes more severe, especially with the presence of melancholic features (loss of pleasure in usual activities, feeling worse in the mornings, insomnia typified by awakening too early in the morning, loss of appetite or weight, excessive guilt, and a quality of mood that is more profound than typical grief). Recent studies have reported that in both depressive and bipolar disorders, treatment with antidepressants or lithium decreases suicide risk—a lot.

• *Schizophrenia.* About 10% of patients with schizophrenia die by suicide, usually in the first few years of illness. Risk is higher in those with paranoia or depressive symptoms, and lower in those with negative symptoms (flat affect, impoverished speech, inability to initiate action). In someone who has made previous attempts, command auditory hallucinations increase risk for another.

• *Substance use.* People with substance dependence have a risk of suicide 2 to 3 times that of the general population (for those who are heroin dependent, it is at least 14 times greater). For those who are alcohol dependent, loss of a close relationship through divorce, separation, death, or interpersonal friction is a common precipitant; risk increases further still if drinking has been recent and heavy.

• *Personality disorder.* The risk of suicide is especially great in antisocial and borderline personality disorders.

• *Other disorders.* Illnesses as varied as PTSD and ADHD may also confer an increased risk for suicide. There is even a risk with panic disorder, especially if major depressive disorder or substance use is also involved. Patients with somatic symptom disorder often attempt suicide; although there are few data, I believe that these people also carry an increased risk for completed suicide. And please remember that having more than one mental disorder greatly increases the risk of attempts and completed suicide.

Individual Factors in Suicide

For many years, numerous social and personal characteristics have been known to increase the risk of suicide:

• *Male gender.* Men have four times the risk of women for *completed* suicide, whereas women are three times as likely to *attempt* suicide.

• *Advancing age.* Suicide rates rise throughout the lifespan to peak in the over-85 group.

- *Skin color.* White people are far more likely to commit suicide than are non-Whites.
- *Employment.* Unemployed and retired persons, and those with long absences from work, may suffer from lower self-esteem and reduced access to support networks—both of which may increase risk.
- *Marital status.* Being single or divorced (divorced is worse) is a risk factor; married people are less likely to commit suicide.
- *Religion.* The risk for Protestants is higher than that for Catholics and Jews. Risk for Muslims is unclear.
- *Family history.* Suicide in a relative increases individual risk, even beyond the presence of mental disorder.
- *Living alone.* Isolation often breeds despair.
- *Gun ownership or access to other lethal means.* And don't forget medications that can be lethal in overdose.
- *Physical disease.* The burden of obstructive lung disease, cancer, epilepsy, chronic pain, and a host of other debilitating conditions predisposes patients to suicide; having multiple illnesses greatly increases the risk.
- *Feelings of hopelessness.* An unrelieved gloomy view of the future has been identified as especially predictive of future suicide.
- *Recent mental hospitalization.* The first few days after discharge are the most dangerous.
- *Financial difficulty.* The image of stock market investors leaping from windows during the Great Depression of the 1930s is no myth: The national suicide rate increased by 20%.
- *Heavy gambling losses.* This factor may be mediated by depression, not gambling disorder per se.
- *Talking about suicide.* The saying "Those who talk about it don't do it" is exactly the opposite of fact: Most people who kill themselves have communicated their intent, often to a care provider.
- *Suicide of others.* The death by suicide of a friend, a relative, or even a total stranger can increase the risk—especially in adolescents, for whom the pull of group behavior is especially powerful.
- *Prior suicide attempt.* This is one of the strongest predictors we can cite. After an attempted suicide, risk for completion persists for up to four decades. In a 2003 study by Beautrais, 9% of those who made a medically serious suicide attempt had died within 5 years; 59% of these had committed suicide. When evaluating an attempt, it is important to consider both medical and psychological seriousness. A medically serious attempt is one that causes unconsciousness, significant loss of blood, or disruption of parts of the body beneath the skin (tendons and arteries are examples). Psycho-

logically serious attempts are those in which the patient expresses regret at surviving, has made efforts to avoid discovery, or states a determination to make another attempt. An attempt that entails either type of seriousness should put you especially on guard.

A number of scales have been devised to measure the degree of suicidal intent and the seriousness of a prior attempt. The "References and Suggested Reading" section (pp. 331–339) lists a website that provides information about such scales.

Violence

Mental health clinicians famously fail to predict violent acts accurately— even within the next few hours or days, let alone far into the future. Over the years, lore has accumulated about factors that supposedly relate to violence. Some of this lore is accurate; some is not. Consider two scenarios:

> Brenda, who is a few months past her 21st birthday, drinks and uses speed. She's even cooked methamphetamine in a lab she helped her boyfriend construct in his grandmother's basement. From age 11 Brenda repeatedly ran away from home, in part to escape the beatings her stepfather administered for years. She is smart, but her poor attention span yielded abysmal grades in school; she dropped out when she was 15. Since then, she's been in and out of juvenile hall. At a rave when she was 16, after consuming alcohol and "other stuff" (she isn't sure just what), she stabbed and nearly killed another girl. Although Brenda was released from custody when she turned 21, her parole officer notes that she's recently resumed drinking. Moreover, she has threatened several times to "finish the job" on the girl she stabbed years ago.

> Brent, also 21, fell ill during his junior year at university. Always a steady, earnest student, both Brent and his family were surprised at how quickly his grades tumbled once the voices he heard began telling him he was the Devil. "Academically, he just seemed to wither away," says the aunt with whom he lived while attending school several hundred miles from where he grew up. After the first few weeks of the fall term, he gradually stopped attending class. He neglected his appearance and refused to go home for Christmas. By the end of April, he wouldn't even leave the house. When questioned, Brent says that

he has come to realize that he is the Antichrist, and through him the world will be destroyed. His aunt tells the clinician that her husband keeps a pistol in an unlocked desk drawer; she doesn't know, but she thinks it might be loaded.

Many people would probably assess Brent's history of psychosis and the fact that he is a young male with apocalyptic delusions as factors rendering him likely to commit a violent offense. However, over the years, traditional clinical methods have proven unreliable in assessing violence potential. A large part of the difficulty lies in the fact that studies of violence are often based on general population samples, whereas we clinicians want to know how likely *our patient* is to commit an act that will harm another person. To that end, in recent years researchers have developed actuarial models that rely less on clinical information and judgment, and more on data from records and demographics. Some of the findings may surprise you.

- *Diagnosis*. Traditionally, violence is associated with a number of diagnoses—schizophrenia, mania, antisocial personality, conduct disorder (in children and adolescents), intermittent explosive disorder, and substance use disorders (especially on days a person actually uses drugs or alcohol). However, the overwhelming majority of mental patients do not perpetrate violence. In fact, a major mental disorder such as bipolar I disorder or Brent's probable schizophrenia carries a lower risk of violence than does personality disorder (see below). A number of physical brain diseases can also lead to violence—head injuries, seizure disorders, Alzheimer's and other dementias, infections, cancer and other mass lesions, toxicity (including drug and alcohol intoxication), and metabolic conditions. Always, the comorbid diagnosis of substance use is an important predictor of violence.
- *Gender*. Men are traditionally regarded as committing the major share of violence. However, among mental patients, women like Brenda are about as likely as men to perpetrate violence, though their victims may be less likely to require medical attention. Women's violence is especially likely to occur in the home.
- *Prior violence*. A history of violent behavior is a traditionally strong predictor. Remarkably, assessment of violence isn't usually a problem; patients are often quite willing to admit to prior offenses. Brenda's prior assault and conviction clearly demonstrated her potential.
- *Abuse*. Childhood physical (but not sexual) abuse history is positively associated with later violence.

• *Antisocial personality disorder.* The risk of violence is greatly increased in people who carry this diagnosis. Although more information would be needed to be sure, Brenda's history should alert us to the possibility of conduct disorder and antisocial personality disorder.

• *Hallucinations.* Command hallucinations that order the person to commit violence increase the risk; other hallucinations are not related. Delusions, such as Brent's ideas about being the Antichrist, do *not* predict violence.

• *Anger and thoughts/fantasies of violence.* Ideas of violence beget violent behavior.

• *Age.* The age for violence, like the age for love and procreation, is youth. No surprise here.

In short, the actuarial model described by Gardner and colleagues predicts that violent mental patients will tend to be those who are hostile, are young, misuse drugs, and have a history of previous violent behavior. And of the two patients described above, it would be Brenda, not Brent, who represents the greater risk. Numerous studies report that discharged mental patients are likely to perpetrate violence only if they use substances. Unfortunately, they are more likely than the general public to misuse substances. When mental patients do reoffend, it usually occurs a relatively short time after discharge from a hospital.

Finally, consider the sobering observation that some of our most notorious violent patients might have slipped past the best of our current predictors: Prosenjit Poddar (who murdered Tatiana Tarasoff, eventually leading to the recognition of a duty to protect known as the *Tarasoff principle*); Mark David Chapman (who killed John Lennon); and John Hinckley, Jr. (who attempted to assassinate Ronald Reagan). Each of these individuals had had intense fantasies, but no prior history of violence. Even with the best in current research and instruments, we can deliver only predictions, not promises.

19 Patients, Patients

With the following case vignettes, you can further explore the methods we've discussed in the previous 18 chapters. I have selected patients varied enough to cover the diagnostic principles and major classes of disorders. Some of these cases are fairly simple; others are remarkably complicated. For each of these historics, I hope you will write down a differential diagnosis, arrange it by the safety principle, and (in your mind, if not on paper) choose the most likely diagnosis and how you would proceed with that patient.

John Clare

John Clare was a working-class man from England's North Country who became famous in the early 1800s for lyrical nature poetry that lives in print today. Throughout his adult life, John drank a great deal (mainly beer). His sexual contacts with a variety of young women, some of whom were probably prostitutes, may have prompted mercury treatment for syphilis. As a young man, he suffered from recurrent depressions, and he may have experienced bursts of activity and writing. In his later life, he had many hallucinations and was chronically delusional—believing, for example, that he had two wives simultaneously, that he was Robert Burns and Lord Byron, and that he was the son of King George III.

Analysis

The available facts, though skimpy, provide enough material for us to practice the construction of a differential diagnosis based on a safety hierarchy. I may not mention the differential diagnosis in every patient vignette, but still we should honor it by using it—every time. Here's how I think about John Clare's psychosis:

- Treatable disorders that can quickly have a profound effect on health:

  Psychosis related to alcohol use
  Psychosis related to syphilis
  Psychosis related to mercury poisoning
- Serious disorders, urgent to treat, though the consequences may be less wide-ranging:

  Bipolar I disorder, with psychosis
  Major depressive disorder, recurrent, with psychosis
- Disorders that are chronic and tend to have a poor prognosis, regardless of treatment:

  Schizophrenia and schizoaffective disorder (untreatable in the early 1800s)
  Alzheimer's dementia with psychosis

John Clare spent most of the last three decades of his life in asylums, ultimately dying when he was 70. Although a recent biographer has suggested that he suffered from a bipolar disorder, the course of his lengthy, chronic psychosis raises serious doubts. Several diagnostic principles drive the selection process—among them, and most important, the admonitions always to consider chemical and general medical causes. With no more information than we have, I'd have to invoke the diagnostic principle of choosing the term *undiagnosed* for the rustic poet who could pen such lines as these:

> I am—yet what I am, none cares or knows;
> My friends forsake me like a memory lost:
> I am the self-consumer of my woes . . .

Marian

When Marian appears for counseling, she feels anxious, and her chronic headaches have worsened. In the course of several weeks, she has managed to worry off about 10 pounds. This is no surprise, since her "appetite has fallen completely off the scale—I haven't eaten a thing for days." She laments that she worries about everything. Her father's health is declining; her sister's marriage is on the rocks. Her job in the county tax assessor's office pays enough to live on, but she believes that she has too little responsibility for her age and experience. She thinks she might quit this job and look elsewhere, as she had done half a dozen other times over the past few years. Now 33 and with her boyfriend scheduled for deployment with the Army Reserves, Marian senses the ticking of her biological clock: "One day I'd like to have a family—but not if I still have this much anxiety." Shoulders slumping, she breaks into tears.

While in high school, Marian had a series of panic attacks. She remembers how, during an algebra midterm exam, her head started to nod uncontrollably and her heart raced as she fought to breathe. Terrified, she'd have gotten up to leave, but with her legs too weak to support her, she could only sit and suffer, unable to cry or concentrate. She scored a D on that test. After several repeat attacks, they began to tail off and eventually disappeared altogether, but the empty, sad feeling that was left behind stayed with her throughout her formal education.

Just before Marian graduated from college, her mother died of breast cancer—the same fate as had met her grandmother and an aunt. Feeling abandoned and emptier than ever, she began drinking. Over the next 10 years, alcohol gained and lost her several lovers. When Jürgen, her current boyfriend, threatened to leave for good if she didn't quit, she finally did. "I haven't touched a drop in the 8 months since," she explains, with a slight smile and steady gaze at the interviewer.

But now, disabling depression has driven her to this appointment. For weeks, she's suffered from low mood that is nearly constant; she also has such difficulty concentrating at work that she fears she'll be fired. She's lost most of her interest in sex ("I haven't dared even hint about that to Jürgen"), and she wonders at the absence of joy in her life. "I even cried for an hour when my cat coughed up a hairball."

Analysis

In assembling a differential diagnosis, I would invoke the following possibilities: mood or anxiety disorder due to metastatic cancer or other physical condition, substance-induced mood or anxiety disorder, major depression, dysthymia, GAD, panic disorder, alcohol dependence, and a personality disorder. Based on what Marian told the interviewer, you could work your way through the decision trees for mood and anxiety disorders, as I would, to arrive at a consideration of both GAD and some form of clinical depression. But, as it turns out, there is more to Marian's case than she could admit at first.

That evening, Marian starts the recommended course of an SSRI. A few nights later, she calls her clinician from the emergency room:

"I'm in the bag," she moans. Without prompting, she admits that right along, she has been drinking and, fearful of losing her boyfriend, has lied about it to everyone.

Life has its surprises, especially if you are a mental health professional; you'll just have to learn how to roll with punches. Of course, the new information beats the older history; it requires both a complete revision of Marian's diagnosis and a therapeutic sea change.

We might wonder: Should Marian's clinician have more diligently investigated her claim that she had stopped drinking? Of course, it is important to trust your patient, as I always try to do. But perhaps the truth process might have been helped along by reminding Marian of the importance to her health and future happiness of a full and accurate history. I sometimes say something like this: "If you feel you can't talk candidly about something, just ask, 'Could we skip that subject right now?'"

It might also help to review the red flags we mentioned in Chapter 4 (see the sidebar "Recognizing Red Flag Information" on pp. 41–42). Is it suspicious that Marian extravagantly claimed to have eaten nothing for days, that she had symptoms of numerous disorders, or that she'd quit a number of jobs? Was the interviewer perhaps lulled by her forthright, seemingly honest manner? How might she have responded had the interviewer requested to meet with Jürgen?

At any rate, the only diagnoses I'd give her at this point would be primary alcohol use disorder and secondary depression of some sort. I'd hold off on any diagnosis of an anxiety disorder until she has achieved several weeks of sobriety—this time, for real.

Ingrid

Ingrid has worked as cashier at a comedy club on Portland's east side for just a few weeks when her boss requests that she seek help. "I was crying all the time, and he said it was bad advertising," she says between sniffles. A few months earlier, after her abusive marriage ended in divorce, Ingrid had moved from rural central Oregon (where she had grown up) to her mother's new home in the city. Despite her mother's presence, for several months she's complained of feeling isolated and "all alone in the world."

To the interviewer, it isn't clear whether her depression is due to the divorce or the move away from her life-long home. Either way, Ingrid replies, she is miserable—unable to sleep or eat, feeling guilty about everything, thinking she'd be better off dead, sometimes *wish-*

ing she were dead already. "Lately, I've felt as bad as I ever did on one of those bridges," she says. "Wait a minute," the clinician interrupts. "*What* bridges?"

When Ingrid was a high school junior, the car in which she and three friends were riding careened right off a bridge into a canyon. The boy at the wheel was drunk and he died, as did her best friend, who was riding in the front passenger seat. Ingrid and the boy in the rear seat miraculously escaped unscathed; forever after, she avoided both drugs and alcohol. With an effort, she forced herself to "get back on the road," and so maintained her ability to drive. Ever since, however, even watching someone else cross a bridge in a movie or on TV causes a tightness in her chest.

Although she is usually healthy and calm, confronting bridges always frightens her, "like the world is ending or something." Usually she has a panic attack—her heart races, she wants to run but feels frozen in place, and she has such shortness of breath she feels about to suffocate. And she'd *never* ride across a bridge; she always imagines what would happen if an earthquake struck. ("Remember the 1989 San Francisco quake that collapsed part of the Bay Bridge and a major freeway? It killed dozens.") There had been no problem when she lived in the dry flatlands, where bridges are rare. "If someone gave them a bridge, they'd have to dig a hole to put it over," she comments. Portland, however, is both earthquake-prone and studded with bridges. That's why she took the comedy club job—it was all she could find on her side of the river.

Ingrid can go shopping just fine (on foot), and though she's never much cared for heights, she denies having any other real phobias. And manias? "Seems like that would be almost nice."

Analysis

The differential diagnosis I'd construct for Ingrid would go as follows: the usual (and terribly important) mood and anxiety disorders due to a (so far, inapparent) medical condition or substance use issue, major depression, dysthymia, somatic symptom disorder, PTSD, GAD, panic disorder, specific phobia, and agoraphobia. Let's start with depression, because it is more dangerous, more acute, and often more readily treated than some of the others. Absence of mania directs us to Figure 11.1; absence of physical disease and substance use, and a history of general good health (and no prolonged grief—there is no evidence that the boy who died was an especially close attachment figure) move us along through steps 1–7 to 11, which tells us we should consider Ingrid for a diagnosis of major depression without psychosis. Note that by using the decision tree, we avoid the temptation to diagnose an adjustment disorder, which we might otherwise justify due to a divorce, a move, living with her mom, or a change of jobs.

The anxiety disorder requires a trip through Figure 12.1. We have already rejected the possibilities of any disorder related to physical or chemical causes, but step 7 brings us up short: Ingrid did have a fear of crossing bridges. That moves us on through steps 11 and 12 to step 13, which suggests that we consider a diagnosis of specific phobia.

Now, which diagnosis—mood or anxiety—do we list first? As is so often the case, major depression is the more urgent to treat, so we should mention it first, even though it appeared second. Anxiety disorders often go unreported for months or years, until another mental disorder—something even more stressful than anxiety—intervenes.

Kat

Kat has complained of ill health all her life. Her fraught medical history began in her early high school years, when the pain of "ulcers" (never proven) often prevented her from participating in gym class. At about that time she also suffered from severe headaches, with which she would take to her bed for several days at a time. Although she refers to these headaches as migraines, she never responded well to the usual migraine prophylaxis or to treatment with triptans.

Her father, a medical doctor, supplied much of Kat's early medical treatment, including a variety of narcotic painkillers. He never exercised much supervision, however, and she had essentially self-medicated her depression, insomnia, anxiety, and suicidal ideas. When depressed, she would sometimes hit her head against the wall, cut herself with knives or scissors, or scratch her forehead with a piece of broken mirror. Later she claimed not to remember hitting her head. Without a trace of irony, she now says, "I must have been bouncing off the walls." She has also tried several antidepressant drugs and at least two mood stabilizers, with little improvement to show for it.

By the time she is evaluated in her early 30s, Kat's medical history includes experiences with aphonia, weakness, heart palpitations, dizziness, hyperventilation, anxiety attacks, marked weight change, nausea, abdominal bloating, constipation, menstrual pain, menstrual irregularity, amenorrhea, menstrual hemorrhaging, lack of interest in sex, inability to experience orgasm, pain on intercourse, pain in extremities, and burning pains in other parts of her body. She has long suffered from premenstrual irritability and she says she is allergic to many foods and medications. When she was 26, she talked a surgeon into removing the tip of her coccyx for "persistent butt pain."

When barely out of her teens, Kat married a man several years older than she. He calls her by her actual name—Katherine—and was more than patient with her, coping with her difficulties with the help of marijuana. The couple has two children, who often require care by one of their grandmothers while their mother's medical problems are being addressed. Kat's family history includes many relatives with emotional problems, including grandparents and great-grandparents with alcoholism and a mother who also had headaches and depressions.

Kat is often whiny and petulant. Yet, when she wants to turn on the charm, she can be attractive, almost seductive. Her personality has been called "borderline" by at least one of her previous clinicians, "histrionic" by others.

Analysis

Kat's history presents a richness of choice that includes physical, mood, anxiety, substance use, personality, and even cognitive disorders. However, we'd like to make the smallest number of diagnoses possible; Occam's razor lives. Using the decision trees for either mood or anxiety disorders, we quickly come to the question of whether the patient had a long history of many unexplained somatic symptoms. Because Kat does have such a history, we are encouraged to consider somatization disorder (with multiple somatic complaints, the DSM-IV term is appropriate here).

Of course, somatization disorder does not rule out the possibility of an independent mood disorder. But Kat has been treated (ineffectively) for clinical depression with a great variety of medications. In my experience, patients with somatization disorder often also have mood or anxiety conditions that rarely respond well to traditional physical therapies.

Fritz

A 17-year Navy lifer, Fritz can't drink during deployments, and while in port he somehow managed to conceal his intoxication at work. But he spends evenings and weekends at the club or in his basement bar. His wife, Cindy, loyally cleans up after him, apologizes for him, rears their children, pays their bills, and manages their legal affairs. "It's always seemed normal—it's how it was with my own parents," she explains the day she finally gets Fritz to counseling.

When he was 40, Fritz developed pancreatitis and almost died. While still recovering, he made friends with an AA member in the next hospital bed and got religion. "Just like the President [then, George W. Bush]," he had informed Cindy—rather smugly, she had thought.

The trouble started during Fritz's first few months of sobriety. Despite his drinking, or maybe because of it, he and Cindy had always gotten along well. She didn't nag him much about his alcohol consumption and he let her alone to manage, which she had always done brilliantly. Once he was no longer chronically intoxicated, that deal was off. Now he expresses opinions about everything, from how to cook a brisket to what school their daughter should attend in the fall. He even enrolls Cindy at a spa to shed some of the weight she's built up over the years.

"I preferred things the way they used to be," she concludes. "From the time I was 10, I've coped with men who're drunk. But now that mine is sober, *I'm* the one at sea."

Analysis

Fritz's alcohol dependence is beyond question; it had affected his family life for many years. By its absence, it has now contributed to a change in his relationship with his wife (step 1 in Figure 17.1). Although Fritz has just survived a major medical illness (pancreatitis), there's no step 2 physiological mechanism through which it could have caused the couple's marital issues. Though the clinician might want to revisit the issue at some point, the brevity of Fritz's change and its nonpervasive nature would speak against a personality disorder as the cause of the current difficulties, so we'll vote "no" at steps 3 and 4. Because Cindy's own upbringing and her acceptance of Fritz's former drinking clearly contributed to the stability their marriage had enjoyed until Fritz's recent reform, we finally arrive at step 5 and the advice to consider a relational problem.

William

While still on active duty, William Minor, a young surgeon for the Union Army during the American Civil War, had begun to imagine that he was being persecuted. He noticed that fellow officers would glance at him suspiciously and mutter; he even challenged one of his best friends to a duel. William carried a concealed revolver while off duty, and he was known to visit prostitutes frequently, almost obsessively. Although he had complained of headaches and dizziness, no physical illness was ever diagnosed. This officer, who had served with distinction on the battlefield, was eventually invalided out of the Army due to "nerves."

At age 33, William was hospitalized as homicidal and suicidal. Released several years later, he continued to feel persecuted by men who, he believed, slipped poison into his mouth while he slept. Ultimately, he went to England to paint and recuperate. There he shot and killed an innocent stranger he imagined was one of the Irishmen who, as he had complained to the police on several occasions, kept sneaking into his room and hiding in the rafters. Found not guilty on grounds of insanity, he was confined to the Broadmoor asylum in England for the next 38 years.

At 40, William remained convinced that intruders were trying to enter his cell at night. He reported that he felt something being pumped into him, that at night he could feel a cold iron being pressed against his teeth. He asked a fellow inmate to cut his throat for him. At age 43, he complained that the marrow of his spine was being pierced, and that instruments of torture were being used to operate on his heart. A year later, he became convinced that electric currents were being passed through him; he also claimed that at night, he would be transported as far away as to Constantinople, where he was made to "perform lewd acts in public." After the Wrights flew at Kitty Hawk in 1903, he believed that this nocturnal transport took place in flying machines. Only once, when he was about 50, did he ever claim to hear a sound that could be a hallucination; it was of the door of his cell being opened at night.

With ample time, and money to spare from his Army pay, William responded to an advertisement for people to help gather quotations for what eventually became the monumental *Oxford English Dictionary*. Over the course of 20 years, he contributed tens of thousands of quotations, becoming the editor's friend and ultimate resource for many hard-to-document words. When so engaged, he would talk coherently and intelligently, and often appeared cheerful. Yet he was ultimately so remorseful for his crime that he offered financial help to the family of his victim. For a time, the widow of the man he had slain even served as his courier, bringing to him at the asylum books he had ordered from London shops.

Toward the end of his life, perhaps to combat the sexual urges of which he had grown ashamed, with surgical skill William cut off his own penis and cast it into the fire. As an old man, released from prison, he returned to the United States, where he was diagnosed with dementia praecox.

Analysis

William's undeniable psychosis suggests the following differential diagnosis: schizophrenia, delusional disorder, psychotic depression, schizoaffective disorder, and psychosis due to a medical condition. Using Figure 13.1, we can summarily reject a substance use factor. Both dementia and somatizing disorders seem terribly remote possibilities for this patient, but we need to think about a possible medical cause for his complaints. Could a tumor or perhaps an endocrine condition have caused both his paranoid thinking and his headaches and dizziness? Confronted today with such a patient, we'd order numerous laboratory tests and an MRI. In the case of William, however, the test of time will have to serve as proxy; decades of psychosis without suggestion of a specific illness allow us to slip past step 1.

At step 6, we come upon the nut of the diagnostic problem: Just what symptoms did William have? Of course, his delusions were extensive and enduring, but did he have any other basic symptoms of psychosis that would affirm the diagnosis of the old term for schizophrenia, *dementia praecox?* His thinking (speech) and his behavior regarding matters that did not pertain to his delusions were unexceptional; rather than showing flattened affect or lack of interest or motivation, if anything, he could be forceful and heated. And nowhere does history suggest that he had pronounced hallucinations, other than one mention that he thought he heard his door opening at night—hardly the sort of auditory hallucination typically experienced by patients with schizophrenia. On the other hand, he did report extensive hallucinations of touch, which are typical of patients with delusional disorder. And that is where we will end up, with a patient who functioned so well apart from his delusions (step 11) that he contributed literally thousands of quotations to the dictionary we still value today.

An important issue has to do with the dangers of trying to diagnose a patient one has never met. It is one thing, as an exercise, to use the historical record to attempt a diagnosis for someone long dead. However, clinicians must be extremely careful about offering their opinions on persons who are still alive, unless these opinions are based on interviews plus all the collateral information it is possible to gather.

Scott

Raised in a strongly religious family, Scott imagined from the age of 6 that Jesus was constantly watching to see whether he would do something naughty. If he should ever be caught, a mark against him would be entered in a long ledger. Consequently, he always sought to make sure that his actions were precise, his behavior unimpeachable.

Little Scott even sought to move and walk "perfectly." He would only cross between rooms by stepping carefully over an imaginary line drawn across the doorway, and he would start climbing any flight of stairs only with his left foot; if he forgot, he would make himself go back and start again. He would count the stairs in a flight, then immediately try to forget the number. He was also careful to arrange his schoolbooks and papers with their margins exactly parallel to his desktop edge. When he was a young child, none of this seemed out of place, but as a teenager, he felt peculiar and ashamed.

Scott started high school feeling all alone. His father had died rather suddenly the year before, and he and his mother continued to live on their small rural acreage outside town. Their quiet lifestyle left him much time to think. What if the house should catch fire— would the volunteer fire department, headquartered miles away, be able to put it out in time? Nearby farmers were growing more and more blueberries—with the constant pumping of water for irrigation, would their own well dry up? These thoughts often intruded on his study time or prevented him from falling asleep at night.

One evening when Scott was 17 and about to graduate from high school, he suddenly "realized" that his life was about to end and that he had nowhere to go. He felt empty, cried to himself, and began to think about suicide. In that era, stories of students who had murdered teachers and classmates were much in the news, and over the next several days Scott felt increasingly compelled to think about ways of inflicting violent death. He had no gun and didn't think he could buy one, but he had access to all the knives he could possibly need. Whenever his mother asked him to peel a potato or dice a carrot, through his mind would flash a scene in which he was stabbing her to death with the knife. Then, he would feel so physically nauseated and shaky that he had to sit on a stool to work in the kitchen. He got an after-school job in the print shop of the local weekly newspaper. He never considered moving away from home.

Although Scott was interested in women, he had no earthly idea how to approach them. He worried that he would never find the woman right for him and would remain unmarried all his life. At night he would masturbate while thinking about the girl who had sat in front of him in senior English class. With release, he would be flooded with shame and the feeling that he had to atone by reading verses from his Bible. When he doubted that he had read every word, he'd go back over them again several times.

When he was 25, his mother started to show signs of forgetfulness. They sought the help of a specialist, who eventually gave them the diagnosis Scott had feared: early-onset Alzheimer's disease. Over the next couple of weeks, his weight fell off as his appetite plummeted, and he stayed up late, feeling guilty and worrying that he might kill himself. On their third visit to the clinician, Scott breaks down in tears and confesses that, at an antique show the week before, he purchased a small, single-shot pistol.

Analysis

Although the differential list we must consider for Scott seems a lot like the one for many other patients, that doesn't make it less important. Remember always that a wide-ranging differential diagnosis is the bedrock of accurate mental health diagnosis. For Scott, I would include general medical and substance use causes of anxiety and depression, major depressive disorder, dysthymia, bipolar disorders, OCD, GAD, and a personality disorder.

Of course, we list this stuff, only to discard much of it. We find no medical or substance use issues that would trip us up at the first three steps of Figure 12.1. With a clear history of both obsessions and compulsions, we strike pay dirt at step 4, which directs us to consider a diagnosis of OCD. OCD is one of those diagnoses so remarkable that clinicians could overlook symptoms of other disorders. However, the diagnostic principle about multiple diagnoses reminds us to ask, "Have we covered all the symptoms?" The answer is "No," for Scott's worries about problems so varied as a dry well, a house afire, and a lonely bachelor life were not explained by OCD. He experienced these ideas not as fears but as worries; they interfered with his sleep and studies; and he had experienced no unusually traumatic event. So at step 6 we must also consider the diagnosis of GAD.

In addition, the step 17 asterisk directs us to carefully consider any symptoms of a mood disorder, and that means a trip through Figure 11.1. Although the information available in the vignette is a bit scanty for any solid diagnosis, major depression seems a good possibility—a nice demonstration of our diagnostic principle always to consider a mood disorder.

OK, which diagnosis should we list first? The mood disorder seems most likely to cause immediate harm, so we'll place major depression at the top of our list for further evaluation and treatment. Next should come OCD, and finally GAD.

Leonard

The first thing Leonard says when he appears for his initial interview is that he'd gotten no help at all from his previous clinician. The second thing, almost, was that he doesn't want anyone to contact previous health care providers.

At 49, Leonard complains he's had anxiety and depression for much of his adult life. Oh, yes, some days he might drink as many as five or six beers, but sometimes entire weeks can go by without any drinking at all. He has used Xanax for many years—only a milligram per day on average, though when he is extra stressed he might take up to three tablets. He is vague about other possible substance use. He occasionally smokes marijuana, but only when at a party, and it never seems to bother him. He has tried numerous antidepressants and other psychotropic drugs; nearly all of them cause profound side effects.

Leonard was born in rural Nebraska, where his parents worked a small truck farm—when they weren't drinking. His father, bright but with little formal education, had resented the burden of children. When he came home from an evening tour of their town's three bars, he'd sometimes haul Leonard out to the watering trough behind the house and "jokingly" whip him with a leather belt until he thought he would pass out. His mother also drank heavily; periodically she became severely depressed, twice attempting suicide. When she was a child, *her* father had leaped to his death from the roof of the highest building in his small town in Iowa.

A skilled artisan, for the last decade Leonard has been self-employed restoring furniture. He had previously worked at a joinery but was fired when discovered having an affair (on company time) with his employer's *au pair*. Although he can make anything with his hands, he has trouble focusing attention on paperwork; consequently, he hasn't paid his taxes for several years. When asked about this, he acts nonchalant, as though it doesn't really matter much at all.

Leonard's anxiety attacks are usually preceded by thinking about his personal problems. Although he describes them as feelings of terror, they are never accompanied by physical symptoms such as pounding heart or shortness of breath. He also complains of nearly constant anxiety that seems unrelated to any specific worry, problem, or emotion. "I'm just not a worrier," he claims. However, he admits to intermittent suicidal ideas, though never with plans or an attempt; these ideas center on the concern that he isn't going anywhere in life. "When I'm 50, if I'm still right where I am now, I'll be a failure. That's when I'll drink the Kool-Aid."

Analysis

Right away, we are concerned that we cannot know enough for a proper diagnosis about someone who intentionally withholds information from the clinician—the ultimate red flag warning that something is amiss (review the sidebar on p. 41). However, despite Leonard's apparent manipulations, we should not leap right to personality disorder as the main diagnosis. Leonard does present symptoms of depression (his clinician had wondered about bipolar II disorder), anxiety (could he have PTSD or GAD?), and substance misuse—all of which we should include in his differential diagnosis. And, of course, he could have a personality disorder. In fact, there isn't enough information for a definite diagnosis in any of the areas we've considered. When that's the case, there's only one sensible remedy: *undiagnosed*.

In this case, as in so many others, *undiagnosed* prevents closure and reminds us that we must continue to inquire into the reasons for a patient's symptoms. Often this means obtaining more information; for example, has Leonard experienced legal difficulties? *Undiagnosed* also discourages us from attempting treatment that is experimental or unusually dangerous. (I have personally known way too many patients who should have been "undiagnosed" entered into randomized drug trials.) And his clinician might even use the lack of a definitive diagnosis as leverage to obtain Leonard's full cooperation with the information-gathering process.

At length, a letter did arrive from a previous physician, who had refused to treat Leonard further with medications because of his drinking. He had driven his SUV into a severe auto accident, caused by alcohol-fueled speeding. The passenger in the other auto had died; the driver was still in a coma. Of course, this information prompted a much fuller investigation.

Gilbert

The Ordeal of Gilbert Pinfold is one of Evelyn Waugh's less weighty creations, but because it was written from personal experience, it provides fodder for our next diagnostic adventure. An insomniac middle-aged writer with no previous mental illness, Gilbert seeks to escape the stresses of his English life by cruising to Ceylon, leaving his sleeping draughts behind. From the very first, he encounters rough sailing: He has trouble understanding a shipping office clerk and the correct procedures for the voyage. He drops things when he first boards the ship and becomes a little disoriented during the first day out. He keeps falling asleep.

Then begin the hallucinations. At first, it's just music; then Gil-

bert hears a dog's feet tripping along the deck; next, a clergyman delivering a sermon; then, crew members swearing. Finally, he begins to
overhear lengthy speeches from many voices. They come to him from
just outside his door, over a wireless device that has been somehow
piped into his cabin, even to his table in the lounge. It becomes clear
to him that he is meant to play a key role in resisting a plot to take
over the ship. In a panic he cries out, "Oh, let me not be mad, not mad,
sweet heaven."

Stepping onto the deck, Gilbert finds it deserted; now the voices
tell him that the plot has been a hoax. He feels that all the passengers
are looking at him and talking about him. The voice of a young woman
declares that she loves him and wants to spend the night with him, but
her mother intervenes. Gilbert lies awake all night as voices urge him
to leap into the ocean. They are, he believes, trying to psychoanalyze
him.

By the end of Gilbert's 14-day adventure, he has escaped his hallucinations and delusions. He is neither depressed nor particularly
anxious, but he is confused about how long he's been at sea—and about
just what he's done there. Although he thinks he's sent a dozen tele-
grams, in reality there was only one.

Analysis

Most clinicians would probably start with a differential diagnosis for psychosis: substance misuse or physical cause of psychosis, mood disorder
with psychosis, schizophreniform psychosis, schizoaffective disorder, and
schizophrenia. (You can see how truly committed I am to a wide-ranging
differential diagnosis; even on first reading, I didn't for a moment believe
that Gilbert had schizophrenia.) Of course, knowing the outcome (rapid,
complete resolution) makes it easy to travel the first couple of steps in
Figure 13.1 to a diagnosis of a psychosis induced by drug withdrawal. We
remember that just before becoming ill, Gilbert had discontinued his long-
time sleeping medication.

OK, so Gilbert had reacted to drug withdrawal. Did he show any symptoms in addition to those of psychosis? A careful reading of the vignette
reveals that he dropped things, was disoriented, and had trouble understanding what a clerk was telling him—all symptoms pointing to a possible
cognitive disorder. Figure 14.1 brings us at once to the definition of delirium,
which fits Gilbert perfectly. The culprits are the sleeping draughts (contain-
ing chloral and bromine) he had been using—unbeknown to his physician,
who had prescribed additional powerful drugs. Indeed, before Gilbert had

left on the voyage he had admitted to his wife that he was "doped to the eyeballs," and he had difficulty writing legibly or even tying his shoelaces. Small wonder that he was having a drug withdrawal delirium—a horse that we too often forget while we are out pursuing zebras.

Norma

"It's a long story," Norma says. "It isn't a happy story." Pieced together from various sources (including a long chat with her grown daughter, Pat), it is a miserable tale indeed.

Norma has a withered leg—a birth defect that has clouded her entire childhood. She wears a brace with a built-up shoe, and when she walks, she must move her foot forward with a kicking motion. "Running is a joke," she reports with a snort. Her childhood anger was fueled by the fact that her older sister, Arlette, was athletic and extremely popular with boys. Although smart and quick-witted, throughout her school years Norma added alienation to her anger, rebelling against authority. With another girl from her high school class, she used to dress provocatively and go down to the naval yard, where they'd welcome sailors home from months at sea. "I had a couple of scares back then," Norma admits, "and penicillin was my best friend." Her mother, guilt-ridden over the congenital damage she feared was her fault, catered to Norma's frequent demands for extra privileges, while severely limiting Arlette's freedom.

Despite her intelligence, Norma swore she'd never go to college. Instead, from high school she moved to Fairbanks and got a job with a company that supplied groceries and clothing to workers constructing the Alaska oil pipeline. It paid well, and it left her the time she needed for recreation, much of which involved men. Through three promotions she stuck with her job long enough to meet her first husband, Kirk. "I knew right from the first that Kirk was gay," Norma said. "But he was so cute—looked like Tony Perkins—I just had to have him. Chased him all around the Arctic Circle one summer. I think he finally married me to be rid of me. Anyway, the marriage was a disaster—no surprise—and after we had two children, he ran off with a priest."

Norma then moved to the lower 48, where it was far cheaper to live; rather than finding another job, however, she ran through her savings. She tried hard to get on disability but was rejected several times. A doctor had gone out of the way to help her, but she turned on him and threatened to blacken his reputation. "I know he lied about me in his report," she complains, "and I told him I was going to report him to the medical board."

Eventually, she solved her insolvency with another wedding. "Whenever my second husband drank, he'd treat me like pond scum— blackened my eye several times, even before we got married," she said. She would call the police when he beat her up, then refuse to press charges. "He always swore he loved me and wouldn't do it again, so we'd have a few beers and make love." When he finally left her for another woman, she was furious; she harassed him by telephone and in person until he got a restraining order. Since her second divorce, she's had several boyfriends, whom she tends to berate until they abandon her. Then she'll cry and say how lonely she is.

Pat and her brother, Danny, had more or less reared themselves while Norma ran a talent agency she started on money she'd borrowed from Arlette. "Mom had lots of energy and creativity," Pat sums up. "But she didn't waste any of it on us."

For months, she'd barely speak to either of her children. "Seven previous counselors have told me it's the kids' fault we don't get along," Norma explains. Danny had broken with her completely. When she had found out he was living with another man, she wrote a letter to several of their relatives, stating that he'd turned out to be "just as queer as his father." Pat had told her, "You give new meaning to the term *family outing.*"

Now Norma stays home and surfs the internet. "I got tired of people looking funny at my leg, thinking up snide comments." Her retirement plan is to inherit money when her mother dies.

Norma finally consents to an assessment "because I've decided I don't know who I am." Although her appetite has been poor, she's recently gained 5 pounds. At times she feels "depressed and empty, but mostly that's when I step on the scales," she admits with a chuckle. She has never been suicidal: "Suicide," she says, "it's for chumps."

Analysis

Everything we know about Norma (even though it is not nearly enough yet) seems to cry out "personality disorder." Here are the hallmarks, based partly on collateral information from her daughter: Her symptoms are lifelong; they affect her in several ways (mood, cognition, interpersonal functioning, and impulse control); they complicate her life and cause her distress in family, interpersonal, and work situations; this pattern has been stable for many years. However, Figure 17.1 and an important diagnostic principle urge us first to carefully consider other possibilities.

From the material we have, her depression appears to be neither intense nor long-lasting, and it certainly hadn't been present throughout her entire adult life, as it would need to be to explain her behavior. At worst, I'd consider it an adjustment to her changing life circumstances, in part brought on by the way she deals with others. Norma's short leg has certainly marked her psyche, but it isn't the sort of step 2 medical problem that would directly cause mental disorders. We'd need to explore further the question of how much she drinks, and I'd want to know about anxiety symptoms, too. But here, for once, is someone I'd consider as possibly having no major (that is, nonpersonality) mental disorder.

Indeed, Norma seems to meet the step 3 entrance requirements for a personality disorder. Her sense of self is impaired (she has empty feelings at times and says she doesn't know who she is—both identity problems), and she doesn't appear to understand or pursue life goals (issues of self-direction). As regards interpersonal issues, though problems with empathy are only implied in the material we have, her lack of close contact with her children certainly suggests issues of intimacy. But would she fully meet criteria for a named personality disorder (step 3)? I wouldn't say so, not on the basis of the current information (though some clinicians might favor a borderline diagnosis). Because her life history is so replete with personality disorder symptoms—which include some borderline, paranoid, histrionic, and perhaps narcissistic features—I would use some of these terms in concocting a step 4 "yes" description of personality disorder traits.

Raymond

When Raymond was growing up in eastern Washington State, he played baritone horn in the high school band. For a small school, the band played pretty well, so it was often invited to bigger cities for parades and competitions. During their bus trips, Raymond usually played penny-ante blackjack. "I always felt a shudder of excitement when I won," he tells his clinician years later. "No matter how often it happened, I never grew bored with it." He had had another fling with gambling—craps—during his early 20s when he served in the Army Reserves, but he'd "had the good sense to get out of the military" before the first Gulf War: "I wasn't *that* high a roller."

Now nearing 30, he takes a job with a civilian contractor working on toxic Superfund site cleanup. Using a forklift, Raymond moves huge drums of radioactive waste into a storage facility. The leisurely pace leaves a lot of time for recreation, so he and some coworkers play poker. They start at dollar pots, but after a few months, whole paychecks can disappear at the turn of a card. When a Native American casino opens down the street from his work, he first tries video poker.

Later he graduates to roulette; a friend covers for him as he takes increasingly long lunch hours. After work, he often walks home rather than take the bus, to save the $1.50 for gambling.

Gambling gives Raymond a lift when he feels depressed (often, it's about his gambling). Though he maxes out seven credit cards, his wife doesn't find out until bill collectors start calling at the house. He tearfully promises her that he will stop, and he does—for a time. At first he attends Gamblers Anonymous meetings, but later he visits the casino instead.

To the intake worker at the mental health clinic, Raymond remarks that his job takes courage. "Misjudge the weight, lose your concentration for a second, and boom! You glow in the dark for the rest of your life, all 7 days of it." It has always seemed strange; at the gaming tables, Raymond has nerves of steel. But to move tons of nuclear waste takes a little of what his grandmother always called "Dutch courage." He tries to limit himself to three or four beers in a day, though several times he has operated his forklift when he is high. When he does drink during the day, no one knows except one close friend at work—and the cop who on two occasions watched him fail field sobriety tests.

Analysis

All those who repeatedly lose more than they can afford have a gambling problem; the question of whether the gambling qualifies as a diagnosable disorder seems almost academic. Much gambling takes place as a social activity with friends; the person is willing to lose up to a specified amount as entertainment, but not to jeopardize the rent or food money in the process. But many of Raymond's gambling behaviors speak to their addictive nature: solitary gambling, concealing it from his wife, feeling uncomfortable if he cannot gamble (reminiscent of the withdrawal symptoms substance users can experience), making repeated attempts to control the behaviors (he failed at Gamblers Anonymous), and gambling instead of working. When push comes to shove, with his wife doing the pushing, even Raymond seems to agree he has a problem. You don't really need Figure 15.1 to arrive at a step 2 diagnosis of gambling disorder.

Well, what about Raymond's drinking? With no history of tolerance or withdrawal (step 1), he isn't obviously alcohol dependent. Even though he doesn't drink all that much, still he has two sorts of problem: two arrests for driving while intoxicated and the use of alcohol in a dangerous situation. Raymond's drinking therefore qualifies as substance use that creates problems for him and for his family. His story also provides stark evidence of the similarity between gambling and substance use, which are highly comorbid. And by the way, though I have not listed a differential diagnosis for Raymond, Table 6.1 suggests that major depression also often accompanies both gambling and substance use.

Which diagnosis should we list first? Both conditions require prompt attention, and they apparently arose more or less together. At least gambling isn't likely to cause Raymond to mishandle a barrel of toxic chemicals, so I'd go with the drinking.

Reynolds

A full professor of chemistry at a Midwestern technical school, at age 57 Reynolds has "never known a sick day," as he later tells his interviewer. One afternoon, standing at his workbench looking at a test tube full of crystals he's just precipitated, he suddenly *knows* that the chairman of his department has marked him for dismissal. The thought causes him to bolt from his lab and carefully collect and burn all of the correspondence in his office files.

Within a few hours, out of the corner of his left eye, Reynolds begins to see swooping blurs of light that trail after objects and gradually fade to black. Over the next 2 weeks, these increase to such an extent that he can barely focus on his work. He misses his first two appointments with the family practitioner who has provided his health care for 30 years. "First I didn't remember making an appointment; then I couldn't remember when it was," he later confesses. By the time he finally appears for the checkup, he's been ill for over a month and is so distraught that he cries throughout the exam. After a thorough workup that finds nothing physically wrong, the doctor writes "Sounds like early schizophrenia" in a letter of referral to a mental health care provider.

Analysis

Even this fragment of a story presents several relevant points. Foremost is the importance of not leaping to conclusions based on appearances; instead, we need historical information as the bedrock for our assessment. Reynolds's primary care physician should have constructed a differential diagnosis and safety hierarchy, which would have included the disorders mentioned in Table 13.1 (p. 188). Working through Figure 13.1, I'd especially worry about exposure to toxic chemicals and delirium (steps 2 and 3). Suppose we don't have access to this history? Then the most conservative diagnosis we can make will be schizophreniform disorder at step 10. Note that Reynolds has visual hallucinations—nontypical for schizophrenia, as is his age; at 57, he is far older than the usual first-onset schizophrenia patient.

What can we predict about the future course of Reynolds's schizophreniform disorder? Of the features that predict a good prognosis (see the sidebar "Prognosis and Schizophreniform Psychosis" on p. 197)—confusion, psychotic features early in the course of the illness, good premorbid functioning, and affect that is not blunt or flattened—Reynolds has them all.

Tonya

"I found out that I'm pregnant. That's what got me here. It made me so anxious—joyful, but anxious." Tonya stares straight forward and laughs, in a sort of rapid giggle that she repeats often during her interview. Her freckles and tousled auburn hair make her seem younger than her 27 years. "It gives me panicky feelings that I'm at last going to do something worthwhile."

Tonya is being interviewed while hospitalized for bipolar I disorder. Just what she was doing previously is a little unclear. Reared in California, in the ninth grade Tonya had left school and ran away to join the carnival. When she was 16, she got married and moved with her husband to the South for several years. "Buddy also worked for the carnival, like me. I started by telling fortunes, but eventually I did pretty much anything. Buddy did cocaine." Another giggle. "Finally, I left him and moved here. This is a great city for the homeless," she adds. This last time she's been homeless for several months, but she says she's lived on the streets "for pretty much my entire adult life."

"In Georgia, I was jumped by three girls I'd turned in for child molestation," Tonya says. "I ended up hurting one pretty bad; she died, but the police called it justifiable homicide, and they didn't hold me." She moistens her lips, but this time she doesn't laugh. She admits that in the hospital she's happier than she's ever been before. "But I don't think I'm too happy—my mood has been pretty midline the last couple of months. My sleep? Oh, that's probably 8 or 9 hours a night."

A year or two ago, while hospitalized in Georgia after an overdose, Tonya was treated with an antidepressant, which she thought had helped her. "I had been drinking some—well, a lot—for a long time. Maybe a pint a day." She says that gin earned her some arrests for a DWI and beating up her husband. "I got so drunk I used to wet myself." She admits to having had the shakes some mornings; then, she might have a "hair of the dog."

Years ago, when she discovered that she'd been sleeping with her half-brother—he had known about the family relationship; she had not—she felt betrayed and made two suicide attempts. First, she cut her wrists; then, she tried to hang herself, but "I couldn't get the knot just right." With neither attempt had she caused herself any serious physical damage. "That's when they told me I'm manic-depressive," she explains.

When Tonya is depressed, her sleep doesn't usually change, and she can focus on reading or watching TV. Her appetite remains mostly unchanged, and she often feels "hyper and restless."

Tonya's mother had been mentally abusive and her father had forced sex on her. "He was a drinker; when I was barely a year old, he did unspeakable things. I remember it all so clearly, even today." Her father's relatives were all "drinkers" like him; her mother's relatives were all "nervous—they had a lot of anxiety and depression." Despite it all, she remembers her childhood as being basically happy. "I had a good time as a kid. I had a girlfriend, and in the sixth grade we had sex together. Afterward, I told the other kids at school about it, so I became more or less the class pariah." Tonya hasn't had sex with women as an adult, but she admits that when she was with the carnival, she did engage in prostitution. "Actually, I've been pretty promiscuous most of my life. I have no idea who my baby's father is. Well, there could be several candidates."

Tonya has also worked as a waitress, as a machinist, and for 3 years as a night clerk at a 7-Eleven; she has never been fired. Although she attended school only until the ninth grade, she later earned a general equivalency diploma. She describes herself as having few friends and "always being a loner, even today." It's one reason she is so glad to be pregnant—now she'll always have a friend. (A slip of paper in the front of her chart notes that her pregnancy test has come back negative, though she hasn't yet been given this information.)

Throughout this interview, she maintains attention and seems to connect well with the interviewer. Other than the giggling, which seems a little forced, her mood is level and appropriate. Alert and quick, she passes the usual tests for orientation, calculations, and memory without difficulty. She denies having previous anxiety or panic attacks; she doesn't feel she is being followed or persecuted, "though a bus once told me, 'Good job!' Yes, it seemed as clear to me as your voice is now. And I wasn't using drugs or alcohol then."

Analysis

In a differential list of possible diagnoses—major depression, bipolar I disorder, panic and other anxiety disorders, psychosis of various sorts, traumatic brain injury, substance use, personality disorder—the one issue that seems pretty clear is Tonya's drinking. By her own admission, she's been a heavy consumer of alcohol, which has led to a number of difficulties, including driving violations and domestic violence. I would consider her as having alcohol dependence (moderate to severe alcohol use disorder), but the extent to which drinking contributes to her other difficulties would need to be sorted out.

Her current clinicians are treating her for bipolar I disorder. Is this wise? Of course, mood disorders reside near the top of any safety hierarchy, and Tonya says she previously responded well to treatment for depression; it's a diagnostic principle that could push us toward such a diagnosis, if we were willing to be pushed. But a great deal of Tonya's history is atypical or even contradictory: She remembers abuse when she was a year old; she couldn't get the knot right for hanging; with depression, her energy level increased and her sleep wasn't much changed; though she was admitted for anxiety and depression, her affect during the interview didn't seem especially depressed. And her claim that the police didn't hold her after she killed someone sounds like fantasy.

Anxiety and even panic symptoms coincided with her "pregnancy," and I don't like to trust information that may be crisis-generated. I would note with interest, but considerable skepticism, the voice of the bus; without more symptoms I would not be pushed very far in the direction of psychosis. Of course, the prostitution and other features of a highly disorganized life would make me consider personality disorder—but, although this seems a good bet, I wouldn't make that diagnosis without a lot more information—preferably from someone who has known Tonya for a long time.

To wrap up, here's an instance where, other than alcohol use disorder, the only safe diagnosis—for now—would be possible mental disorder, undiagnosed type.

Hannah

Hannah is pushing 40, and she's come to the mental health clinic for the first time in nearly two decades. The occasion this time? She's worried.

When a teenager, she was evaluated for gender dysphoria. Back then it was called gender identity disorder, but her symptoms were classic for gender dysphoria: Though born an apparent male, from the time she entered middle school she felt like a girl. She hated boys' games ("they are always so rough"), loved girls' clothing, and always pretended she was a girl when engaged in fantasy play. When she explained to her mother how her penis disgusted her, she was told to wait, that she might feel differently in a few years.

But the passing years had no effect. By the time she started high school, Hannah *knew* she was a girl: "I was locked in this horrific prison of my anatomy. I knew if I didn't take action, I'd go mad." As soon as she turned 18, she began the consultations that would eventually lead first to dressing exclusively as a girl, next to hormone therapy, then to the surgery that provided her final release.

And now her worry is . . . just what?—the interviewer wants to know. "Actually, it's Arthur who's so concerned," she responds. "Arthur is my husband; we've been married for almost 5 years. He's awakened in the night several times to find me calling out, having a bad dream. It's always the same dream, from the time when I was a kid and the other children would tease me—bully me, really. I was so different from other kids! But I haven't worried about that for years. I can go weeks without even thinking about it."

Hannah asks that Arthur join their consultation. He sits close, takes her hand. "Maybe I'm being too cautious," he says, "but she has such a history of being tormented, especially when she was in elementary school. Kids can be so cruel, and they are quick to turn on anyone they view as different."

"I certainly was that," Hannah agrees. "And no one would take my part. The boys pointed and made gross jokes while the girls froze me out. My teachers seemed oblivious, though now I wonder, did they just not know what to say? So I put my energy into study and bided my time."

Hannah made excellent use of her time. She did extraordinarily well in her studies and graduated near the top of her class, both in high school and in college, where she majored in philosophy. "I have a strong interest in ethics, which is what I teach now—same college. My personal history gives me strong perspective on struggle, on right and wrong."

Since she completed her transition ("top surgery, bottom surgery—all with good results"), she has thrived. But the dreams? "They don't really bother me, not now. I'm here because they worry Arthur. But I just go back to sleep for the remaining couple of hours until it's time to get up."

"That doesn't feel exactly right, either. It's so confusing, being me!" A cascade of tears leaves a dark patch on the front of Hannah's broadcloth shirt.

By way of review, Hannah tells the clinician about drinking beer "rarely" and perhaps an occasional glass of wine—in company, and never to the point of intoxication. "And I've never used drugs. Well, I did try a hit off a joint when I was in college. It made me feel weird and uncomfortable, so I never did it again."

Other than those dreams, she sleeps "pretty well, most nights" and her appetite is good, her weight steady.

Analysis

Using several diagnostic principles, our differential diagnosis should include some of the usual suspects—mood disorder, anxiety disorder, physical illness, gender dysphoria. Ordinarily, I'd add in substance use as a possibility, but there seems to be zero compatible history of the use of anything illegal, or even unhealthful. Personality disorder? Pursuant to yet another diagnostic principle, we should postpone that one until near the end of our quest, but honestly, I don't see anything here that would tempt me in that direction.

Indeed, I've gotta say, Hannah stands out as having a profound absence of symptoms. Even the dreams that drove her to the sleep disorders clinic are underwhelming. Had it not been for Arthur's concern, she'd probably have stayed home. She awakens and remembers the dream content, but she doesn't seem particularly upset by it. She certainly doesn't seem distressed, even to a clinically *in*significant degree. I'd say nightmare disorder is off the table. And, she's explicitly denied the mood and anxiety symptoms that might encourage us to look for other emotional issues.

What about nightmare disorder? Disturbed sleep was what got her here, but she wasn't the one concerned: It was her husband. The DSM-5-TR criteria are silent on this point, but I'm pretty sure that it's the person having the nightmare who is supposed to be distressed or impaired socially, interpersonally, or occupationally. And Hannah is pretty clear: She'd not have come but for Arthur's concern.

Technically, you could say that at one time Hannah qualified for gender dysphoria, with the specifier that she is many years posttransition. OK, her history conforms in every respect to the requirements for gender dysphoria, first as a child, then as an adult. But that's all been definitively resolved, so none of the criteria apply to her current adult self. And there is one major criterion that she certainly lacks: distress or impairment in some life area. Twenty or 30 years ago? Of course, she was distressed beyond belief. But now? Not at all.

Whereas we could of course say that she has a history of gender dysphoria, does it need saying now? What benefit would it confer? If she had had bipolar disease, but no episodes for 20 years, there would be a benefit to noting her long-ago history: It might alert a future clinician to watch for a recurrence. But a recurrence of gender dysphoria in a patient nearly 20 years posttransition? That seems well beyond the bounds of plausibility. I think I'm going to exercise my clinician prerogative and leave this diagnosis out of consideration.

In thinking through the rest of Hannah's story, I find myself tossing out all diagnosis . . . but one. And that is perhaps my very favorite of all time, which I've enshrined in a diagnostic principle: Consider the possibility of no mental disorder. Sure, Hannah has had a lot of issues that needed sorting out at one time or another, but they appear largely behind her and they certainly don't define who she is now. Neither should they direct the course of her life going into the future. That's what I'd tell her, and tell Arthur, and inform the rest of her family, should they ever ask (and should Hannah give me permission to speak with them).

What a pleasure, then, to conclude the evaluation with: "To me, you seem a healthy, adult woman who has no mental disorder." It's about the best feeling a clinician can have!

Appendix
Diagnostic Principles

Throughout this book, I've described the principles that for years have guided my evaluation of thousands of mental health patients. Here I've collected them all, arranged into four broad categories. I'll be the first to admit that these 24 principles sometimes overlap and sometimes conflict with one another. The principles are listed here in the order that might be needed when evaluating a patient; it's a little different from their order in the text. I've also sometimes shortened the text versions here. Finally, to facilitate use I've added letters for easy reference and page numbers for full discussion in the text.

Create a Differential Diagnosis

A. Arrange your wide-ranging differential diagnosis according to a safety hierarchy (p. 16).
B. Family history can help guide diagnosis, but because we often cannot trust reports, clinicians should attempt to rediagnose each family member (p. 30).
C. Physical disorders and their treatment can cause or worsen mental symptoms (p. 101).
D. Consider somatic symptom (somatization) disorder whenever symptoms don't jibe or treatments don't work (p. 111).
E. Substance use, including prescribed and over-the-counter medications, can cause a variety of mental disorders (p. 114).
F. Because of their ubiquity, potential for harm, and ready response to treatments, always consider mood disorders (p. 129).

When Information Sources Conflict

G. History beats current appearance (p. 25).
H. Recent history beats ancient history (p. 27).
I. Collateral information sometimes beats the patient's own (p. 27).
J. Signs beat symptoms (p. 28).
K. Be wary when evaluating crisis-generated data (p. 29).

L. Objective findings beat subjective judgment (p. 29).
M. Use Occam's razor—choose the simplest explanation (p. 31).
N. Horses are more common than zebras; prefer the more frequently encountered diagnosis (p. 32).
O. Watch for contradictory information (p. 37).

Resolve Uncertainty

P. The best predictor of future behavior is past behavior (p. 50).
Q. Having more symptoms of a disorder increases its likelihood as your diagnosis (p. 51).
R. Typical features of a disorder increase its likelihood as your diagnosis; faced with nontypical features, look for alternatives (p. 51).
S. Previous typical response to treatment for a disorder increases its likelihood as your current diagnosis (p. 52).
T. Use the word *undiagnosed* whenever you cannot be sure of your diagnosis (p. 52).
U. Consider the possibility that the patient should be given no mental diagnosis at all (p. 54).

Multiple Diagnoses

V. When symptoms cannot be adequately explained by a single disorder, consider multiple diagnoses (p. 62).
W. Avoid personality disorder diagnoses when your patient is acutely ill with a major mental disorder (p. 63).
X. Arrange multiple diagnoses to list first the one that is most urgent, treatable, or specific. Whenever possible, also list diagnoses chronologically (p. 64).

References and Suggested Reading

I've included here citations for a number of studies and papers mentioned throughout the book, as well as some of the important papers written about diagnostic method. Some of the classic papers date back several decades or more; despite their age, they still have much to teach us. Wherever possible, I've tried to cite resources that can be read in their entirety free at PubMed.gov. Though not individually noted, you can read the abstract of many other articles free at PubMed.

General References on Interviewing and Diagnosis

American Psychiatric Association: *Diagnostic and Statistical Manual of Mental Disorders* (5th ed., text rev.). Arlington, VA: Author, 2022.—The most recent revision of this important document.

American Psychiatric Association: *Diagnostic and Statistical Manual of Mental Disorders* (4th ed., text rev.). Washington, DC: Author, 2000.—I include DSM-IV-TR here because I recommend continuing to follow it for the diagnosis of somatization disorder, the Global Assessment of Functioning (GAF), and the Global Assessment of Relational Functioning (GARF).

Beidel DC, Frueh C (Eds.): *Adult Psychopathology and Diagnosis* (8th ed.). Hoboken, NJ: Wiley, 2018.—Aimed at graduate students in psychology, counseling, and social work, this nearly 900-page text covers the spectrum of diagnostic conditions.

Montgomery K: *How Doctors Think*. New York: Oxford University Press, 2005.—A professor of humanities and medicine (who is not a physician herself) discusses clinical judgment and the practice of medicine.

Morrison J: *DSM-5-TR Made Easy*. New York: Guilford Press, 2023.—Here, I use patient vignettes to illustrate and, at times, critique the classic, standard manual; this edition reflects recent changes in diagnostic criteria.

Morrison J: *The First Interview* (4th ed.). New York: Guilford Press, 2014.—An introduction to the art and science of mental health interviewing.

Morrison J: *When Psychological Problems Mask Medical Disorders* (2nd ed.). New York: Guilford Press, 2015.—It provides a mental health slant on 60 medical conditions.

Roberts LW (Ed.): *The American Psychiatric Publishing Textbook of Psychiatry*

(7th ed.). Washington, DC: American Psychiatric Publishing, 2010.—Highly authoritative text, addressing all aspects of mental health diagnosis and treatment in over 1,300 pages.

Sadock BJ, Sadock VA, Ruiz P (Eds.): *Kaplan and Sadock's Comprehensive Textbook of Psychiatry* (10th ed.). Philadelphia: Lippincott Williams & Wilkins, 2017.— This behemoth (nearly 5,000 pages) covers all aspects of mental health illness and treatment.

Diagnostic Method

Allen VG, Arocha JF, Patel VL: Evaluating evidence against diagnostic hypotheses in clinical decision making by students, residents and physicians. *Int J Med Informatics* 1998; 51:91–105.

Andreasen NC: Editorial: Vulnerability to mental illness. *Am J Psychiatry* 2005; 162:211–213.

Biturajac M, Jurjako M: Reconsidering harm in psychiatric manuals within an explicationist framework. *Med Health Care Philos* 2022; 25:239–249. Free at PubMed.

Coderre S, Mandin H, Harasym PH, Fick GH: Diagnostic reasoning strategies and diagnostic success. *Med Educ* 2003; 37:695–703.

Dunphy L, Penna M, El-Kafsi J: Somatic symptom disorder: A diagnostic dilemma. *BMJ Case Rep.* 2019; 12:e231550. Free at PubMed.

Faust D, Nurcombe B: Improving the accuracy of clinical judgment. *Psychiatry* 1989; 52:197–208.

Fava M, Farabaugh AH, Sickinger AH, Wright E, Alpert JE, Sonawalla S, Nierenberg AA, Worthington JJ 3rd: Personality disorders and depression. *Psychol Med* 2002; 32:1049–1057.

Hall KH: Reviewing intuitive decision-making and uncertainty: The implications for medical education. *Med Educ* 2002; 36:216–224.

Hall RC, Popkin MK, Devaul RA, Faillace LA, Stickney SK: Physical illness presenting as psychiatric disease. *Arch Gen Psychiatry* 1978; 35:1315–1320.

Heilig M, Forslund K, Asberg M, Rydberg U: The dual-diagnosis concept used by Swedish social workers: Limited validity upon examination using a structured diagnostic approach. *Eur Psychiatry* 2002; 17:363–365.

Henig RM: At war with their bodies, they seek to sever limbs. *The New York Times*, March 22, 2005; *www.nytimes.com/2005/03/22/health/psychology/22ampu.html*

Heuss SC, Schwartz BJ, Schneeberger AR: Second opinions in psychiatry: A review. *Psychiatr Prac* 2018; 24:434–442. Free at PubMed.

Honig A, Pop P, Tan ES, Philipsen H, Romme MA: Physical illness in chronic psychiatric patients from a community psychiatric unit: The implications for daily practice. *Br J Psychiatry* 1989; 155:58–64.

Keel PK, Dorer DJ, Eddy KT, Franko D, Charatan DL, Herzog DB: Predictors of mortality in eating disorders. *Arch Gen Psychiatry* 2003; 60(2):179–183.

Kennedy N, Boydell J, Kalidindi S, Fearon P, Jones PB, van Os J, Murray RM:

Gender differences in incidence and age at onset of mania and bipolar disorder over a 35-year period in Camberwell, England. *Am J Psychiatry* 2005;
162:257–262.

Kessler RC, Berglund P, Demler O, Jin R, Merikangas KR, Walters EE: Lifetime
prevalence and age-of-onset distributions of DSM-IV disorders in the National
Comorbidity Survey replication. *Arch Gen Psychiatry* 2005; 62:593–602.

Kessler RC, McGonagle KA, Zhao S, Nelson CB, Hughes M, Eshleman S, Wittchen
HU, Kendler KS: Lifetime and 12-month prevalence of DSM-III-R psychiatric
disorders in the United States. *Arch Gen Psychiatry* 1994; 51:8–19.

Koran LM, Sheline Y, Imai K, Kelsey TG, Freedland KE, Mathews J, Moore M:
Medical disorders among patients admitted to a public-sector psychiatric inpa-
tient unit. *Psychiatr Serv* 2002; 53:1623–1625.

Krueger RF: The structure of common mental disorders. *Arch Gen Psychiatry*
1999; 56:921–926.

Mark DB: Decision-making in clinical medicine. In Kasper DL, Braunwald E, Fauci
A, Hauser S, Longo D, Jameson JL (Eds.): *Harrison's Principles of Internal
Medicine* (16th ed.). New York: McGraw-Hill, 2004.

Roberts B: A look at psychiatric decision making. *Am J Psychiatry* 1978; 135:1384–
1387.

Schildkrout B: Complexities of the diagnostic process. *J Nerv Ment Dis* 2018;
206:488–490.

van der Feltz-Cornelis CM, Allen SF, van Eck van der Sluijs JF: Misdiagnosis of an
underlying medical condition as conversion disorder/functional neurological
disorder (CD/FND) still occurs. *Gen Hosp Psychiatry* 2020; 65:43–46. Free
at PubMed.

Welner A, Liss JL, Robins E: A systematic approach for making a psychiatric diagnosis. *Arch Gen Psychiatry* 1974; 31:193–196.

Witztum E, Grinshpoon A, Margolin J, Kron S: The erroneous diagnosis of malingering in a military setting. *Mil Med* 1996; 161:225–229.

Zimmerman M: What should the standard of care for psychiatric diagnostic evaluations be? *J Nerv Ment Dis* 2003; 191:281–286.

Anxiety and Fear

Alomari NA, Bedaiwi SK, Ghasib AM, Kabbarah AJ, Alnefaie SA, Hariri N, Altam-
mar MA, Fadhel AM, Altowairqi FM: Social anxiety disorder: Associated conditions and therapeutic approaches. *Cureus* 2022; 14:e32687.

Bruce SE, Machan JT, Dyck I, Keller MB: Infrequency of "pure" GAD: Impact of
psychiatric comorbidity on clinical course. *Depress Anxiety* 2001; 14:219–225.

Carvajal C: Posttraumatic stress disorder as a diagnostic entity—clinical perspec-
tives. *Dialogues Clin Neurosci* 2018; 20:161–168. Free at PubMed.

Eaton WW, Bienvenu OJ, Miloyan B: Specific phobias. *Lancet Psychiatry* 2018;
5:678–686.

Fava GA, Rafanelli C, Grandi S, Conti S, Ruini C, Mangelli L, Belluardo P: Long-term outcome of panic disorder with agoraphobia treated by exposure. *Psychol Med* 2001; 31:891–898.

Lee DO, Helmers SL, Steingard RJ, DeMaso DR: Case study: Seizure disorder presenting as panic disorder with agoraphobia. *J Am Acad Child Adolesc Psychiatry* 1997; 36:1295–1298.

Locke AB, Kirst N, Shultz CG: Diagnosis and management of generalized anxiety disorder and panic disorder in adults. *Am Fam Physician* 2015; 91:617–624.

Newman MG, Llera SJ, Erickson TM, Przeworski A, Castonguay LG: Worry and generalized anxiety disorder: A review and theoretical synthesis of evidence on nature, etiology, mechanisms, and treatment. *Annu Rev Clin Psychol* 2013; 9:275–297. Free at PubMed.

Penninx BW, Pine DS, Holmes EA, Reif A: Anxiety disorders. *Lancet* 2021; 397:914–927. Free at PubMed.

Stein DJ, Costa DLC, Lochner C, Miguel EC, Reddy YCJ, Shavitt RG, van den Heuvel OA, Simpson HB: Obsessive-compulsive disorder. *Nat Rev Dis Primers* 2019; 5:52. Free at PubMed.

Cognitive Disorders

Folstein MF, Folstein SE, McHugh PR: Mini-Mental State: A practical method for grading the cognitive state of patients for the clinician. *J Psychiatr Res* 1975; 12:189–198.

Marcantonio ER: Delirium in hospitalized older adults. *N Engl J Med* 2017; 377:1456–1466. Free at PubMed.

Sachdev PS, Blacker D, Blazer DG, Ganguli M, Jeste DV, Paulsen JS, Petersen RC: Classifying neurocognitive disorders: The DSM-5 approach. *Nat Rev Neurol* 2014; 10:634–642. Free at PubMed.

Depression and Mania

Brockington I: Postpartum psychiatric disorders. *Lancet* 2004; 363:303–310.

Clayton PJ, Lewis CE: The significance of secondary depression. *J Affect Disord* 1981; 3:25–35.

Cook BL, Shukla S, Hoff AL, Aronson TA: Mania with associated organic factors. *Acta Psychiatr Scand* 1987; 76:674–677.

de Kemp EC, Moleman P, Hoogduin CA, Broekman TG, Goedhart A, Schaap CP, van den Berg PC: Diagnosis at the first episode to differentiate antidepressant treatment responses in patients with mood and anxiety disorders. *Psychopharmacology (Berl)* 2002; 160:67–73.

Garvey MJ, Tuason VB: Mania misdiagnosed as schizophrenia. *J Clin Psychiatry* 1980; 41:75–78.

Ghaemi SN, Sachs GS, Chiou AM, Pandurangi AK, Goodwin K: Is bipolar disorder still underdiagnosed? Are antidepressants overutilized? *J Affect Disord* 1999; 52:135–144.

Harrison PJ, Geddes JR, Tunbridge EM: The emerging neurobiology of bipolar disorder. *Trends Neurosci* 2018; 41:18–30. Free at PubMed.

Hirschfeld RM, Lewis L, Vornik LA: Perceptions and impact of bipolar disorder: How far have we really come? Results of the National Depressive and Manic–Depressive Association 2000 survey of individuals with bipolar disorder. *J Clin Psychiatry* 2003; 64:161–174.

Klein DN, Taylor EG, Harding K, Dickstein S: Double depression and episodic major depression: Demographic, clinical, familial, personality, and socioenvironmental characteristics and short-term outcome. *Am J Psychiatry* 1988; 145:1226–1231.

Leader JB, Klein DN: Social adjustment in dysthymia, double depression and episodic major depression. *J Affect Disord* 1996; 37:91–101.

Lin CC, Bai YM, Hu PG, Yeh HS: Substance use disorders among inpatients with bipolar disorders and major depressive disorder in a general hospital. *Gen Hosp Psychiatry* 1998; 20:98–101.

McCullough JP Jr., Klein DN, Borian FE, Howland RH, Riso LP, Keller MB, Banks PL: Group comparisons of DSM-IV subtypes of chronic depression: Validity of the distinctions, part 2. *J Abnorm Psychol* 2003; 112:614–622.

Miller IW, Norman WH, Keitner GI: Combined treatment for patients with double depression. *Psychother Psychosom* 1999; 68:180–185.

Eating Disorders

Aviv R: *Strangers to Ourselves: Unsettled Minds and the Stories That Make Us.* New York: Farrar, Straus & Giroux, 2022.

Hay P: Current approach to eating disorders: A clinical update. *Intern Med J* 2020; 50:24–29. Free at PubMed.

Sanjay K, Nitin K, Jubbin J: Orthorexia nervosa. *J Pak Med Assoc* 2020; 70:1282–1284. Free at PubMed.

Treasure J, Duarte TA, Schmidt U: Eating disorders. *Lancet* 2020; 395:899–911.

Gender Dysphoria

Crocq M-A: How gender dysphoria and incongruence became medical diagnoses—a historical review. *Dialogues Clin Neurosci* 2022; 23:44–51. Free at PubMed.

Personality and Relationship Problems

Black DW: The natural history of antisocial personality disorder. *Can J Psychiatry* 2015; 60:309–314. Free at PubMed.

Ekselius L: Personality disorder: A disease in disguise. *Ups J Med Sci* 2018; 123:194–204. Free at PubMed.

Lee R: Mistrustful and misunderstood: A review of paranoid personality disorder. *Curr Behav Neurosci Rep* 2017; 4:151–165. Free at PubMed.

Rosell DR, Futterman SE, McMaster A, Siever LJ: Schizotypal personality disorder: A current review. *Curr Psychiatry Rep* 2014; 16:452. Free at PubMed.

Vanwoerden S, Stepp SD: *The Diagnostic and Statistical Manual of Mental Disorders, Fifth Edition*, alternative model conceptualization of borderline personality disorder: A review of the evidence. *Personal Disord* 2022; 13:402–406. Free at PubMed.

Psychosis

Arciniegas DB: Psychosis. *Continuum* (Minneap Minn) 2015; 21:715–736. Free at PubMed.

Evans JD, Heaton RK, Paulsen JS, McAdams LA, Heaton SC, Jeste DV: Schizoaffective disorder: A form of schizophrenia or affective disorder? *J Clin Psychiatry* 1999; 60:874–882.

Gurland B: Aims, organization, and initial studies of the Cross-National Project. *Int J Aging Hum Dev* 1976; 7:283–293.

Kasanin J: The acute schizoaffective psychoses. *Am J Psychiatry* 1994; 151(Suppl. 6):144–154.—A reprint of a 1933 article in the same journal.

Lammertink M, Lohrer F, Kaiser R, Hambrecht M, Pukrop R: Differences in substance abuse patterns: Multiple drug abuse alone versus schizophrenia with multiple drug abuse. *Acta Psychiatr Scand* 2001; 104:361–366.

Maj M, Pirozzi R, Formicola AM, Bartoli L, Bucci P: Reliability and validity of the DSM-IV diagnostic category of schizoaffective disorder: Preliminary data. *J Affect Disord* 2000; 57:95–98.

Marneros A: The schizoaffective phenomenon: The state of the art. *Acta Psychiatr Scand* 2003; 106(Suppl. 418):29–33.

Parker G: How well does the DSM-5 capture schizoaffective disorder? *Can J Psychiatry* 2019; 64:607–610. Free at PubMed.

Sacks, O. *Hallucinations*. New York: Knopf, 2012.

Schwartz JE, Fennig S, Tanenberg-Karant M, Carlson G, Craig T, Galambos N, Lavelle J, Bromet EJ: Congruence of diagnoses 2 years after a first-admission diagnosis of psychosis. *Arch Gen Psychiatry* 2000; 57:593–600.

Tsuang D, Coryell W: An 8-year follow-up of patients with DSM-III-R psychotic depression, schizoaffective disorder, and schizophrenia. *Am J Psychiatry* 1993; 150:1182–1188.

Wilson JE, Nian H, Heckers S: The schizoaffective disorder diagnosis: A conundrum in the clinical setting. *Eur Arch Psychiatry Clin Neurosci* 2014; 264:29–34.

Zisook S, McAdams LA, Kuck J, Harris MJ, Bailey A, Patterson TL, Judd LL, Jeste DV: Depressive symptoms in schizophrenia. *Am J Psychiatry* 1999; 156:1736–1743.

Substance Misuse and Other Addictions

Aly SM, Omran A, Gaulier JM, Allorge D: Substance abuse among children. *Arch Pediatr* 2020; 27:480–484. Free at PubMed.

Khan S: Concurrent mental and substance use disorders in Canada. *Health Rep* 2017; 28:3–8. Free at PubMed.

Prom-Wormley EC, Ebejer J, Dick DM, Bowers MS: The genetic epidemiology of substance use disorder: A review. *Drug Alcohol Depend* 2017; 180:241–259. Free at PubMed.

Schuckit MA, Smith TL, Danko GP, Bucholz KK, Reich T, Bierut L: Five-year clinical course associated with DSM-IV alcohol abuse or dependence in a large group of men and women. *Am J Psychiatry* 2001; 158:1084–1090.

Sleep Disorders

Cohen ZL, Eigenberger PM, Sharkey KM, Conroy ML, Wilkins KM: Insomnia and other sleep disorders in older adults. *Psychiatr Clin North Am* 2022; 45:717–734.

Smith MT, McCrae CS, Cheung J, Martin JL, Harrod CG, Heald JL, Carden KA: Use of actigraphy for the evaluation of sleep disorders and circadian rhythm sleep-wake disorders: An American Academy of Sleep Medicine clinical practice guideline. *J Clin Sleep Med* 2018; 14:1231–1237. Free at PubMed.

Wang Y, Salas RME: Approach to common sleep disorders. *Semin Neurol* 2021; 41:781–794. Free at PubMed.

Somatic Symptom Disorders

Löwe B, Levenson J, Depping M, Hüsing P, Kohlmann S, Lehmann M, Shedden-Mora M, Toussaint A, Uhlenbusch N, Weigel A: Somatic symptom disorder: A scoping review on the empirical evidence of a new diagnosis. *Psychol Med* 2022; 52:632–648.

Scamvougeras A, Howard A: Somatic symptom disorder, medically unexplained symptoms, somatoform disorders, functional neurological disorder: How DSM-5 got it wrong. *Can J Psychiatry* 2020; 65:301–305.

Suicide and Violence

Beautrais AL: Subsequent mortality in medically serious suicide attempts: A 5-year follow-up. *Aust NZ J Psychiatry* 2003; 37:595–599.

Boudreaux ED, Camargo CA Jr, Arias SA, Sullivan AF, Allen MH, Goldstein AB, Manton AP, Espinola JA, Miller IW: Improving suicide risk screening and detection in the emergency department. *Am J Prev Med* 2016; 50:445–453. Free at PubMed.

Brockington I: Suicide and filicide in postpartum psychosis. *Arch Womens Ment Health* 2017; 20:63–69. Free at PubMed.

Fenton WS, McGlashan TH, Victor BJ, Blyler CR: Symptoms, subtype, and suicidality in patients with schizophrenia spectrum disorders. *Am J Psychiatry* 1997; 154:199–204.

Gardner W, Lidz CW, Mulvey EP, Shaw EC: Clinical versus actuarial predictions of violence of patients with mental illnesses. *J Counseling Clin Psychol* 1996; 64:602–609.

Harkavy-Friedman JM, Kimhy D, Nelson EA, Venarde DF, Malaspina D, Mann JJ: Suicide attempts in schizophrenia: The role of command auditory hallucinations for suicide. *J Clin Psychiatry* 2003; 64:871–874.

Posner K, Brown GK, Stanley B, Brent DA, Yershova KV, Oquendo MA, Currier GW, Melvin GA, Greenhill L, Shen S, Mann JJ: The Columbia-Suicide Severity Rating Scale: Initial validity and internal consistency findings from three multisite studies with adolescents and adults. *Am J Psychiatry* 2011; 168:1266–1277. Free at PubMed.

Werth JL Jr., Cobia DC: Empirically based criteria for rational suicide: A survey of psychotherapists. *Suicide Life-Threat Behav* 1995; 25:231–240.

Real-Life People

These entries are placed in alphabetical order by the persons' last names, followed by the chapters in which the persons are mentioned and then by the bibliographical information. Check Wikipedia for information on some of the more notorious people mentioned throughout the book, including Marshall Applewhite (Chapter 13), Kenneth Bianchi (Chapter 4), Ted Bundy (Chapter 17), and John Hinckley, Jr. (Chapters 13 and 18).

Rigoberto Alpizar (Chapter 18): Goodnough A: Fretful passenger, turmoil on jet and fatal shots. *The New York Times*, Dec. 9, 2005.

Doug Bruce (Chapter 14): *The New Yorker*, Feb. 27, 2006, 27–30.

John Clare (Chapter 19): Bate J: *John Clare: A Biography*. New York: Farrar, Straus & Giroux, 2003.

Camille Claudel (Chapter 13): Ayral-Clause O: *Camille Claudel: A Life*. New York: Abrams, 2002.

Samuel Taylor Coleridge (Chapter 15): Holmes R: *Coleridge: Early Visions, 1772–1804*. New York: Pantheon, 1999; Holmes R: *Coleridge: Darker Reflections, 1904–1834*. New York: Pantheon, 1989.

Charles Darwin (Chapter 12): Barloon TJ, Noyes R Jr.: Charles Darwin and panic disorder. *JAMA* 1997; 277:138–141.

Phineas Gage (Chapter 17): *www.uakron.edu/gage*

Carolyn Heilbrun (Chapter 11): Grigoriadis V: A death of one's own. *New York*, Dec. 8, 2003; *nymag.com/nymetro/news/people/n_9589*

Effrain Marrero (Chapter 9): Wilson D: Steroids are blamed in suicide of young athlete. *The New York Times*, March 10, 2005.

William Minor (Chapter 19): Winchester S: *The Professor and the Madman*. New York: HarperCollins, 1998.

Joe Namath (Chapter 8): *http://usatoday30.usatoday.com/sports/football/nfl/2004-10-14-namath_x.htm*

Opal Petty (Chapter 7): Lehmann-Haupt C: Opal Petty, 86, patient held 51 years involuntarily in Texas. *The New York Times*, March 14, 2005, Section C, page 15.

Jim Piersall (Chapter 12): Piersall J, Hirshberg A: *Fear Strikes Out: The Jim Piersall Story*. Boston: Little, Brown, 1957; Piersall J, Whittingham R: *The Truth Hurts*. Chicago: Contemporary Books, 1984.

Daniel Paul Schreber (Chapter 13): Freud S: Psycho-analytic notes on an autobiographical account of a case of paranoia (dementia paranoids). In Strachey J (Ed. & Trans.): *The Standard Edition of the Complete Psychological Works of Sigmund Freud* (Vol. 12). London: Hogarth Press, 1958 (orig. pub. 1911).

Elizabeth Shin (Chapter 17): Sontag D: Who was responsible for Elizabeth Shin? *The New York Times*, June 2, 2002, Section 6, page 10.

Virginia Woolf (Chapter 10): Lee H: *Virginia Woolf*. New York: Knopf, 1997.

Andrea Yates (Chapter 11): O'Malley S: *"Are You There Alone?": The Unspeakable Crime of Andrea Yates*. New York: Simon & Schuster, 2004.

Index

Note. **Boldface** indicates a case example; *italics* a definition; *t* a table